STRESS AND COPING IN CHILD HEALTH

ADVANCES IN PEDIATRIC PSYCHOLOGY
Sponsored by the Society of Pediatric Psychology

Stress and Coping in Child Health
Annette M. La Greca, Lawrence J. Siegel, Jan L. Wallander, and C. Eugene Walker, Editors

Stress and Coping in Child Health

Annette M. La Greca
Lawrence J. Siegel
Jan L. Wallander
C. Eugene Walker
EDITORS

THE GUILFORD PRESS / New York / London

© 1992 The Guilford Press
A Division of Guilford Publications, Inc.
72 Spring Street, New York, N.Y. 10012

Printed in the United States of America

This book is printed on acid-free paper.

Last digit is print number: 9 8 7 6 5 4 3 2 1

Library of Congress Cataloging-in-Publication Data

Stress and coping in child health / edited by Annette M. La Greca . . .
 [et al.].
        p.   cm.—(Advances in pediatric psychology)
    Includes bibliographical references and index.
    ISBN 0-89862-112-7
    1. Pediatrics—Psychological aspects.   2. Sick children—
Psychology.   3. Teenagers—Diseases—Psychological aspects.
4. Stress in children.   5. Stress in adolescence.   I. La Greca,
Annette M. (Annette Marie)   II. Series.
    [DNLM: 1. Adaptation, Psychological—in adolescence.
2. Adaptation, Psychological—in infancy & childhood.   3. Stress,
Psychological—in adolescence.   4. Stress, Psychological—in infancy
& childhood.   WS 105.5.A8 S915]
RJ475.S77   1992
618.92′0001′9—dc20
DNLM/DLC
for Library of Congress   91-38224
                                                                      CIP
                                                                      r91

Contributors

Frank Andrasik, PhD, Department of Psychology, University of West Florida, Pensacola, Fla.

Lawrence H. Cohen, PhD, Department of Psychology, University of Delaware, Newark, Del.

Christopher Combs, MA, Department of Psychology, Temple University, Philadelphia, Pa.

Bruce E. Compas, PhD, Department of Psychology, University of Vermont, Burlington, Vt.

Lynnda M. Dahlquist, PhD, Department of Psychiatry and Behavioral Sciences, Baylor College of Medicine, Houston, Tex.; Pediatric Psychiatry Consultation—Liaison Service, Texas Children's Hospital, Houston, Tex.

Alan M. Delamater, PhD, Department of Pediatrics, University of Miami School of Medicine, Miami, Fla.

Sydney Ey, BA, Department of Psychology, University of Vermont, Burlington, Vt.

Tiffany Field, PhD, The Touch Research Institute, Department of Pediatrics, University of Miami School of Medicine, Miami, Fla.

Doreen J. Gagnon, MA, Department of Psychology, University of West Florida, Pensacola, Fla.

William T. Garrison, PhD, Department of Psychology, Children's National Medical Center, Washington, D.C.

Jeffrey Gillman, PhD, Department of Pediatrics, Ohio State University, Columbus, Ohio; Department of Psychology, Children's Hospital, Columbus, Ohio

Cindy L. Hanson, PhD, Diabetes Research Group, California School of Professional Psychology, San Diego, Calif.

Cynthia Harbeck, PhD, Department of Pediatrics, Ohio State University, Columbus, Ohio; Department of Psychology, Children's Hospital, Columbus, Ohio

Leslie Hudnall, MA, Department of Psychology, University of West Florida, Pensacola, Fla.

Anne E. Kazak, PhD, Department of Pediatrics, University of Pennsylvania School of Medicine, Philadelphia, Pa.; Division of Oncology, Children's Hospital of Philadelphia, Philadelphia, Pa.

Lenora G. Knapp, PhD, Department of Child and Family Psychiatry, Rhode Island Hospital/Brown University Program in Medicine, Providence, R.I.

Linda Kruus, BA, Department of Psychology, Temple University, Philadelphia, Pa.

Mary Jo Kupst, PhD, Department of Pediatrics, Medical College of Wisconsin, Midwest Children's Cancer Center, Milwaukee, Wi.

Annette M. La Greca, PhD, Department of Psychology, University of Miami, Coral Gables, Fla.

Barbara G. Melamed, PhD, Ferkauf Graduate School of Psychology, Yeshiva University, Bronx, N.Y.

Suzanne M. Miller, PhD, Department of Psychology, Temple University, Philadelphia, Pa.

Larry L. Mullins, PhD, Department of Pediatric Psychology, University of Oklahoma Health Sciences Center, Oklahoma City, Okla.

Joseph K. Murphy, PhD, Department of Psychiatry and Human Behavior, The Miriam Hospital/Brown University Program in Medicine, Providence, R.I.

Crystal Park, MA, Department of Psychology, University of Delaware, Newark, Del.

Alexandra L. Quittner, PhD, Department of Psychology, Indiana University, Bloomington, Ind.

Howard D. Sherman, MA, Department of Psychology, Temple University, Philadelphia, Pa.

Lawrence J. Siegel, PhD, Ferkauf Graduate School of Psychology, Yeshiva University, Bronx, N.Y.

Anthony Spirito, PhD, Department of Child and Family Psychiatry, Rhode Island Hospital/Brown University Program in Medicine, Providence, R.I.

Lori J. Stark, PhD, Department of Child and Family Psychiatry, Rhode Island Hospital/Brown University Program in Medicine, Providence, R.I.

James W. Varni, PhD, Behavioral Pediatrics Program, Orthopaedic Hospital, Los Angeles, Calif.; Department of Psychology, University of Southern California, Los Angeles, Calif.

C. Eugene Walker, PhD, Department of Pediatric Psychology, University of Oklahoma Health Sciences Center, Oklahoma City, Okla.

Jan L. Wallander, PhD, Civitan International Research Center, University of Alabama at Birmingham, Birmingham, Ala.

Nancy L. Worsham, MS, Department of Psychology, University of Vermont, Burlington, Vt.

Preface

It is with pleasure that the Society of Pediatric Psychology (Section V of the Division of Clinical Psychology, American Psychological Association) presents this volume. Such sponsorship recognizes the scholarly significance of the volume and the care taken in the development of the chapters on scientific and professional issues. Recognized experts in the field of pediatric psychology were solicited to contribute chapters. This was followed by a careful peer review process for each chapter. As a special project of the Society of Pediatric Psychology, this book has not been considered by the American Psychological Association Council of Representatives and does not represent official policy of the American Psychological Association as a whole.

This volume inaugurates a series of edited books devoted to contemporary topics in pediatric and child health psychology and sponsored by the Society of Pediatric Psychology (SPP). The goal of this series is to provide "snapshots" of research in pediatric psychology by focusing each volume on a current area of interest and importance within the field, and by including contributors who are active researchers in pediatric psychology and affiliated professions. Within each volume, investigators will have the opportunity to describe their current work and to comment upon the state of their field. The series is not intended to provide a comprehensive picture of the breadth and scope of pediatric psychology as much as to present an in-depth examination of selected topics and issues.

The idea for this series was borne out of extensive discussions among members of the SPP Executive Committee, who wished to encourage, promote, and recognize the activities of pediatric researchers. In particular, the SPP Ad Hoc Committee on Publications (of which we are members) was instrumental in developing the format and plan for the series, and in guiding and editing the first volume.

As can be seen from the table of contents, this volume is divided into three main sections. The first section covers general issues pertinent to the broad field of stress and coping, such as conceptual, developmental, and methodological issues; the role of temperament in understanding coping with pediatric conditions; psychophysiological aspects of stress; and the importance of considering contextual factors in children's coping responses. In the second main section, chapters are focused primarily on youngsters' and families' coping responses in the face of specific medical stressors (e.g., invasive medical procedures, anesthesia induction, dental procedures) or chronic illnesses (e.g., diabetes, cancer, etc.). Several chapters in this section also illustrate the use of conceptual, multivariate approaches to stress and coping with chronic pediatric conditions. The third and last section is devoted to research relevant to clinical interventions for stressful medical conditions and procedures. Prior to each section of the text, we provide a brief introduction that sets the stage for subsequent chapters.

We appreciate the considerable expertise of the contributors, whose work is at the forefront of pediatric psychology. The chapters herein should provide the reader with a stimulating, interesting, and scholarly view of children's stress and coping with pediatric problems.

Annette M. La Greca
Lawrence J. Siegel
Jan L. Wallander
C. Eugene Walker
May 1991

Contents

SECTION II: CURRENT RESEARCH PERSPECTIVES

SECTION III: CURRENT PERSPECTIVES ON INTERVENTION

STRESS AND COPING IN CHILD HEALTH

CONCEPTUAL AND GENERAL ISSUES

Overview

LAWRENCE J. SIEGEL
Yeshiva University

The concepts of stress and coping are ubiquitous in our society today. Despite the wide use of these terms in the psychological literature, there is a lack of consensus as to their exact definitions. Generally, the literature in this area has been hampered by the use of the word "stress" to refer to a number of different constructs. An additional source of confusion has been the extent to which the concept of "stress" refers to a property that is inherent in the individual or in the person's environment. Similarly, the term "coping" is often used to describe a vague, all-inclusive construct. For example, the literature frequently fails to differentiate the methods or types of coping, the functions of coping, and the outcomes of coping.

The concepts of stress and coping go hand in hand. A discussion of stress is not complete without an understanding of how an individual responds in regards to a stressful experience—that is, the individual's coping behaviors.

As demonstrated by the various chapters in this book, stress and coping are topics of considerable interest in the field of pediatric psychology. The epidemiology of psychosocial stress has demonstrated a consistent relationship between exposure to a wide range of stressors and virtually every type of childhood morbidity. This finding has been observed in diverse pediatric populations and settings.

Developmental considerations are of paramount importance in understanding factors that influence stress and coping in children. Until recently, much of the child literature in this area has been guided almost exclusively by conceptual and theoretical models developed with adults. Research on stress and coping with pediatric problems has begun to recognize the importance of assessing children's coping responses with stress within the context of a developmental framework. A child's cognitive appraisal of potentially stressful experiences, for example, will clearly depend on his or her level of understanding of that event.

Stress is often described in terms of specific life events. Many investigators have focused on major life events as antecedents of psychological and physical problems. This approach to stress assumes that stress originates primarily in the individual's environment, rather than from sources within the individual. More recently, researchers have begun to examine the role of minor life events or "daily hassles" as factors in childhood morbidity.

The impact of stress on pediatric populations is not uniform across patients. Individual-difference factors can influence both a child's response to stress and his or her use of coping strategies. Attention to individual differences in children's behavioral, emotional, and physiological responsiveness to their environment can provide a useful perspective in understanding the effects of stress on children's health-related problems. For research on psychosocial stress to elucidate patterns of childhood morbidity, it is important to explain why certain children are susceptible to the pathogenic effects of stressors while others are more resilient.

A number of factors may mediate the impact of stress on a given child. Patterns of physiological reactivity constitute one important but often neglected factor that may mediate a child's response to stress. Recent research suggests that there may be some physiological specificity in response to particular stressful events. There is also a growing body of evidence for a relationship between children's exaggerated biobehavioral responses to stress and a greater risk for health-related problems. Cardiovascular reactivity has received particular attention in this regard.

Another aspect of psychobiological responsivity that may be particularly important in influencing a child's response to stress is temperament or behavioral style. Children differ in their sensitivity to the environment, with some exhibiting signs of arousal and distress to a wider range of stimuli than others. Temperament may define a range of responsivity to stress, and thereby may influence a child's coping responses.

Social support has also been identified as a primary mediator of the impact of stressful events on an individual. A substantial amount of research documents the psychological and physical benefits of social support. Research suggests that an individual's perceptions of the adequacy of support are more important than the number of persons who are available in that individual's social network. Importantly, social support may be viewed not only as a moderator between stress and coping responses, but also as a form of coping in itself. Furthermore, it has been suggested that social support may be an individual-difference resource, in that some individuals have better skills for making use of potential sources of social support than others.

The first section of this book addresses a number of substantive theoretical, conceptual, and developmental issues that are relevant to the areas of stress and coping with pediatric conditions. Several intrapersonal and contextual factors that are important in understanding stress and coping in children are reviewed.

In Chapter 1, Compas, Worsham, and Ey discuss a number of issues central to the study of children's coping with stress associated with illness, injury, and aversive medical procedures. They provide a conceptual framework for understanding the function and process of coping in pediatric populations within a developmental and family perspective. Two subtypes of coping strategies, "emotion-focused" and "problem-focused" strategies, are used throughout the chapter to illustrate the various points addressed by the authors. A distinction is also made between models that emphasize coping as a trait and models that emphasize coping as a process varying across situations. Moreover, the authors observe that a linear model that focuses only on the consequences of coping *or* the determinants of coping is not sufficient to describe the coping process. They argue instead for a transactional model that examines aspects of coping both across time and in specific situations. A study of children's and adolescents' coping with a parent with cancer is presented to demonstrate the conceptual model of coping proposed in this chapter.

Conceptual and methodological issues in life stress research in children and adolescents are reviewed by Cohen and Park in Chapter 2. The authors present a distinction between life stress as a stimulus, as a response, and as a transactional process involving the appraisal of threat or loss of an event or experience. Issues in the measurement of life stress in children are briefly discussed. In addition, the etiological role of life stress in pediatric disorders, as well as in illness-related and preventive health behaviors, is reviewed. Cohen and Park note that a lack of theory-driven research and confusion over various statistical models have contributed to equivocal findings in this area. A discussion of the mediating and/or moderating influence of a number of variables that may be associated with children's vulnerability or resistance to the impact of life stress events is also presented. Finally, the authors suggest that some pediatric conditions may represent chronic stressors for children and their families, and as a result other major or minor life events may not have the same effect on these children as on children who do not have a chronic illness or disability. Future research is needed to address this issue.

In Chapter 3, Murphy reviews the research on physiological responses to stress in children and adolescents, with a specific focus on cardiovascular reactivity. Reactivity studies that have been conducted in laboratory and natural settings are discussed for the purpose of identifying possible etiological factors in pediatric conditions that may contribute to our understanding of prevention and treatment of such conditions.

The major portion of the chapter is devoted to a review of a number of biological and psychosocial variables that may mediate the relationship between stress reactivity and the later onset of pathophysiological conditions such as hypertension. Murphy concludes that although many of the studies in this area present inconsistent and conflicting results, there is sufficient evidence to support a consistent association between reactivity and future blood pressure levels. Additional longitudinal research in this area is needed to clarify these findings with children.

In Chapter 4, Garrison argues for the importance of studying the construct of temperament, in order to facilitate our understanding of various clinical outcomes in pediatric populations. The child's temperament or behavioral style is viewed as a mediator of the child's response to stress and coping efforts. Following a brief discussion of various theoretical approaches to temperament, Garrison reviews several core dimensions of temperament that have been identified in the literature. He specifically addresses these dimensions within the context of their relevance to children's coping with various pediatric conditions, and he notes the importance of studying these dimensions within a theoretical framework.

The final chapter in this section, by Quittner, examines the role of social support as a mediator of stress in pediatric conditions. A major thesis of Chapter 5 is the need to take into consideration situational factors that can affect the conditions under which social support influences adaptation to stress. Specifically, Quittner proposes a model of social support in children with chronic illnesses and their families that evaluates support within the context of such factors as these: the temporal and normative aspects of the stressor, the tasks and demands imposed by the pediatric condition, developmental and family life cycle issues, and social roles of family members as impacted by the pediatric condition. Finally, the author reports the findings of two studies that illustrate a contextual framework for investigating the relationship between and among maternal stress, social support, and psychological distress in mothers of children who are hearing-impaired or who have a seizure disorder.

Conceptual and Developmental Issues in Children's Coping with Stress

BRUCE E. COMPAS, NANCY L. WORSHAM,
and SYDNEY EY
University of Vermont

The concept of "coping" is central to theory, research, and clinical practice in the field of pediatric psychology. Patterns of coping with the stress of everyday life and with infrequent major life disruptions can serve either as sources of risk for or as protection from a variety of pediatric conditions, including acute and chronic illnesses and injuries. Furthermore, the ways in which children and adolescents cope with their own illnesses and injuries, as well as with aversive aspects of medical treatment, can significantly affect the short- and long-term outcomes of medical interventions.

Given the significance of coping for this field, the advancement of theory, research, and interventions related to coping processes is a high priority for pediatric psychology. Although a strong body of literature has accumulated on characteristics of coping in pediatric populations, further advancement in this area of research and practice can be informed by the broader literature on children's and adolescents' coping with stress. The purpose of this chapter is to highlight the implications for pediatric psychology of several aspects of theory and research on children's and adolescents' coping with stress. The chapter discusses three major themes: (1) issues in the conceptualization of the coping process, (2) developmental changes and continuities in coping throughout childhood and adolescence, and (3) the importance of understanding individual coping efforts within the context of the family.

COPING WITH THE CONCEPT OF COPING

Few concepts in the behavioral and health sciences have proven as difficult to define and operationalize as the constructs of "stress" and "coping." Various conceptual models are available to describe and explain the nature of stressful events, their impact on individuals, and processes of coping and adjustment. Furthermore, numerous instruments are available to measure aspects of stress and coping, although the majority of these measures are not theoretically based. Four issues seem especially pertinent in conceptualizing coping in pediatric populations: (1) delineation of subtypes of coping, (2) trait versus process conceptualizations of coping, (3) coping as an independent versus a dependent variable, and (4) the focus or target of coping efforts (i.e., coping with what?).

Subtypes of Coping

Several conceptual models have been used to guide research on the ways in which children and adolescents cope with stress (see Compas, 1987, and Compas, Malcarne, & Banez, in press, for reviews). These include the cognitive appraisal model of Lazarus and Folkman (1984); the two-dimensional model of primary and secondary control (Rothbaum, Weisz, & Snyder, 1982; Weisz, Rothbaum, & Blackburn, 1984); Murphy and Moriarty's (1976) ego-psychological model; and the monitoring–blunting model (Miller, 1980). In spite of the apparent diversity of these models, all of these approaches emphasize a basic distinction between two fundamental types of coping—a distinction that centers around the intention or function of coping efforts. The first type of coping refers to efforts to change or master some aspect of the person, the environment, or the relation between these two elements that is perceived as stressful. For example, a child suffering from Type I insulin-dependent diabetes mellitus (IDDM) may carefully monitor his or her diet in an effort to control the illness. This type of coping has been labeled "problem-focused coping" (Lazarus & Folkman, 1984), "primary-control coping" (Band & Weisz, 1988), "Coping I" (Murphy & Moriarty, 1976), "approach coping" (Altshuler & Ruble, 1989), "problem solving" (Wertlieb, Weigel, & Feldstein, 1987), "active coping" (Peterson, 1989), or "monitoring" (Miller, 1980). The second type of coping refers to efforts to manage or regulate the negative emotions associated with the stressful episode. For example, a child with IDDM may take steps to relax himself or herself before self-administering insulin. This type of coping has been labeled "emotion-focused coping" (Lazarus & Folkman, 1984), "secondary-control coping" (Band & Weisz, 1988), "Coping II" (Murphy & Moriarty 1976), "emotion manipulation," "tension reduction," "avoidance" (Altshuler & Ruble, 1989), "emotion management" (Wertlieb et al., 1987), "avoidant coping" (Peterson, 1989), or "blunting" (Miller, 1980).

In general, the results of studies of coping in pediatric populations have favored the efficacy of more active, problem-focused efforts over more passive, emotion-focused coping. For example, in a review of coping of children undergoing stressful medical procedures, Peterson (1989) concluded that active (problem-focused) coping was associated with more beneficial responses on a variety of different outcome measures related to behavioral, emotional, and somatic functioning. Similarly, studies of coping with IDDM have indicated that primary-control or instrumental (problem-focused) coping is associated with more positive control of diabetes symptoms and fewer behavioral problems (e.g., Band, 1990; Band & Weisz, 1990).

These findings notwithstanding, it may be premature to conclude that emotion-focused or secondary-control coping is generally an ineffective strategy for pediatric patients to use. Finer distinctions among subtypes of emotion-focused coping are likely to prove important in identifying those types of coping that may be maladaptive under virtually all circumstances, as opposed to other strategies that may be quite beneficial under certain circumstances. For example, in coping with a chronic illness such as IDDM, it may be highly maladaptive to attempt to deny the significance of the disorder by telling oneself, "I don't care about this problem," or "it just isn't important to me" (Band & Weisz, 1990). On the other hand, emotion-focused coping efforts such as positively reframing the problem, feeling a sense of accomplishment in mastering the daily tasks of dealing with IDDM, or trying to maintain a positive attitude may have a direct effect on maintaining emotional well-being and an indirect effect on management of the disease by facilitating better problem-focused coping (Band & Weisz, 1990; Lazarus & Folkman, 1984).

We are pursuing analyses of subtypes of problem- and emotion-focused coping in our current research on the ways in which parents and children cope when a mother or father has cancer. From the time of diagnosis, each family member responds to a series of individual structured interviews every 4 months over a period of 1 year; these include questions concerning the ways in which the family member is coping with the cancer experience at that point in time. In our analyses of the interview responses, problem-focused coping is further delineated as (1) planful problem solving or (2) confrontive coping. Emotion-focused coping is classified as (1) denial/avoidance, (2) distraction/minimization, (3) wishful thinking, (4) self-control of feelings, (5) seeking meaning, (6) self-blame, and (7) expressing and sharing feelings. These data will provide the opportunity to examine developmental differences in the use of these subtypes of coping in a sample of children, adolescents, and adults who are coping with a common family health crisis. In addition, we see analyses of finer-grained distinctions among subtypes of coping of this type as an important next step in understanding the effectiveness of various coping efforts.

Coping as a Trait or a Process

Coping efforts are influenced by both characteristics of the person and characteristics of the situation in which he or she is coping. However, different models of coping give relatively greater emphasis to personal as opposed to situational factors, leading some to be more trait-oriented (personal) and others to be more process-oriented (situational). That is, conceptualizations of coping differ in the degree of cross-situational and temporal consistency or variability that is expected in an individual's coping. The relevance of this issue for pediatric psychologists is twofold. First, pediatric patients can be expected to cope in similar or varied ways with different illnesses and qualitatively different types of medical procedures. Second, pediatric patients can be expected to cope in consistent or varied ways with the same illness or medical procedure over the course of time.

Studies of coping in college students and adults have provided a solid body of information on cross-situational and temporal stability of coping. The results of several studies provide support for a process model as opposed to a trait model of coping. For example, Folkman and Lazarus (1985) examined temporal aspects of coping in a study of undergraduates' efforts at coping with an examination at three points in time: before the exam (time 1), after the exam but before grades were returned (time 2), and after grades were returned (time 3). This prospective design allowed for an analysis of the degree to which students' reports of coping remained consistent or changed over the three stages of the exam process. Support was found for a process-oriented model of coping, as significant changes occurred in coping over time. Problem-focused coping (seeking social support, emphasizing the positive, and self-isolation) decreased from time 1 to time 2, whereas distancing increased. Wishful thinking and distancing decreased from time 2 to time 3.

Compas, Forsythe, and Wagner (1988), also using a college student sample, examined both temporal and cross-situational change and consistency in coping with stress in the domains of academic achievement and interpersonal relationships. Students reported on an ongoing stressor or hassle in each domain once a week for a period of 4 weeks. Patterns of coping were characterized by moderate consistency in response to the same stressor over time and low consistency across the interpersonal and academic stressors. There was very little consistency in the use of seven subtypes of coping (e.g., distraction, situation redefinition, direct action) across the two different stressors, with most correlations below .20 and failing to reach significance. The correlations for the use of the subtypes of coping in response to the same stressor over time were higher, with most of these reaching significance and falling between .30 and .50. Furthermore, temporal stability of coping was predicted by individuals' initial levels of negative affect. Those individuals who reported higher levels of initial anxious, depressive, and angry emotions were more stable in their coping over the following 3 weeks. This pattern suggests that coping is influenced by both personal and situational factors, with personal factors exerting relatively greater influence when the situation remains stable.

Unfortunately, there are precious few data on coping patterns of children or adolescents across situations or over time in the same context. Most studies have sampled children's and adolescents' coping in a single context at a given point in time. Assessment of situational and temporal consistency versus variability has been further clouded by the use of measures that ask participants to report on the ways they cope "in general." The use of such instruments prohibits the analysis of situational or temporal processes by asking the respondents to aggregate their own coping efforts and to report on an ill-defined central tendency in their own thoughts and actions. The few studies that have addressed consistency and variability in coping in younger populations have suggested that children may be more consistent in their coping across different situations than adults are. For example, both Wills (1986) and Compas, Malcarne, and Fondacaro (1988) reported significant correlations that were moderate in magnitude for young adolescents' use of coping strategies across different situations. These findings lead to the hypothesis that coping becomes more differentiated with development. It is expected that this increased differentiation will be reflected in greater variability in response to the demands of different stressful situations. This hypothesis, however, has not yet been directly tested.

In summary, research supports the conceptualization of coping as a process that is responsive to the varying demands of different situations and changes in the same stressful encounter as it unfolds over time. The adoption of a process-oriented model of coping has two important implications for pediatric psychology. First, the assessment of coping needs to be sensitive to situational and temporal changes. It will be at best insufficient and at worst misleading to ask pediatric patients how they cope in general. Second, optimally adaptive coping may differ across types of illnesses and medical procedures, and at different points in the course of an illness episode or treatment.

Coping as an Independent Variable;
Coping as a Dependent Variable

Embracing a process-oriented model of coping also requires adopting a more general conceptual model of the nature of stress and coping. Linear models in which coping is viewed either as an independent or as a dependent variable will be inadequate to capture the evolving character-istics of the coping process. The broader framework must be a transac-tional one, in which factors that contribute to coping and outcomes that result from coping are assessed. Most previous research has not reflected a transactional perspective. Instead, studies have been divided between those that have examined the consequences of coping (i.e., coping as an independent variable) and those that have examined the determinants of coping (i.e., coping as a dependent variable).

Coping is often studied as an independent variable that is used to predict other outcomes, most frequently psychological and somatic symp-toms. Coping responses can serve as sources of protection from stress and thus can decrease the risk of individuals to illness or accidents. Alternatively, certain coping responses themselves represent significant health risk behaviors. For example, smoking and alcohol and drug use are employed by some youths as efforts to manage stress, and these behaviors are linked to a variety of negative health outcomes (e.g., Wills, 1986). In an effort to alter the use of smoking and substance use as ways of coping with stress, interventions have been developed to facilitate the use of more adaptive coping skills (e.g., Botvin, Baker, Dusenbury, Tortu, & Botvin, 1990).

Other studies have treated coping as an outcome or dependent variable in the search for factors that determine or influence the types of coping strategies employed. Factors that have been examined as potential determinants of coping have included the type of stressful event, cogni-tive appraisals of the stressor, social support resources available for coping, developmental level or age, and gender.

A more comprehensive picture of coping will depend on the acquisi-tion of data in which the determinants *and* the consequences of coping are examined together. This will require longitudinal designs in which possible reciprocal relations between coping and other variables can be examined. For example, it is likely that the relation between coping and emotional distress is bidirectional. Initial levels of anxiety in the face of threat may elicit the use of emotion-focused coping strategies. In turn, attempts to distract oneself or to use relaxation techniques may reduce the initial anxiety. Similar reciprocal relations are likely to be found between aspects of the environment that are sources of stress and the use of problem-focused coping.

The Focus of Coping Efforts: Coping with What?

Pediatric populations are faced with a variety of stressful circumstances that require coping responses, including stressful events that contribute to illness or injury, the stress of the illness or injury itself, aversive aspects of treatment, and the correlates or consequences of various pediatric conditions. These stressful situations vary along a number of dimensions. For example, illnesses may be distinguished in terms of nature of onset, chronicity, severity of current symptoms, prognosis, and degree of physical impairment. The ways in which coping of children and adolescents may vary as a function of any of these dimensions needs to be delineated. Furthermore, the effectiveness of problem- and emotion-focused coping may vary as a function of these factors.

The nature of stressful conditions also varies as a function of the individual's cognitive appraisals of his or her relationship with the environment. That is, the individual is coping not only with the "objective" aspects of the situation, but even more centrally with his or her appraisal of the situation. In this regard, appraisals of control have received the most attention in previous research. The association between perceptions of control and coping processes are central in cognitive appraisal models of stress and coping, as well as in various models of perceived control. Folkman (1984) has outlined a complex set of relations among control beliefs, appraisals of threat and challenge, and the use of problem- and emotion-focused coping. Among these is the notion that problem-focused efforts are more adaptive when they are directed toward aspects of the person-environment relationship that are perceived as changeable, whereas emotion-focused efforts are more adaptive when a situation is recognized as uncontrollable. Along this line, Weisz (1986) has suggested that a key developmental task involves learning to distinguish between situations where persistence (which can be seen as similar to continued problem-focused coping efforts) pays off and situations where it does not. Perceptions of control are seen as playing the central role in this judgment process. Similarly, Weisz (1986) has noted the need for research examining whether behavior that involves acceptance (a form of emotion-focused coping) has different correlates, depending on whether it is associated with a sense of loss of control or a sense of secondary control.

Although there is some evidence to support the notion that both problem- and emotion-focused coping are tied to perceptions of control (e.g., Folkman & Lazarus, 1980), other findings suggest that problem- and emotion-focused coping are actually matched to separate sets of cues.

That is, problem-focused coping efforts may be regulated in conjunction with increases and decreases in perceived control over a stressful situation, whereas emotion-focused coping efforts may be linked instead to internal cues of emotional arousal and distress. Studies with adolescents and with college students have found positive correlations between perceived control and problem-focused coping, no association between emotion-focused coping and control, and positive correlations between emotion-focused coping and symptoms of emotional distress (Compas, Forsythe, & Wagner, 1988; Forsythe & Compas, 1987). This pattern is consistent with the original formulation of the different functions served by problem- and emotion-focused coping. For example, Folkman (1984) has proposed that emotion-focused efforts should increase as threat appraisals and associated emotions (fear, anxiety) increase; as these emotions increase, more coping efforts have to be directed toward emotion regulation. Although the relations between problem-focused coping and control and between emotion-focused coping and emotional distress are most likely reciprocal in nature, longitudinal data to test this possibility have not been reported.

The relation between perceived control and coping in children and adolescents is less clear. The majority of studies of children's and adolescents' coping have not assessed their perceptions of control over stress (e.g., Altshuler & Ruble, 1989; Band & Weisz, 1988; Curry & Russ, 1985; Wertlieb et al., 1987). Findings from three studies that did measure perceived control have been inconsistent. Compas, Malcarne, and Fondacaro (1988) found higher reports of problem-focused coping (but not emotion-focused coping) in situations rated as controllable, whereas Band (1990) found no relation between ratings of control and either problem- or emotion-focused coping. More recently, Compas, Banez, Malcarne, and Worsham (1991) found that problem-focused coping, but not emotion-focused coping, was correlated with control beliefs in a sample of 6- to 12-year-old children. Thus, whether or not control beliefs and coping are related in childhood, and how this relationship may remain stable or change with development, are unclear.

DEVELOPMENT OF COPING DURING CHILDHOOD AND ADOLESCENCE: IT CHANGES *AND* IT STAYS THE SAME

The tremendous variability in the developmental level of pediatric populations represents a substantial challenge for pediatric psychologists (Burbach & Peterson, 1986; Maddux, Roberts, Sledden, & Wright, 1986). Because children and adolescents differ in their levels of cognitive, social, emotional, and biological development, they present pediatric psychologists with much wider variation than is encountered by health psychologists working with adults. As a consequence, it is imperative that pediatric psychologists take a developmental approach in their research and practice.

The general literature on children's and adolescents' coping has identified some important developmental patterns. Specifically, five recent studies of the ways in which children and adolescents cope with a wide range of stressors have examined developmental changes and stabilities in problem- and emotion-focused coping (Altshuler & Ruble, 1989; Band & Weisz, 1988; Compas, Malcarne, & Fondacaro, 1988; Curry & Russ, 1985; Wertlieb et al., 1987). All five of these studies have found at least some evidence of a positive relation between reports of emotion-focused coping and age or some other marker of developmental level (e.g., cognitive-developmental level). Evidence for this developmental change has been found in samples of children ranging from 5½ to 10½ years of age (Altshuler & Ruble, 1989; Curry & Russ, 1985; Wertlieb et al., 1987), in children and adolescents ages 6 to 17 (Band, 1990; Band & Weisz, 1988), and in older children and young adolescents ages 10 to 14 (Compas, Malcarne, & Fondacaro, 1988). This developmental increase in emotion-focused coping has been found in reports of coping with medical or dental stressors (Altshuler & Ruble, 1989; Band & Weisz, 1988; Curry & Russ, 1985) and interpersonal stressors (Compas, Malcarne, & Fondacaro, 1988).

In contrast to this consistent finding of developmental increases in emotion-focused coping, no consistent developmental changes have been found in problem-focused coping, with three studies finding no change with age (Altshuler & Ruble, 1989; Compas, Malcarne, & Fondacaro, 1988; Wertlieb et al., 1987) and two studies finding a decrease in problem-focused coping with age (Band & Weisz, 1988; Curry & Russ, 1985). The two findings of decreases in problem-focused coping were both noted in reference to medical or dental stressors, whereas no changes in problem-focused coping were found in relation to a wider range of stressors.

In the broader literature on the development of children's problem-solving skills, which can be considered germane to the study of coping (see Compas, 1987), there is evidence for increases with age in certain types of abilities. For example, Spivack, Shure, and colleagues found that the capacity to generate multiple solutions to interpersonal problems emerges at about age 4 or 5, whereas the ability to use means–ends thinking (i.e., identifying the sequence of steps needed to solve a problem) does not appear until about ages 8 to 10 (Spivack & Shure, 1982). Interventions designed to improve children's problem-solving skills have been successful in increasing both of these skills (Spivack & Shure, 1982). More recently, Compas et al. (1991) examined reports of coping with interpersonal stress in a sample of 6- to 12-year-old children. The use of problem-focused coping increased with age ($r = .45$, $p < .01$), whereas emotion-focused coping was unrelated to age ($r = .02$).

We are also investigating developmental differences in reports of problem- and emotion-focused coping with the diagnosis and treatment of cancer in a mother or father in a sample of children (ages 6–10), adolescents (ages 11–18), and young adults (ages 19–35). Although this differs from research on pediatric populations in that parental cancer does not represent a personal illness of the child, it does provide the opportunity to examine developmental changes in coping with a health-related stressor across a much wider range of developmental levels than in previous studies. As part of the study, we ask each family member to report on the ways in which he or she has coped with the cancer and his or her own intentions in using each coping strategy. That is, participants indicate whether they were trying to change something about the stressful situation (problem-focused), to manage their feelings (emotion-focused), or to accomplish both of these objectives with a single coping act (both problem- and emotion-focused). Preliminary analyses (Compas & Worsham, 1991) indicate that emotion-focused coping increases with age across these three groups, $F (2, 101) = 5.27$, $p = .007$. Reports of problem-focused coping do not differ across the groups, although all age groups have reported using very little strictly problem-focused coping. Reports of the use of strategies to achieve both problem- and emotion-focused intentions also increase with age, $F (2, 101) 5.66$, $p = .004$. By allowing respondents to describe coping strategies that they have used to try to address both problem- and emotion-focused objectives, we have obtained a somewhat different picture of the development of problem-solving skills. The use of complex strategies that serve multiple intentions appears to increase with developmental age in a manner similar to the age-related increase in emotion-focused coping.

In summary, studies of coping in children and adolescents suggest that problem-focused and emotion-focused coping skills emerge at different points in development. Problem-focused skills appear to be acquired earlier, with some evidence for the acquisition of problem-solving skills apparent by the preschool years. One reason for the earlier development of these skills may be that they are more readily acquired through modeling of adult behaviors, as many of these coping strategies involve overt behavior and are observable even to young children. Emotion-focused coping skills appear to develop in later childhood and early adolescence. This may be the result of several factors, including younger children's having less access to their internal emotional states, their failure to recognize that their emotions can be brought under self-regulation, and the fact that emotion-focused coping efforts of others are less observable and therefore less easily learned through modeling processes.

Recent studies with pediatric populations have generated findings quite consistent with the developmental patterns found in community samples of children and adolescents. For example, studies of children and adolescents coping with IDDM have found an increase with age or cognitive developmental level in the use of emotion-focused or secondary-control coping (Band, 1990; Band & Weisz, 1990; Hanson et al., 1989). Band (1990; Band & Weisz, 1990) classified a sample of preadolescents (mean age = 8.8 years) and adolescents (mean age = 14.6 years) with IDDM as either pre-formal-operational or formal-operational in their thinking on the basis of a Piagetian cognitive task. The researchers found that higher levels of cognitive development were associated with the use of more secondary-control coping. That is, although both pre-formal-operational and formal-operational children used a greater proportion of primary-control (problem-focused) coping than secondary-control (emotion-focused) coping, the formal-operational group used more secondary-control coping than did the pre-formal-operational group. Similarly, in a study of preadolescent and adolescent IDDM patients (mean age = 14.5 years), Hanson et al. (1989) found that age was positively correlated with greater use of two types of emotion-focused coping: avoidance and ventilation of feelings.

It is noteworthy that the association between emotion-focused coping and more advanced cognitive development does not imply that these methods are more effective. As noted above, several studies have shown that these types of coping are associated with poorer health outcomes and more emotional and behavioral problems. This is similar to findings from studies with nonpediatric populations. For example, Compas, Malcarne, and Fondacaro (1988) found that reports of use of emotion-focused coping with interpersonal stressors were associated with more self-reported and mother-reported emotional and behavioral problems. These findings suggest that, at least during early adolescence, the types of emotion-focused coping skills that are learned are relatively less sophisticated methods of managing feelings (e.g., inappropriate ventilation of feelings, blaming others for problems, trying to minimize the significance of a problem). This again underscores the need to examine subtypes of emotion-focused coping to determine the developmental sequence in the acquisition of these skills and the consequences of their use.

COPING DURING CHILDHOOD AND ADOLESCENCE: IT'S A FAMILY AFFAIR

Theoretical and empirical treatments of the coping process have a history of examining how *individuals* manage stress in their lives. However, pediatric psychologists have long been aware that the ways in which children and adolescents cope with health- and illness-related stress cannot be understood solely in individual terms (Roberts & Maieron, 1989; Wright, 1967). Coping with general life stress, coping with aversive medical treatments, and coping with chronic illness all occur in a social context. Contextual factors serve both as resources that aid and facilitate effective coping, and as impediments or blocks to adequate adjustment. Although children and teens function in a variety of proximal contexts (family, school, peer group) and more distal settings (neighborhoods, cities, societies), the family stands out as pre-eminent in understanding coping processes in pediatric populations.

Family characteristics and processes may be related to coping in a variety of ways. First, family members can serve as resources for children and adolescents who are coping with an illness or its treatment through the provision of social support and information (Davies, 1988). Second, at the opposite end of the continuum of the provision of social support, family members can be impediments to the coping process by interrupting or constraining the coping efforts of a child or teen, or by turning to the child or adolescent for help in coping for themselves in ways that exceed the youngster's developmental capacity. Third, family members, especially parents, can serve as models for coping strategies that may be employed by a child. Fourth, families generate rules and enact regulatory processes that influence the coping strategies used by individual family members. Finally, families operate as systems in which the coping efforts of individual family members may affect and be affected by the coping efforts of other family members in addressing a common problem.

Social support from family members has been identified as an important resource for children and adolescents in coping with stress. Such support is thus a logical starting point for understanding the ways that families contribute to coping in pediatric populations. It appears that family support in pediatric populations has a direct relation to adjustment, whereas evidence for social support as a buffer against stress has been inconsistent. For example, Varni, Wallander, and colleagues have examined social support from family members, as well as from friends and teachers, among chronically ill and handicapped children (e.g., Varni, Rubenfeld, Talbot, & Setoguchi, 1989; Wallander & Varni, 1989). Social support from parents was related to lower levels of depressive symptoms in children with congenital and acquired limb deficiencies (Varni et al., 1989), and to lower levels of externalizing (but not internalizing) behavior problems in chronically ill and handicapped children (Wallander & Varni, 1989).

It is also possible that family members, in addition to providing valuable support, can in some instances impede the coping of the pediatric patient. Although this issue has not been addressed directly in studies of pediatric patients and their families, there is substantial evidence documenting the adverse effects of pediatric illnesses on the parents and siblings of a patient. Parents experience increased levels of depressive symptoms and other indicators of psychological distress. Similarly, siblings experience behavioral and other developmental problems associated with illness of the child patient. An important next step will be the examination of the impact of these problems on the parents' and siblings' ability to provide support to the patient.

It is widely assumed that the family provides the primary context in which children naturally acquire ways of coping with stress. From a viewpoint of general social learning theory, parents serve as models for coping who influence the children's coping behavior through observational learning processes. Unfortunately, there are no data available on parents and children that bear on the question. Modeling and direct instruction are frequently combined in interventions to teach problem-solving skills and emotion management techniques to pediatric patients (e.g., Manne et al., 1990). If similar processes operate in families on a natural basis, it is likely that parents' active problem-focused coping strategies are more readily observable to children than are emotion-focused coping techniques. Problem-focused coping is more likely to involve behavioral strategies that the child can observe and emulate, whereas many important emotion-focused coping skills involve covert cognitive processes and are unlikely to be verbalized by parents. To the extent that parents do serve as important models of coping for their children, this would underscore the importance of helping parents acquire effective coping skills and enlisting them in teaching these skills to their children (e.g., Jay & Elliott, 1990). This certainly represents a high priority for future research.

In addition to processes of modeling and observational learning, it is assumed that families affect the coping behaviors of their members through rules and regulatory mechanisms. Drawing on the work of Reiss and his colleagues (Reiss, 1981; Reiss, Oliveri, & Curd, 1983), Fiese and Sameroff (1989) have discussed the importance of family paradigms, stories, and rituals in regulating the family and in shaping the experiences and behaviors of individual family members. Most pertinent to the process of coping with pediatric conditions, these family regulatory mechanisms provide rules for acceptable or preferred coping behavior in the family. These rules may be as specific as defining prescribed coping behaviors and roles for individual family members. For example, in some families children may be encouraged to share their feelings with an ill family member, whereas in others emotional expression may be prohibited. It also appears that mothers and fathers take on different roles in coping with children's cancer (e.g., Mulhern, Crisco, & Camitta, 1981) and IDDM (Hauser et al., 1986).

Finally, the broadest perspective on the role of the family in coping with pediatric conditions, and perhaps a perspective that encompasses all of the other aspects of family functioning discusses above, is the notion of the family as a system. The potential significance of family systems theory for pediatric psychology has been discussed (e.g., Kazak, 1989). Our intent here is to highlight the ways in which a systemic perspective may enhance our understanding of children's, adolescents', and families' coping with illness and injury. Questions regarding family coping can be asked in two ways. First, researchers may ask, "How is this *family* coping with an illness or injury in a child?" In this case, the coping process is operationalized at the level of the family, and corresponding measures of family functioning are obtained. For example, the Family Environment Scale (Moos & Moos, 1986) and other measures of family functioning are frequently used to assess the responses of families to pediatric conditions (Davies, 1988). This approach provides useful information on characteristics of families that are associated with good versus poor psychological and medical outcomes in pediatric patients. However, aggregate-level measures of family functioning have two limitations as measures of family coping. First, these are measures of perceived family functioning that are appropriate only for adults and are completed only by parents (virtually always mothers). Second, they describe the functioning of the family as a whole without reference to the actions of specific family members.

A second approach to analyzing coping in a family system involves the examination of reports or observations of coping of each family member. Systemic processes and interpretations are then derived from the aggregated data on all family members. For example, Hauser et al. (1986) observed interactions of families with children recently diagnosed with IDDM and families with children with acute illnesses or injuries. Families were observed while they tried to achieve resolution on a standard set of family problems. Diabetic children and their parents displayed significantly more behaviors that could be considered reflective of effective coping (enabling behaviors), as well as behaviors that could adversely affect coping (constraining behaviors) (Hauser et al., 1986). Observational methods of this type are particularly useful for assessing coping behaviors that involve direct interactions among family members.

Family processes may also affect the coping behaviors of family members outside of direct family interactions. That is, the tendency for a parent or child to use various problem- or emotion-focused strategies in his or her personal efforts to cope with a pediatric problem may be influenced by family roles and by the individual coping behaviors of others in the family. We are pursuing this possibility in our analyses of parents' and children's responses to individual coping interviews concerning parental cancer. Preliminary analyses indicate that there may well be significant relations among the ways in which family members choose to cope with a parent's cancer (Ey, Worsham, & Compas, 1991). For example, the use of emotion-focused coping by the patient is significantly correlated with the use of more emotion-focused coping by the spouse, r (74) = .23, p = .054. In contrast, patients' use of coping strategies that have a dual focus (i.e., that address both problem- and emotion-focused functions in a single coping effort) are inversely related to children's use of emotion-focused coping, r (16) = −.44, p < .08, and inversely related to children's use of dual-focus coping, r (16) = −.47, p < .06. Although the direction of influence of one family member's coping behavior on another's must await future analyses of our longitudinal data from these families, these preliminary analyses suggest the potential links between the coping efforts of spouses and of parents and children. Obtaining data of this type requires the use of individual indices of each family member's coping behavior on measures that are developmentally appropriate for children and adults, but that also yield comparable data across different individuals.

SUMMARY

Recent research on coping in children, adolescents, and families has generated a solid foundation for future investigations of coping in a variety of special populations. Foremost among these special groups are pediatric patients and their families. On the basis of this research, we would like to close by considering the definition of coping from a developmental and familial perspective. The viewpoint that has guided the vast majority of recent research has been that of Lazarus and Folkman (1984), who define coping as "constantly changing cognitive and behavioral efforts to manage specific external and/or internal demands that are appraised as taxing or exceeding the resources of the person" (p. 141). In building on this definition, it will be essential to consider that coping efforts change not only as a function of situational and temporal factors related to the stressor, but as a function of the developmental level of the individual as well. Furthermore, both appraisals of stress and appraisals of coping resources are influenced not only by the cognitive processes of the individual, but by the perceptions of other family members who are affected by the stressful circumstances. Consideration of developmental and family contributions to the coping process will make this concept even more focal and more useful to the field of pediatric psychology.

Acknowledgment

Preparation of this chapter was supported in part by National Institute of Mental Heath Grant No. MH43819.

REFERENCES

Altshuler, J. L., & Ruble, D. N. (1989). Developmental changes in children's awareness of strategies for coping with uncontrollable stress. *Child Development, 60,* 1337-1349.

Band, E. B. (1990). Children's coping with diabetes: Understanding the role of cognitive development. *Journal of Pediatric Psychology, 15,* 27-41.

Band, E. B., & Weisz, J. R. (1988). How to feel better when it feels bad: Children's perspectives on coping with everyday stress. *Developmental Psychology, 24,* 247-253.

Band, E. B., & Weisz, J. R. (1990). Developmental differences in primary and secondary control coping and adjustment to juvenile diabetes. *Journal of Clinical Child Psychology, 19,* 150-158.

Botvin, G. J., Baker, E., Dusenbury, L., Tortu, S., & Botvin, E. M. (1990). Preventing adolescent drug abuse through a multimodal cognitive-behavioral approach: Results of a 3-year study. *Journal of Consulting and Clinical Psychology, 58,* 437-446.

Burbach, D. J., & Peterson, L. (1986). Children's concepts of physical illness: A review and critique of the cognitive-developmental literature. *Health Psychology, 5,* 307-325.

Compas, B. E. (1987). Coping with stress during childhood and adolescence. *Psychological Bulletin, 101,* 393-403.

Compas, B. E., Banez, G. A., Malcarne, V. L., & Worsham, N. (1991). *Perceived control, coping with stress, and depressive symptoms in school-aged children.* Burlington, VT: University of Vermont.

Compas, B. E., Forsythe, C. J., & Wagner, B. M. (1988). Consistency and variability in causal attributions and coping with stress. *Cognitive Therapy and Research, 12,* 305-320.

Compas, B. E., Malcarne, V. L., & Banez, G. A. (in press). Coping with psychosocial stress: A developmental perspective. In B. Carpenter (Ed.), *Personal coping: Theory, research and application.* New York: Praeger.

Compas, B. E., Malcarne, V. L., & Fondacaro, K. M. (1988). Coping with stressful events in older children and young adolescents. *Journal of Consulting and Clinical Psychology, 56,* 405-411.

Compas, B. E., & Worsham, N. (1991, April). *When Mom or Dad has cancer: Developmental differences in children's coping with family stress.* Paper presented at the conference of the Society for Research on Child Development, Seattle, WA.

Curry, S. L., & Russ, S. W. (1985). Identifying coping strategies in children. *Journal of Clinical Child Psychology, 14,* 61-69.

Ey, S., Worsham, N. L., & Compas, B. E. (1991). *When mom or dad has cancer: III. Patterns of coping in families.* Burlington, VT: University of Vermont.

Fiese, B. H., & Sameroff, A. J. (1989). Family context in pediatric psychology: A transactional perspective. *Journal of Pediatric Psychology, 14,* 293-314.

Folkman, S. (1984). Personal control and stress and coping processes: A theoretical analysis. *Journal of Personality and Social Psychology, 46,* 839-852.

Folkman, S., & Lazarus, R. S. (1980). An analysis of coping in a middle-aged community sample. *Journal of Health and Social Behavior, 21,* 219-239.

Folkman, S., & Lazarus, R. S. (1985). If it changes it must be a process: A study of emotion and coping during three stages of a college examination. *Journal of Personality and Social Psychology, 48,* 150-170.

Forsythe, C. J., & Compas, B. E. (1987). Interaction of stressful events and coping: Testing the goodness of fit hypothesis. *Cognitive Therapy and Research, 11,* 473-485.

Hanson, C. L., Cigrang, J. A., Harris, M. A., Carle, D. L., Relyea, G., & Burghen, G. A. (1989). Coping styles in youths with insulin-dependent diabetes mellitus. *Journal of Consulting and Clinical Psychology, 57,* 644-651.

Hauser, S. T., Jacobson, A. M., Wertlieb, D., Weiss-Perry, B., Follansbee, D., Wolfsdorf, J. I., Herskowitz, R. D., Houlihan, J., & Rajapark, D. C. (1986). Children with recently diagnosed diabetes: Interactions with their families. *Health Psychology, 5,* 273-296.

Jay, S. M., & Elliott, C. H. (1990). A stress inoculation program for parents whose children are undergoing painful medical procedures. *Journal of Consulting and Clinical Psychology, 58,* 799-804.

Kazak, A. E. (1989). Families of chronically ill children: A systems and social-ecological model of adaptation and change. *Journal of Consulting and Clinical Psychology, 57,* 25-30.

Lazarus, R. S., & Folkman, S. (1984). *Stress, appraisal and coping.* New York: Springer.

Maddux, J. E., Roberts, M. C., Sledden, E. A., & Wright, L. (1986). Developmental issues in child health psychology. *American Psychologist, 41,* 25-34.

Manne, S. L., Redd, W. H., Jacobsen, P. B., Gorfinkle, K., Schorr, O., & Rapkin, B. (1990). Behavioral intervention to reduce child and parent distress during venipuncture. *Journal of Consulting and Clinical Psychology, 58,* 565-572.

Miller, S. M. (1980). When is a little information a dangerous thing? Coping with stressful life-events by monitoring vs. blunting. In S. Levine & H. Ursin (Eds.), *Coping and health* (pp. 145-169). New York: Plenum.

Moos, R. H., & Moos, B. S. (1986). *Family Environment Scale manual.* Palo Alto, CA: Consulting Psychologists Press.

Mulhern, R. K., Crisco, J. J., & Camilla, B. M. (1981). Patterns of communication among pediatric patients with leukemia, parents, and physicians: Prognostic disagreements and misunderstandings. *Journal of Pediatrics, 99,* 480-483.

Murphy, L. B., & Moriarty, A. E. (1976). *Vulnerability, coping and growth.* New Haven, CT: Yale University Press.

Peterson, L. (1989). Coping by children undergoing stressful medical procedures: Some conceptual, methodological, and therapeutic issues. *Journal of Consulting and Clinical Psychology, 57,* 380-387.

Reiss, D. (1981). *The family's construction of reality.* Cambridge, MA: Harvard University Press.

Reiss, D., Oliveri, M. E., & Curd, K. (1981). Family paradigm and adolescent social behavior. In H. D. Grotevant & C. R. Cooper (Eds.), *New directions for child development: Vol. 22. Adolescent development in the family.* (pp. 77-91). San Francisco: Jossey-Bass.

Roberts, M. C., & Maieron, M. J. (1989). Editorial: Family issues in pediatric psychology. *Journal of Pediatric Psychology, 14,* 153-156.

Rothbaum, F., Weisz, J. R., & Snyder, S. S. (1982). Changing the world and changing the self: A two-process model of perceived control. *Journal of Personality and Social Psychology, 42,* 5-37.

Spivack, G., & Shure, M. B. (1982). The cognition of social adjustment: Interpersonal cognitive problem-solving thinking. In B. B. Lahey & A. E. Kazdin (Eds.), *Advances in clinical child psychology* (Vol. 5, pp. 323-372). New York: Plenum.

Varni, J. W., Rubenfeld, L. A., Talbot, D., & Setoguchi, Y. (1989). Stress, social support, and depressive symptomatology in children with congenital/acquired limb deficiencies. *Journal of Pediatric Psychology, 14,* 515-530.

Wallander, J. L., & Varni, J. W. (1989). Social support and adjustment in chronically ill and handicapped children. *American Journal of Community Psychology, 17,* 185-201.

Weisz, J. R. (1986). Understanding the developing understanding of control. In M. Perlmutter (Ed.), *Minnesota Symposium on Child Psychology: Vol. 18. Cognitive perspectives on children's social and behavioral development* (pp. 219-275). Hillsdale, NJ: Erlbaum.

Weisz, J. R., Rothbaum, F. M., & Blackburn, T. C. (1984). Standing out and standing in: The psychology of control in America and Japan. *American Psychologist, 39,* 955-969.

Wertlieb, D., Weigel, C., & Feldstein, M. (1987). Measuring children's coping. *American Journal of Orthopsychiatry, 57,* 548-560.

Wills, T. A. (1986). Stress and coping in early adolescence: Relationships to substance abuse in urban school samples. *Health Psychology, 5,* 503-529.

Wright, L. (1967). The pediatric psychologist: A role model. *American Psychologist, 22,* 323-325.

CHAPTER 2

Life Stress in Children and Adolescents: An Overview of Conceptual and Methodological Issues

LAWRENCE H. COHEN and CRYSTAL PARK
University of Delaware

The conceptualization and measurement of life stress and its relation to psychological and medical problems are among the most popular research topics today. Although most of this research has focused on adult and college student populations, there is a rapidly growing literature specifically concerned with child and adolescent life stress, with a sizable segment of that literature directly relevant to pediatric issues.

The purpose of this chapter is to review the major issues confronting research on child and adolescent life stress, broadly defined. Because the life stress field is characterized by differing opinions over basic concerns such as measurement and etiological research design, this chapter focuses on the important issues facing the field, rather than describing empirical studies, many of which have produced contradictory results. However, research projects are described when appropriate for illustrative purposes. Whenever possible, issues unique to pediatric life stress are highlighted.

DEFINITIONAL ISSUES

The conceptualization and measurement of life stress are inseparable topics in principle, but for clarity's sake we treat them as relatively independent. "Life stress" can be conceptualized as a stimulus (an event or accumulation of events); as a response (a psychophysiological reaction); or as a transactional process, in which a person and an environment interact to produce an appraisal of threat or loss. The second (response-based) definition is rarely used today, but there is considerable controversy over the advantages and disadvantages of the first (stimulus-based) versus the third (appraisal-based) definition of stress.

Bruce Dohrenwend and George Brown are the best-known contemporary advocates of the stimulus-based approach to life stress research, whereas Richard Lazarus and Susan Folkman are the major proponents of the appraisal-based approach. Dohrenwend and Shrout (1985) and Brown and Harris (1989) argue that reliance on respondents' subjective evaluations of event valence, broadly defined, results in a potential confound between respondents' dispositional status and life stress scores. For example, an adolescent might rate the event "sibling moved out of the house" as extremely negative because of some characteristic of that adolescent, rather than because of some "objective" characteristic of the event. Lazarus and Folkman (e.g., Lazarus, DeLongis, Folkman, & Gruen, 1985) acknowledge the methodological impurity of subjective evaluations, but also contend that event appraisal is *the* critical component of life stress (Lazarus & Folkman, 1984). For them, the event "sibling moved out of the house" has no objective characteristics, but becomes negative or stressful only if it is so appraised by the adolescent.

To measure adolescent life stress, both Dohrenwend and Brown advocate self-reports (or others' reports) of the occurrence of life events, with separate and independent assessment of valence, broadly defined. Dohrenwend's method of valence assessment is "normative-empirical," based on judges' ratings of the readjustment required of "typical" adolescents who experience a given event. Brown's method of valence assessment is "clinical-empirical," based on the interviewer/researcher's evaluation of the meaning (contextual threat) of an event for a particular individual. In contrast, Lazarus and Folkman advocate self-reports of both the occurrence and valence of adolescents' life events.

The child and adolescent literature has examples of both subjective and independent assessments of life event valence, although, for obvious reasons, self-reported valence is more common for adolescent than for child populations. Although the controversy over subjective versus independent assessment of life event valence has important theoretical implications, the pragmatic implications appear to be trivial. For *major* events, normative and clinical valence ratings usually match subjective ratings. As a result, the independent and subjective measurement strategies produce highly comparable life stress scores that are equally predictive of outcome criteria. Moreover, in general, negative event scores that are weighted by degree of event severity are highly comparable to unit scores (simple counts) of negative events, at least for populations with a low occurrence base rate of severe events (e.g., Cohen, 1988). In our research, therefore, we typically ask adolescents to self-report the valence (negative, neutral, or positive) of experienced events, and we simply count the number of self-rated negative events for an index of recent life event stress.

In addition to the issue of valence appraisal, life events researchers are faced with decisions concerning the scope and temporal context of life stress. Our own research, and that of most American life stress researchers, has focused on the accumulation of relatively discrete events during a brief period of time (e.g., the past 6 months or year). This focus stems from the seminal work of Holmes and Rahe (1967), who developed the first instrument (the Schedule of Recent Experiences) for the quantitative assessment of life event stress. Their research, and most subsequent studies, have been based on an erosion model of life stress. Put simply, the erosion model posits that an accumulation of life events can lead to psychiatric and/or medical problems because of an erosion over time in one's resistance resources (e.g., self-concept, immune system).

However, a number of other perspectives can be taken when conceptualizing the life stress construct, for both children and adults. These other perspectives include (1) the study of a single major life event (e.g., divorce, parental death); (2) the study of a single, major, chronic life circumstance (e.g., physical disability); (3) the study of an accumulation of small daily events (hassles and uplifts, such as losing a wallet or doing well on a specific exam, respectively); and (4) the study of chronic stressful processes (e.g., dysfunctional family interactions). The child and adolescent literature furnishes examples of each of these perspectives, but in this chapter we focus on the accumulation-of-major-events approach.

In any case, the aforementioned perspectives are interrelated, differing primarily on the size of the temporal window through which life stress is viewed. For example, a chronic circumstance (e.g., a child's disability) can produce a chronic process (family conflict), which can produce a major event (divorce); this can produce other major events (moving), which can then produce a host of hassles. In fact, this temporal chain is an extreme oversimplification of the stress process, which is comprised of a dialectical transaction among patterns of major and minor stressors, disturbances in daily mood, and extended patterns of health (Lazarus & Folkman, 1984). Of course, in some contexts, minor events, major events, and chronic stressors do operate independently. Our point is that an appreciation of the transactional nature of the stress process is required.

MEASUREMENT OF CHILD AND ADOLESCENT LIFE STRESS

Cohen (1988) has recently reviewed the major issues related to the measurement of life event stress, and most of these issues are applicable to child and adolescent populations (see Compas, 1987, and Johnson, 1986, for recent reviews of measurement of life stress in these populations). A comprehensive discussion of these issues is beyond the scope of this chapter, but it is important to highlight some of the more important measurement problems. Problems associated with life event questionnaires are emphasized.

Item Composition

Items on life events questionnaires should be relevant to the population under study. Measures for children will differ from those for adolescents; the former will be comprised primarily of family-based events, whereas the latter will have some balance between family-based events and those that reflect a more active involvement with the environment. The most widely used child and adolescent measures include that by Coddington (1972), which is based on Holmes and Rahe's (and Dohrenwend's) normatively scored readjustment approach, and those by Compas, Davis, Forsythe, and Wagner (1987), Swearingen and Cohen (1985), and Johnson and McCutcheon (1980), all of which adhere to an appraisal approach (Compas et al.'s also allows for separate assessment of small events). Other scales of note include an early adolescent hassles measure (Kanner, Feldman, Weinberger, & Ford, 1987); specific life events scales for children of divorce (Sandler, Wolchik, Braver, & Fogas, 1988) and children of alcoholics (Roosa, Sandler, Gehring, & Beals, 1988); a measure of family life stress (Patterson & McCubbin, 1983); and a semistructured interview based in part on Brown and Harris's (1989) model of contextual threat (Goodyer, Kolvin, & Gatzanis, 1985).

Items that are obvious manifestations of pathology (e.g., sleep difficulties, drug use) should be excluded from a life stress measure, to avoid a contamination between the independent and dependent variables. There is some controversy over the extent and impact of item–criterion contamination in the extant life stress literature. Fortunately, recent research with adolescents suggests that the significant relationship between life stress and maladjustment persists even after deletion of life event items that appear to be confounded with pre-existing psychopathology (e.g., Rowlison & Felner, 1988).

Basic Psychometric Analyses

A life events measure for children or adolescents, like any measure, should be subjected to basic psychometric tests. Our work with Swearingen and Cohen's (1985) adolescent scale illustrates psychometric development. The current version is comprised of 46 items (mostly negative; 6-month time frame) and is scored according to subjects' own reports of occurrence and valence (bad, neutral, or good). Psychometric analyses have included the following (Burdge & Cohen, 1991; Cohen, Burt, & Bjorck, 1987; Swearingen & Cohen, 1985):

1. Intercorrelations of all possible scoring approaches (e.g., unit vs. weighted scores; judge-based weights vs. subjective weights). As with most adult life stress scales, the various scoring approaches produce highly comparable scores (r's > .90).
2. Comparisons of the life stress scores' relations to outcome criteria, such as anxiety and depression. As in previous research, the various scoring approaches produce highly comparable correlations with criteria (r's = about .40).
3. Correlations between the scoring approaches and a measure of a socially desirable response set (all r's= about .15).
4. Two-week test–retest reliability, for quantitative scores as well as for the reporting of specific life events (r's > .90).
5. Kuder–Richardson internal reliability (about .60).
6. Corroboration of event occurrence (and valence), with about 65–70% of adolescents' self-reported life events receiving corroboration from mothers.

The issue of internal reliability is an interesting one in the construction of life stress scales. For most tests, a high (e.g., > .80) Cronbach's alpha or Kuder–Richardson reliability is desirable, because it indicates that responses to a scale's items are highly interrelated and that the test is uniform in its assessment of the specific construct. For a life events measure, however, a high internal reliability is usually undesirable, because it suggests that any given event influences the occurrence of other events, which is inconsistent with a measurement strategy for *discrete* life experiences. In this regard, a life events scale represents a survey rather than a test.

The issue of event corroboration by significant others is also quite interesting. It represents a strategy for the *validation* of a self-report life events measure. Our confirmation rate with Swearingen and Cohen's (1985) adolescent scale is comparable to that obtained in other corroboration studies involving life events questionnaires (e.g., Compas et al., 1987; Lakey & Heller, 1985), but it is substantially lower than that obtained for interview assessments of adult life events (e.g., Brown & Harris, 1989). For adolescents, of course, one would not expect a particularly high mother–adolescent confirmation rate, because one of the developmental tasks of adolescence is the establishment of some autonomy from parents.

Our research group has recently completed a study of about 250 adolescent–mother pairs, in an attempt to study mothers' awareness of their adolescents' life events as a function of the latter's age, sex, and psychosocial characteristics (family environment, alienation, adjustment, etc.) (Burdge & Cohen, 1991). One interesting, and expected, finding was that across the range of adolescence, mothers were more knowledge-able about girls' life events than about boys' life events. The data suggest that parents' life event knowledge is important not only from a method-ological standpoint, but on a theoretical level as well.

We have not yet tested the Swearingen and Cohen (1985) scale's vulnerability to a concurrent mood-related response bias. This issue concerns the effects of concurrent mood on subjects' responses on a life events measure. For example, a sad mood at the time of testing may influence respondents' recollection of negative and positive experiences, or respondents' valence ratings of remembered events.

A recent experiment by Cohen, Towbes, and Flocco (1988) demon-strated a methodology to test for mood-related response biases on life stress questionnaires. College students were randomly assigned to an elated, depressed, or neutral mood condition, produced by Velten's (1968) mood induction procedure. They then completed measures of life events and of perceived and received social support. There was a signifi-cant mood effect on the number of self-reported negative life events, with subjects in the elated condition reporting fewer negative events than those in the neutral and depressed conditions. Mood had no effect on the number of self-reported positive life events or the rated intensity of negative and positive events. Perceived social support (but not received support) was affected by the mood manipulation, with subjects in the depressed condition scoring the lowest.

A mood-related response bias of the kind reported by Cohen et al. (1988) poses a serious challenge to the interpretation of a significant relation between self-reported recent life stress (and perceived social support) and concurrent psychological symptomatology. Such a response bias may be a particularly serious problem with life event questionnaires that rely on subjective scoring, in which respondents evaluate the valence of experienced events.

Scoring

Cohen (1988) has reviewed the scoring options for adult life events questionnaires, and, in general, the issues are applicable to child and adolescent measures. It is important to compute separate scores as a function of event valence (negative vs. positive), although the determina-tion of event valence remains a controversial issue—subjective ratings versus judge-based ratings versus researcher-based clinical judgments. Not surprisingly, negative event scores are more predictive of distress than are positive event scores, although intriguing data suggest that for adolescents, positive events can serve as a life stress buffer in the prediction of self-esteem (e.g., Cohen et al., 1987) and can lead to physical illness for those with a low self-concept (Brown & McGill, 1989).

Classification of Life Events

In addition to valence, there are several other dimensions for classifying child and adolescent life events. The most important of these is occurrence controllability. This dimension is important for etiological research, in which it is necessary to quantify environmental input that is relatively independent of a respondent's dispositional or clinical status (e.g., Cohen et al., 1987). Determination of occurrence controllability is usually based on ratings by judges, who may or may not be the researchers. Unfortunately, with the exception of obvious and usually low-frequency events (e.g., death of a parent), this determination is often quite difficult and imprecise (Monroe & Peterman, 1988). Moreover, occurrence controllability and valence are often confounded, with uncontrollable events usually seen as negative.

Another important life event dimension is the actual content or theme of the event. There have been several attempts to link specific types of events to specific child and adolescent disorders, with mixed success (e.g., Goodyer et al., 1985). A more promising approach is the study of distress or disease onset as a function of a vulnerability-based match between person variables (e.g., personality, developmental issues) and event type and its attendant demands. For example, a recent study showed that for the prediction of distress, family stress was the most important for early adolescents, peer stress for middle adolescents, and academic stress for older adolescent college students (Wagner & Compas, 1990).

Some life events happen directly to parents and have less direct effects on children and adolescents. Examples include job changes, accidents, and legal problems. Therefore, life events can be classified on the basis of whether they represent primarily parents' or children's experiences. A number of child and adolescent studies have quantified parents' life stress and used this score, either alone or in combination with the children's or adolescents' scores, in etiological predictions (e.g., Cohen et al., 1987; Compas, Howell, Phares, Williams, & Ledoux, 1989). In principle, however, parental stress is a separate (although obviously related) construct, and we do not discuss it further in this chapter unless it was specifically tested in a study as a causal link in the child or adolescent stress process.

Time Frame for Life Events Measurement

The time frame for life events assessment can range from 1 day (in daily event-monitoring studies; e.g., Ham & Larson, 1990) to several months (e.g., Cohen et al., 1987) to several years (e.g., Gersten, Langner, Eisenberg, & Simcha-Fagan, 1977). In theory, one's time frame should be chosen on the basis of expectations concerning the delay between life stress occurrence and criterion display. More often than not, however, time frame is probably chosen on the basis of methodological convenience; this is not that surprising, in the absence of articulated theories or conclusive data on the temporal lag between life event occurrence and distress or illness onset. In this context, data recently obtained by Goodyer, Kolvin, and Gatzanis (1987) are interesting: They found that a *clustering* of stressful life events was related to the onset of psychiatric problems in children and adolescents several weeks later. This result is similar to the earlier findings of Brown and Harris (1989) with respect to the onset of adult depression and schizophrenia.

EFFECTS OF CHILD AND ADOLESCENT LIFE EVENTS

There is a rapidly growing literature on the relations between child and adolescent life stress and psychological, medical, and behavioral outcomes. Psychological outcomes can include psychiatric status and subclinical distress. Medical outcomes can include disease onset, disease course, disease control, and subclinical illness. Behavioral outcomes can include some sports injuries, as well as initiation and maintenance of smoking and alcohol and drug use. They can also include preventive health behaviors, such as condom use and diet.

This empirical literature is extremely difficult to evaluate, and to do so fairly would require many more pages than have been allotted. The complexity of this literature is due to a number of factors. First, there is a lack of consistency in the specific measures of life stress and outcomes, including the time frame for life events assessment. Second, most of the studies are based on a cross-sectional methodology—that is, concurrent measurement of life stress and criterion variables, which precludes causal inferences. Finally, even those studies that have incorporated a longitudinal component have relied on quite disparate statistical models.

It is our opinion that "the jury is still out" on the etiological role of child and adolescent life stress. To summarize a complex literature, our conclusions are as follows:

1. There are inconsistent data on the prospective (etiological) effects of adolescent life stress, and very few data at all on these effects for child life stress (e.g., Johnson & Bradlyn, 1988).

2. There are some data to suggest that for adolescents (and adults), life stress can be the *result* of initial criterion status (e.g., Cohen et al.,

1987; Roosa, Beals, Sandler, & Pillow, 1990). For example, depression at time 1 can lead to the subsequent (time 2) occurrence of negative life events.

3. Very few studies have attempted to incorporate the various components of the stress process (major events, small events, chronic stressors, parental events, etc.).

4. Very few studies have differentiated between the prediction of criterion onset and the prediction of criterion maintenance (e.g., Monroe & Peterman, 1988). In other words, life events might relate to the *onset* of depression in initially healthy respondents, and/or they might relate to the *continuation or exacerbation* of depression in initially depressed respondents.

5. A number of studies have used criterion measures with unknown reliability and validity, and have relied too exclusively on self-reports.

6. Very few studies have attempted to control for confounding variables that might influence both life stress and outcomes (e.g., negative affectivity).

On a general level, one major problem is the lack of articulated theories on the specific role of child and adolescent life events in the onset (or maintenance) of psychiatric, medical, or behavioral outcomes. One exception is Wallander and Varni's (Chapter 13, this volume) model for pediatric life stress.

A related problem is an inconsistency in statistical models. For illustrative purposes, let us assume that we have a community sample of 500 young adolescents, and that we administer life stress and depression measures on two occasions, separated by about 6 months. Let us also assume that we rely on a regression model to analyze our data. How do we test for the "longitudinal" or etiological role of negative events? The options include the following:

1. Examination of the relation between time 2 negative events and time 2 depression, controlling for the effects of time 1 depression. This strategy tests the relation between time 2 negative events and time 1–time 2 change in depression. Conceptually, this is a good strategy, but it is possible that the time 1–time 2 change in depression will have "caused" the time 2 negative events. One safeguard is inclusion of only uncontrollable events, because, by definition, occurrence of these events should be unaffected by criterion status.

2. The exact model above, with the additional statistical control of time 1 negative events. This strategy tests the relation between time 1–time 2 change in negative events and time 1–time 2 change in depression, and it assumes that *change* in stress level is the etiological agent.

3. Examination of the relation between *time 1* negative events and time 2 depression, statistically controlling for time 1 depression.

The third option above is sometimes called a "true prospective analysis," and the temporal lag between the independent and dependent variables rules out reverse causation as a viable explanation of the data. It is clearly the most conservative model. But it is also a model that is difficult to justify conceptually. A significant prospective effect for time 1 negative events means that these events have produced a time 1-time 2 change in depression. Because these events have occurred before the assessment of time 1 depression, this effect signifies that these events not only have caused time 1 depression (assuming a significant cross-sectional effect), but also have produced an additional increase in depression from time 1 to time 2. This finding makes sense if one's model posits a *lagged* or delayed effect for child and adolescent life stress. More often than not, this finding is probably due to some stability in time 1-time 2 negative event scores, such that the real etiological agent is time 2 life stress, with the time 1 score serving as a proxy for the sake of methodological purity. However, a high correlation between time 1 and time 2 life stress suggests an environment characterized by chronic stress, or a personality variable related to the chronic occurrence of negative experiences—variables that are quite different from an accumulation of discrete events, the supposed focus of the study. We have no profound resolution to these issues, but present them to illustrate the difficulties associated with testing the causal role of life stress.

Major versus Minor Life Events

In an influential paper, Kanner, Coyne, Schaefer, and Lazarus (1981) tested the relative importance of major versus minor events in the prediction of adults' distress. They found that an accumulation of small negative events (hassles) was more predictive than an accumulation of major negative life events. Since then, several similar studies have been conducted with both adult and child populations. The usual approach is to test the relationship between hassles and maladjustment, with major life stress controlled, and to test the relationship between major life stress and maladjustment, with hassles controlled. In the adolescent literature, a few studies have used this methodology to support the predictive superiority of minor compared to major life events (e.g., Rowlison & Felner, 1988).

We do not believe that this kind of statistical comparison will prove fruitful in the long run. First, the comparison is confounded with a number of methodological problems, including those of event controllability and event-outcome contamination. Rowlison and Felner (1988) present a good review of some of these problems. The second issue is conceptual: In some cases (samples, time frames, life circumstances), small events and major events are intrinsically interrelated, whereas in other cases they represent conceptually distinct sources of life stress. Statistical comparisons in the absence of an appreciation and assessment of context will probably result in contradictory findings.

Positive Effects of Life Stress

It is generally assumed that negative life events lead to negative outcomes, but it is possible that specific negative events, or an accumulation of negative events, can lead to positive outcomes over time. For some children and adolescents, there may be a "steeling" effect, in which early stressful experiences serve to develop and bolster coping resources that will be important later in life. Elder (1979) studied the long-term effects of economic deprivation on children who grew up during the Great Depression. Some of the children from deprived families grew up to become more competent than did their counterparts from less deprived families. One possible explanation of this finding involves the added responsibilities that the former had to assume as children. The literature also includes occasional reports of personal growth resulting from the occurrence of specific medical and psychosocial tragedies. The reader is directed to Schaefer and Moos (in press) for an excellent literature review and conceptual model for the relationship between life crises and personal growth.

In our own research, we discovered the depression-*reducing* effects of uncontrollable life stress for Protestant college students with an intrinsic religious orientation (Park, Cohen, & Herb, 1990). Apparently, the internalized and deeply held faith of these students allowed them to attach meaning and a sense of control to their uncontrollable negative experiences, resulting in a reduction of sadness over time.

Beyond Main Effects of Life Stress

In theory, children differ in their vulnerability to the deleterious effects of life stress. Resistance factors may include "personality" variables, such as locus of control, self-concept, intelligence, temperament, and instrumentality. These factors may also include "environmental" variables, such as family stability, social class, and peer support.

There is, in fact, a growing body of relatively recent research on variables that serve as buffers for child and adolescent life stress. By way of definition, a "life stress buffer" is a variable that protects an individual from the negative effects of a high level of life stress. As a moderator variable, a stress buffer is represented statistically by an interaction with life stress in the prediction of a criterion. Typically, researchers compute life stress–criterion regression lines for various levels (e.g., high, average, and low) of the moderator variable. In general, theory would predict that the stress–criterion regression line will become less positive at higher (more desirable) levels of the moderator variable. S. Cohen and Edwards (1989) present an excellent overview of conceptual and statistical issues related to research on life stress moderation.

A personality or environmental variable can function as a life stress buffer in a number of ways. First, it can influence appraisals of negative events—specifically, evaluations of the meaning of events (i.e., degree of threat or loss). Second, it can influence evaluations of the effectiveness of coping resources. Finally, it can serve as a stress moderator by influencing the reliance on specific coping strategies (S. Cohen & Edwards, 1989).

The child and adolescent literature contains a number of recent studies that have reported intriguing results for a variety of stress-moderating variables. Most of this research has focused on the prediction of psychological adjustment. Specifically, there is some support for the stress-buffering role of social support, broadly defined, both for children (e.g., Dubow & Tisak, 1989; Pryor-Brown & Cowen, 1989) and for adolescents (e.g., Barrera, 1981). Towbes, Cohen, and Glyshaw (1989) found that instrumentality served as a life stress buffer for middle adolescent girls. Brown and Siegel (1988) found that exercise served as a life stress buffer in the prediction of adolescents' physical health. Wertlieb, Weigel, and Feldstein (1988) found a stress × temperament interaction in the prediction of children's utilization of medical services.

In a cross-sectional study, Murch and Cohen (1989) found that a positive family environment served as a life stress buffer for adolescents with spina bifida. Specifically, the positive relationship between negative events and depression was stronger for those adolescents with heightened perceptions of conflict and control in their family. Perceptions of independence in the family played a different role for these handicapped teenagers. At *low* levels of life stress, high scores on family independence were protective with respect to anxiety and depression, but at *high* levels of life stress, high independence scores were associated with increased levels of anxiety and depression.

Although the specific effects for family independence were not expected, they can be easily explained in retrospect. One might assume that for these adolescents, achieving and maintaining a sense of independence was stressful in and of itself. During periods of low stress, these adolescents may have been able to maintain a relatively high level of family independence. During stressful times, however, it may have been necessary for them, in light of their physical limitations, to depend more on family members for support and assistance. At such times, a family that was perceived as placing a high value on independence may have caused a teenager with spina bifida to feel that he or she was being pushed beyond his or her capabilities.

Some recent studies show that life stress moderation is a more complex issue than was originally thought. For example, Towbes et al. (1989) found that the personality trait of instrumentality served as a life stress buffer in the longitudinal prediction of anxiety, but only for middle adolescent girls—not for middle adolescent boys or for early adolescents of either sex. Even for the middle adolescent girls, the stress-moderating effect of instrumentality was obtained only in the context of a high level of relationship stress. Another example concerns the stress-buffering effect of perceptions of a positive family climate. As discussed above, Murch and Cohen (1989) found such an effect in the cross-sectional prediction of the psychological adjustment of adolescents with spina bifida; however, Burt, Cohen, and Bjorck (1988) failed to find similar effects with a nonclinical sample of adolescents. In a college student study, we (Park et al., 1990) found that intrinsic religiousness served as a life stress buffer in the prospective prediction of Protestants', but not Catholics', depression. These findings suggest that increased specificity is required in future research on life stress moderation. For example, rather than asking whether temperament serves as a stress buffer for children, a more appropriate question is as follows: What kind of temperament serves as a life stress moderator for which children, for what kinds of life events, and for the prediction of which outcomes?

In addition, most stress-buffering studies of children and adolescents have assumed that the specific moderator variable operates directly on a child or adolescent. However, it is quite possible that beneficial effects are mediated by interactional processes with parents. This may be true even for traditional personality variables. For example, a child's temperament may influence parents' reactions to a negative event, which then affects the child's adjustment to that event.

Stress moderators specify *when* life stress effects will occur—for example, when social support or instrumentality is low. On the other hand, stress mediators specify *how* life stress effects will occur—for example, as a *result* of lowered social support. Stress moderation is usually tested by a regression model, whereas stress mediation is usually tested by a path-analytic model that requires a temporal ordering of the variables. For example, Compas et al.'s (1989) study of adolescents' adjustment to major life events tested a number of potential life stress mediators, including the parents' major events and adjustment, as well as the small events of the adolescents and their parents. Another example is a recent study by Quittner, Glueckauf, and Jackson (1990), which tested the stress-mediating role of social support in the prediction of the psychological distress of mothers of hearing-impaired children.

ISSUES UNIQUE TO PEDIATRIC LIFE STRESS

All of the issues mentioned previously in this chapter have heuristic applicability to any child or adolescent population, be it pediatric, psychiatric, or nonclinical. Of course, some conceptual and methodological problems are unique to pediatric life stress research—a topic to which we now turn.

Life Stress Measurement

Use of a standard life events measure permits a comparison of distinct populations—for example, pediatric patients versus psychiatric patients versus healthy controls. Despite its advantages, measurement uniformity imposes limits on measurement sensitivity. For example, Murch and Cohen (1989) found that 6-month life stress scores of adolescents with spina bifida were comparable to those of normal adolescents. However, we do not really believe that the two groups experienced an equivalent "number" of negative life experiences. The obtained equivalence was probably due to the insensitivity of our adolescent events scale to the unique experiences of physically handicapped children.

Prediction of Illness Onset Versus Illness Maintenance

It is important to make explicit whether life stress is conceptualized as a cause of a pediatric condition, or whether it is viewed instead as contributing to the course or severity of an already existing condition. If the latter is the case, the effects of life stress on compliance with medical treatment must be disentangled from its more direct effects on the disorder itself. In any case, effects on illness onset, course, or severity can be mediated by life events' impact on emotional functioning.

A number of studies have compared diagnosis-based groups of children—for example, organic versus functional abdominal pain patients, or pediatric versus psychiatric versus nonclinical samples. Similar to psychiatric research, this type of pediatric research must assess and control for potentially important confounding variables, such as the sex, age, intelligence, and social class of the respondents.

In our opinion, a recent study by Walker and Greene (1991) is an example of relatively sophisticated research on the role of life stress for a pediatric population. Walker and Greene sampled three groups of children and adolescents: (1) those with recurrent abdominal pain with no identifiable organic etiology (functional group), (2) those with an organic cause for recurrent abdominal pain (organic group), and (3) a healthy comparison sample. The groups were comparable on such indices as age, race, sex, and social class. Measures included Johnson and McCutcheon's

(1980) life events scale, and self-report scales for pain, somatization symptoms, anxiety, and depression. The study allowed for longitudinal analyses, as the measures were administered on two occasions, separated by a 3-month interval.

In summary, Walker and Greene's (1991) results showed that at the time of the clinic visit (time 1), life events did not discriminate between the pediatric patients with and without an organic basis for abdominal pain, or between these patients and the healthy comparison respondents. However, for the functional patients, a high level of life stress prior to or following the clinic visit was predictive of continued abdominal pain. For these functional patients, high life stress subsequent to the clinic visit was associated with the maintenance of anxiety and somatization symptoms. Life stress was not predictive of illness course for the organic patients. In sum, Walker and Greene concluded that negative life events did not aid in the differential diagnosis of children and adolescents with and without an organic basis for abdominal pain, and that life stress was not predictive of outcome in the organic patients. The important finding, however, was that life stress was useful in predicting the prognosis of the functional patients.

Despite its inclusion of comparison groups and a longitudinal design, Walker and Greene's (1991) study is not without its limitations. Most notable are its sole reliance on self-report measures and its relatively short 3-month time frame.

Chronic Stress

One issue that is especially relevant to research on pediatric populations is the role of chronic stress. For some conditions, the illness itself emerges as a salient and chronic stressor, for a child as well as an entire family. For children and families attempting to cope with the chronic burdens of serious neurological and developmental problems, an accumulation of minor and/or major events of the kind typically included on checklists may have relatively little impact over time. In other words, discrete events may not have the same salience for populations whose lives are in constant upheaval, compared to populations whose lives are more stable. Cohen et al. (1987) presented a similar view in their interpretation of nonsignificant prospective effects for discrete life events experienced by young adolescents. In a recent cross-sectional survey of adults, McGonagle and Kessler (1990) found that the experience of chronic stress served to dampen the deleterious effects of discrete negative events. This finding is difficult to interpret, but the authors discuss the potential roles of anticipation and reappraisal. It is possible that a similar process operates for some pediatric conditions, although obviously a large number of medical and ecological variables must be considered. In any case, it is our opinion that future research on pediatric life stress should be conducted with a greater appreciation for the potential role of chronic stress.

Acknowledgment

We thank Rita Yopp Cohen, Bruce Compas, Roger Kobak, and James Johnson for providing helpful comments on an earlier version of this chapter.

REFERENCES

Barrera, M. (1981). Social support in the adjustment of pregnant adolescents: Assessment issues. In B. Gottlieb (Ed.), *Social networks and social support* (pp. 69-96). Beverly Hills, CA: Sage.

Brown, G., & Harris, T. (Eds.). (1989). *Life events and illness.* New York: Guilford Press.

Brown, J., & McGill, K. (1989). The cost of good fortune: When positive life events produce negative health consequences. *Journal of Personality and Social Psychology, 57,* 1103-1110.

Brown, J., & Siegel, J. (1988). Exercise as a buffer of life stress: A prospective study of adolescent health. *Health Psychology, 7,* 341-353.

Burdge, C., & Cohen, L. H. (1991). *Mothers' knowledge of adolescents' life events.* Manuscript in preparation.

Burt, C., Cohen, L. H., & Bjorck, J. (1988). Perceived family environment as a moderator of young adolescents' life stress adjustment. *American Journal of Community Psychology, 16,* 101-122.

Coddington, R. (1972). The significance of life events as etiological factors in the diseases of children: I. A survey of professional workers. *Journal of Psychosomatic Research, 16,* 7-18.

Cohen, L. H. (1988). Measurement of life events. In L. H. Cohen (Ed.), *Life events and psychological functioning: Theoretical and methodological issues* (pp. 11-30). Newbury Park, CA: Sage.

Cohen, L. H., Burt, C., & Bjorck, J. (1987). Life stress and adjustment: Effects of life events experienced by young adolescents and their parents. *Developmental Psychology, 23,* 583-592.

Cohen, L. H., Towbes, L., & Flocco, R. (1988). Effects of induced mood on self-reported life events and perceived and received social support. *Journal of Personality and Social Psychology, 55,* 669-674.

Cohen, S., & Edwards, J. (1989). Personality characteristics as moderators of the relationship between stress and disorder. In R. Neufeld (Ed.), *Advances in the investigation of psychological stress* (pp. 235-283). New York: Wiley.

Compas, B. (1987). Stress and life events during childhood and adolescence. *Clinical Psychology Review, 7,* 275-302.

Compas, B., Davis, G., Forsythe, C., & Wagner, B. (1987). Assessment of major and daily events during adolescence: The Adolescent Perceived Events Scale. *Journal of Consulting and Clinical Psychology, 55,* 534–541.

Compas, B., Howell, D., Phares, V., Williams, R., & Ledoux, N. (1989). Parent and child stress and psychological symptoms: An integrative analysis. *Developmental Psychology, 25,* 550–559.

Dohrenwend, B. P., & Shrout, P. (1985). "Hassles" in the conceptualization and measurement of life stress variables. *American Psychologist, 40,* 780–785.

Dubow, E., & Tisak, J. (1989). The relation between stressful life events and adjustment in elementary school children: The role of social support and social problem-solving skills. *Child Development, 60,* 1412–1423.

Elder, G. (1979). Historical change in life patterns and personality. In P. Baltes & O. Brim (Eds.), *Life span development and behavior* (Vol. 2, pp. 117–159). New York: Academic Press.

Gersten, J., Langner, T., Eisenberg, J., & Simcha-Fagan, O. (1977). An evaluation of the etiologic role of stressful life-change events in psychological disorder. *Journal of Health and Social Behavior, 18,* 228–244.

Goodyer, I., Kolvin, I., & Gatzanis, S. (1985). Recent undesirable life events and psychiatric disorder in childhood and adolescence. *British Journal of Psychiatry, 147,* 517–523.

Goodyer, I., Kolvin, I., & Gatzanis, S. (1987). The impact of recent undesirable life events on psychiatric disorders in childhood and adolescence. *British Journal of Psychiatry, 151,* 179–184.

Ham, M., & Larson, R. (1990). The cognitive moderation of daily stress in early adolescence. *American Journal of Community Psychology, 18,* 567–585.

Holmes, T., & Rahe, R. (1967). The Social Readjustment Rating Scale. *Journal of Psychosomatic Research, 11,* 213–218.

Johnson, J. (1986). *Life events as stressors in childhood and adolescence.* Newbury Park, CA: Sage.

Johnson, J., & Bradlyn, A. (1988). Life events and adjustment in childhood and adolescence. In L. H. Cohen (Ed.), *Life events and psychological functioning: Theoretical and methodological issues* (pp. 64–95). Newbury Park, CA: Sage.

Johnson, J., & McCutcheon, S. (1980). Assessing life stress in older children and adolescents: Preliminary findings with the Life Events Checklist. In I. Sarason & C. Spielberger (Eds.), *Stress and anxiety* (Vol. 7, pp. 111–125). Washington, DC: Hemisphere.

Kanner, A., Coyne, J., Schaefer, C., & Lazarus, R. (1981). Comparison of two modes of stress measurement: Daily hassles and uplifts versus major life events. *Journal of Behavioral Medicine, 4,* 1–39.

Kanner, A., Feldman, S., Weinberger, D., & Ford, M. (1987). Uplifts, hassles, and adaptational outcomes in early adolescents. *Journal of Early Adolescence, 7,* 371–394.

Lakey, B., & Heller, K. (1985). Response biases and the relation between negative life events and psychological symptoms. *Journal of Personality and Social Psychology, 49,* 1662–1668.

Lazarus, R., DeLongis, A., Folkman, S., & Gruen, R. (1985). Stress and adaptational outcomes: The problem of confounded measures. *American Psychologist, 40,* 770–779.

Lazarus, R., & Folkman, S. (1984). *Stress, appraisal and coping.* New York: Springer.

McGonagle, K., & Kessler, R. (1990). Chronic stress, acute stress, and depressive symptoms. *American Journal of Community Psychology, 18,* 681–706.

Monroe, S., & Peterman, A. (1988). Life stress and psychopathology. In L. H. Cohen (Ed.), *Life events and psychological functioning: Theoretical and methodological issues* (pp. 31–63). Newbury Park, CA: Sage.

Murch, R., & Cohen, L. H. (1989). Relationships among life stress, perceived family environment, and the psychological distress of spina bifida adolescents. *Journal of Pediatric Psychology, 14,* 193–214.

Park, C., Cohen, L. H., & Herb, L. (1990). Intrinsic religiousness and religious coping as life stress moderators for Catholics versus Protestants. *Journal of Personality and Social Psychology, 59,* 562–574.

Patterson, J., & McCubbin, H. (1983). The impact of family life events and changes on the health of a chronically ill child. *Family Relations, 32,* 255–264.

Pryor-Brown, L., & Cowen, E. (1989). Stressful life events, support, and children's school adjustment. *Journal of Clinical Child Psychology, 18,* 214–220.

Quittner, A., Glueckauf, R., & Jackson, D. (1990). Chronic parenting stress: Moderating versus mediating effects of social support. *Journal of Personality and Social Psychology, 59,* 1266–1278.

Roosa, M., Beals, J., Sandler, I., & Pillow, D. (1990). The role of risk and protective factors in predicting symptomatology in adolescent self-identified children of alcoholic parents. *American Journal of Community Psychology, 18,* 725–741.

Roosa, M., Sandler, I., Gehring, M., & Beals, J. (1988). The Children of Alcoholics Life Events Schedule: A stress scale for children of alcohol-abusing parents. *Journal of Studies on Alcohol, 49,* 422–429.

Rowlison, R., & Felner, R. (1988). Major life events, hassles, and adaptation in adolescence: Confounding in the conceptualization and measurement of life stress and adjustment revisited. *Journal of Personality and Social Psychology, 55,* 432–444.

Sandler, I., Wolchik, S., Braver, S., & Fogas, B. (1988). Life events, life settings and social support. In S. Wolchik & P. Karoly (Eds.), *Children of divorce: Empirical perspectives on adjustment* (pp. 191–220). New York: Wiley.

Schaefer, J., & Moos, R. (in press). Life crises and personal growth. In B. Carpenter (Ed.), *Personal coping: Theory, research, and applications.* New York: Praeger.

Swearingen, E., & Cohen, L. H. (1985). Measurement of adolescents' life events: The Junior High Life Experiences Survey. *American Journal of Community Psychology, 13,* 69–85.

Towbes, L., Cohen, L. H., & Glyshaw, K. (1989). Instrumentality as a life stress moderator for early versus middle adolescents. *Journal of Personality and Social Psychology, 57,* 109–119.

Velten, E. (1968). A laboratory task for induction of mood states. *Behaviour Research and Therapy, 6,* 473–482.

Wagner, B., & Compas, B. (1990). Gender, instrumentality, and expressivity: Moderators of the relation between stress and psychological symptoms during adolescence. *American Journal of Community Psychology, 18,* 383–406.

Walker, L., & Greene, J. (1991). Negative life events and symptom resolution in pediatric abdominal pain patients. *Journal of Pediatric Psychology, 16,* 341–360.

Wertlieb, D., Weigel, C., & Feldstein, M. (1988). The impact of stress and temperament on medical utilization by school-age children. *Journal of Pediatric Psychology, 13,* 409–421.

CHAPTER 3

Psychophysiological Responses to Stress in Children and Adolescents

JOSEPH K. MURPHY
The Miriam Hospital/Brown University Program in Medicine

> *". . . all life is an experiment."*
> —Oliver Wendell Holmes, Jr. (1919)

In the context of this quotation, psychophysiological responses to stress may play a prominent role in our understanding of health and illness. Indeed, both noninvasive and intra-arterial ambulatory monitoring demonstrate that each of us has thousands of significant and insignificant changes in both blood pressure (BP) and heart rate (HR) each day. Both cardiovascular and hormonal variables demonstrate circadian variations as well (Portaluppi et al., 1990). Thus, a better understanding of psychophysiological reactivity may enhance the prevention, diagnosis, and treatment of pediatric conditions.

By design, this chapter concentrates on cardiovascular variables and provides only tangential mention of studies of adults. Readers interested in biological reactivity to stress in other pediatric disorders are referred to other chapters in this volume. Other resources include recent reviews of clinical applications of pediatric psychophysiology (e.g., Beidel, 1989), as well as entire volumes concerning cardiovascular disease (Chesney & Rosenman, 1985; Houston & Snyder, 1988; Matthews, Weiss, et al., 1986; Schmidt, Dembroski, & Blumchen, 1986; Schneiderman, Weiss, & Kaufmann, 1989). Finally, readers who study and work with children and adolescents will be aware that this age group is an understudied one. With the notable exception of congenital disorders, this age group is generally free of cardiovascular symptoms and disease. Consequently, invasive studies are often unjustified, and studies that might be performed in adults cannot be performed in children. Within these limitations, this chapter reviews the psychophysiological responding of children and adolescents; it may, perhaps, stimulate future research that will address the associated questions raised by this review.

The rationale for studying reactivity is straightforward: A dynamic study (e.g., of BP during a video game) will provide information that cannot be obtained by a static study (e.g., BP during a physical examination), and this information will be useful in understanding the precursors or pathophysiology of disease or in guiding intervention and treatment. Though further documentation must be obtained if reactivity testing is to become a diagnostic test, parallel dynamic–static studies have become accepted clinical procedures for several disorders, such as diabetes (glucose tolerance testing vs. fasting glucose) and asthma (methacholine challenge testing vs. spirometry). Although most reactivity studies have been performed in laboratories, the laboratory may not be representative of the natural environment. Therefore, several investigators have performed their studies outside the laboratory, most notably in schools. In addition, investigators have developed devices that permit ambulatory physiological monitoring. In recent years, ambulatory BP monitoring in children has become an acceptable, though infrequently used, clinical method (e.g., Daniels, Loggie, Burton, & Kaplan, 1987). Ambulatory recordings may be likened to assessing reactivity to "real-life" stressors, and they have been used primarily in research rather than clinical settings. Where appropriate, these studies are discussed in the present review.

The earliest systematic studies of children's stressor responses were conducted by Hines and Brown with the cold pressor in the 1930s (Hines, 1937a, 1937b; Hines & Brown, 1932, 1933, 1936). Their cold-pressor procedure, used with subjects ranging from 6 to 91 years of age, required immersing the hand in ice water for 1 minute. BP measurements were performed at 30 seconds and at the conclusion of the 1-minute period. The greater of the two readings was defined as the response. The purposes of these studies were (1) to classify individuals according to the magnitude of this response, (2) to determine whether individuals predisposed to hypertension had excessive responses, and (3) to permit study of the effects of drugs and other regimens upon vasomotor responses (Hines & Brown, 1932). They hypothesized that hyperreactivity would be associated with the development of hypertension.

PREDICTION OF FUTURE BLOOD PRESSURE

In the major childhood study by Hines (1937a), 400 healthy school children between the ages of 6 and 19 years were examined. Based upon previous studies, a hyperreactive response was defined as a systolic BP (SBP) increase of 22 mm Hg accompanied by a diastolic BP (DBP) increase of 18 mm Hg. By this definition, 18% ($n = 72$) of children were hyperreactors. Subsequent follow-up studies at 27 years (Barnett, Hines, Schirger, & Gage, 1963) and 45 years (Wood, Sheps, Elveback, & Schirger, 1984) after initial testing generally supported the importance of hyperreactivity. By the 27-year follow-up, only four subjects had become hypertensive; all had been initially hyperreactive (now defined as SBP and DBP increases of 25 and 20 mm Hg, respectively). At the 45-year follow-up, 34 of the 48 hyperreactors who were located, or 71%, exhibited hypertension (SBP greater than 140 mm Hg or DBP greater than 90 mm Hg). Although the Wood et al. (1984) study has been criticized on methodological grounds (Horwitz, 1984), this sample is the only one whose members were initially studied as healthy children and followed until the development of clinical endpoints.

Studies by Falkner and colleagues (Falkner, Kushner, Onesti, & Angelakos, 1981; Falkner, Onesti, & Hamstra, 1981) supported the association between reactivity and clinical endpoints (i.e., hypertension), but focused upon adolescents (ages 10–18 years) already exhibiting borderline hypertension (between the 90th and 95th percentiles). Using a 10-minute mental arithmetic task with follow-ups at 4 and 5 years, Falkner and colleagues observed that borderline hypertensives who progressed to fixed hypertension (above the 95% percentile) and those whose BP remained in the borderline range exhibited greater reactivity as well as stronger family histories of hypertension than normotensive controls. Comparisons between fixed and borderline hypertensives were not reported. Potentially, hypertensive–normotensive differences were affected by pre-existing differences attributable to borderline hypertension.

Additional studies from the Bogalusa Heart Study (Parker et al., 1987), the Muscatine Study (Mahoney, Schieken, Clarke, & Lauer, 1988), and the Juvenile Health Study (Murphy, Alpert, Walker, & Willey, in press) indicated that BP reactivity among healthy children was associated with future BP levels. In a 2-year follow-up of children between the ages of 6 and 15 at the initial examination, Parker et al. (1987) reported that partial correlations (controlling for initial BP, age, and weight) between reactivity and subsequent BP ranged between .13 and .20 (accounting for between 1.6% and 4% of the variance). Correlations for orthostasis, handgrip, and cold pressor were comparable, and SBP correlations were somewhat greater than DBP correlations. In a 3½-year follow-up of 274 children ages 6–15 years, Mahoney et al. (1988) reported that SBP reactivity to maximal cycle ergometry explained an additional 4.7% of the variance in follow-up SBP. In addition, DBP reactivity explained 4.9% of the variance in follow-up left ventricular mass, an important predictor of cardiovascular morbid events (Devereux, 1989). The associations with follow-up SBP and ventricular mass were independent of the initial levels of SBP and ventricular mass. Finally, a 1-year follow-up (Murphy, Alpert, Walker, & Willey, in press) reported that reactivity to a video game was independently associated with subsequent SBP for both black children and white children, and with later DBP for white children. Reactivity explained from 3% to 32% of the variance in follow-up BP. Results were comparable at a 2-year follow-up (Murphy, Alpert, Walker, & Niaura, 1991).

However, the evidence supporting reactivity is not entirely consistent. Two reports from The Netherlands (Hofman & Valkenburg, 1983; Visser, Grobbee, & Hofman, 1987) reported that cold-pressor reactivity was not related to changes in BP ($n = 462$; age range $= 5$-19 years). In addition, cold-pressor responses of children showing large increases in resting SBP ($n = 25$; mean $= 29.6$ mm Hg) over the 7-year follow-up were comparable to those of children showing small increases ($n = 78$; mean $= 13.8$ mm Hg). A final European study examined the association between reactivity during mental arithmetic and submaximal exercise and subsequent ambulatory BP in 63 prepubertal boys (mean age $= 11.5$ years) (Eiff, Gogolin, Jacobs, & Neus, 1985). Using a median split of HR and SBP changes during reactivity testing, the investigators found that high-HR reactors to mental arithmetic exhibited a significantly greater increase in ambulatory SBP (7 mm Hg) at a 1-year follow-up. At a 2-year follow-up, this difference was not present.

In summary, a number of U.S. studies indicate that the magnitude of a child's reactivity is associated with later BP or the development of hypertension. However, only one cohort has been followed for more than 5 years. In addition, European studies have not shown this association. Reasons for differences between U.S. and European studies are not readily apparent. Only one sample was gender specific (Eiff et al., 1985), and studies that have both supported and failed to support the reactivity hypothesis have examined children across both wide and restricted age ranges. It should also be noted that although the majority of longitudinal studies of college students and young adults have supported the reactivity hypothesis, these data, like the childhood data, are mixed (e.g., Gillum, Taylor, Anderson, & Blackburn, 1981; Harlan, Oberman, Mitchell, & Graybiel, 1973; Menkes et al., 1989; Thomas et al., 1985).

Overall, the preponderance of evidence indicates that reactivity is associated with future BP. Discrepant results point to the need for greater precision in identifying the individuals and/or conditions that may augment or diminish the association with future BP. Such studies may determine whether reactivity is an epiphenomenon, a marker, or a mechanism. Logically, methodological, biological, and psychosocial variables may mediate the association between reactivity and a study's dependent variable(s), and thereby the association with later pathophysiology. This chapter now examines a number of potential mediators.

RELIABILITY/STABILITY

Because prediction is limited by reliability, psychophysiological measurements must be reliable to be useful. In general, children's reactivity demonstrates satisfactory stability. In the longest follow-up study, 27 years, Hines and colleagues reported that 31 of 31 children were still hyperreactive to the cold pressor in adulthood (Barnett et al., 1963). Correspondingly, 99 of 120 (82.5%) children remained normoreactive.

Other investigators, treating reactivity as a continuous variable (as opposed to a dichotomous classification), have shown reactivity to a variety of stressors to demonstrate stability generally comparable to that of resting BP and HR (e.g., Mahoney et al., 1988; Matthews, Rakaczky, Stoney, & Manuck, 1987). This statement seems to be truer when reactivity is measured as an absolute level (e.g., SBP of 120 mm Hg) than when measured as a simple change value (e.g., 10 mm Hg). For example, Sallis et al. (1989) reported a correlation of 0.56 for SBP level but a correlation of −.05 for SBP change. We (Murphy, Alpert, Walker, & Willey, in press) found that both HR and BP reactivity when measured as absolute levels were as stable as resting values. In a subsequent 2-year follow-up report, absolute levels were often significantly more stable than change values (Murphy, Alpert, & Walker, 1991c). In addition, stability was not significantly affected by race (black or white), gender, body mass (light or heavy), or performance (low or high). Using multiple-regression procedures in a 4-year follow-up, Matthews, Woodall, and Stoney (1990) reported that from 42% to 80% of the variance in follow-up reactivity could be accounted for primarily by the initial reactivity and follow-up baseline measurements. Inconsistent correlates included gender, performance, age, and initial baseline measurements.

In summary, studies of the stability of children's reactivity are fairly consistent in reporting correlation coefficients for absolute levels in the range of .40–.70. Generally, HR reactivity is more stable than BP reactivity; SBP reactivity exhibits greater stability than DBP reactivity.

LONGITUDINAL TRACKING OF REACTIVITY

Although I have concluded in the preceding discussion of stability that reactivity is a stable characteristic, the magnitude of the correlation suggests that for some children reactivity is quite stable and that for other children it demonstrates little stability. Maintaining rank order over time has been referred to as "tracking." Longitudinal studies of children's resting BP have shown that only a small percentage of children demonstrate well-defined tracking—for example, resting BP in the highest decile that remains in that decile over multiple annual measurements (e.g.,

Lauer, Clarke, & Beaglehole, 1984). As noted earlier, Barnett et al. (1963) reported that all hyperreactors were still hyperreactors at the 27-year follow-up; that is, they tracked.

Data from our longitudinal study also suggest that tracking occurs but only for a small percentage of children (Murphy, Alpert, & Walker, 1991a). In this study, 396 children had BP and HR reactivity measured during a television video game on three annual examinations. Each year's video game measurements were averaged, and quartiles of mean arterial pressure (⅓ SBP + ⅔ DBP) reactivity were calculated. Cross-tabulation of annual data indicated that 28 children (17 boys and 11 girls) were consistently in the highest quartile, and 24 children (11 boys and 13 girls) were consistently in the lowest quartile. Mean ages of hyper- and hypo-reactors were comparable (9.4 and 9.1 years, respectively). Consistently, hyperreactors had greater resting BP (see Table 3.1) than hyporeactors. From year 1 to year 3, the increase in resting BP was greater for hyperreactors. In addition, both SBP and DBP divergence increased annually, suggesting that hyperreactivity may be a marker or mechanism in the development of high BP.

GENERALIZABILITY

Logically, the case for reactivity's being associated with subsequent BP would be strengthened by the demonstration that reactivity in the laboratory is associated with reactivity in the natural environment. Although this area has received limited systematic study, research does support such an association. Matthews, Manuck, and Saab (1986) studied reactivity during three laboratory stressors (serial subtraction, star tracing, and handgrip) and during a natural stressor (a 5-minute speech in English class). After performing a median split of subjects based upon each lab-

Table 3.1. Mean Resting BPs (± *SD*; in mm Hg) of Hyperreactors (Highest Quintile) and Hyporeactors (Lowest Quintile) by Year

	Systolic		Diastolic	
Year	Hyperreactors	Hyporeactors	Hyperreactors	Hyporeactors
1	112.2 ± 10.2	98.8 ± 10.1	65.1 ± 7.7	54.9 ± 6.4
2	120.4 ± 9.1	104.4 ± 7.3	69.5 ± 6.6	58.4 ± 7.1
3	121.8 ± 9.7	103.4 ± 9.9	68.1 ± 8.3	56.6 ± 6.6

Note. From *A Longitudinal Comparison of Hyper- and Hyporeactive Children* by J. K. Murphy, B. S. Alpert, and S. S. Walker, 1991, manuscript in preparation.

oratory tasks and each hemodynamic variable, the investigators compared reactors and nonreactors during the class speech. Results indicated that the association between laboratory reactivity and speech reactivity varied according to the laboratory task. In general, the reactivity during the subtraction task was most strongly associated with speech task reactivity.

More recently, we (Harshfield, Alpert, Murphy, Willey, & Somes, 1990) used ambulatory BP and HR monitoring to compare children who were hyper- or hyporeactive in the laboratory. Children were classified according to quartiles of SBP and HR reactivity to a television video game. Ambulatory measures were performed every 20 minutes between 6 A.M. and midnight, and every hour between midnight and 6 A.M. When defined by HR reactivity, hyperreactors (highest quartile; $n = 48$) demonstrated greater SBP both while awake and while asleep than the hyporeactors (lowest quartile; $n = 48$). The two groups had similar ambulatory DBP and HR. Differences between hyper- and hyporeactive children were more pronounced among black children. Reactivity status according to SBP was not associated with ambulatory data. HR reactivity was hypothesized to be a better discriminator of ambulatory SBP than SBP reactivity because of its greater stability.

Parallel results were provided in another ambulatory BP study that dichotomized children (median split) according to HR during mental arithmetic (Langewitz et al., 1985). Specifically, high-HR reactors demonstrated a steady increase in ambulatory BP over repeated ambulatory assessments. A final ambulatory BP study indicated that high-SBP reactors had greater ambulatory SBP and DBP (Coates, Parker, & Kolodner, 1982). A later analysis of the Coates et al. data that treated reactivity as a continuous variable indicated that laboratory and ambulatory measures of SBP were significantly correlated, whereas DBP and HR measures were not (Southard et al., 1986). In summary, the evidence indicates that some measures of laboratory reactivity are generalizable to the natural environment.

A second aspect of generalizability is the comparison of reactivity across different laboratory procedures. Although many childhood investigations have used multiple stressors, only a few have specifically examined stressor–stressor generalizability. Matthews et al. (1987) reported correlation coefficients for BP and HR reactivity (change values) to serial subtraction, mirror-image tracing, and isometric handgrip that were more often than not significant; coefficients were usually between .30 and .60. Among the sample of girls (boys did not undergo identical protocols), interstressor correlations tended to increase over the mean follow-up period of 10.4 months. The Bogalusa Heart Study (Parker et al., 1987), reported interstressor correlations for BP reactivity (maximal values) that were highly significant, ranging from .53 to .84.

In contrast, Strong, Miller, Striplin, and Salehbhai (1978) reported only modest correlations for reactivity to isometric and dynamic exercise. However, isometric reactivity was defined as the measured value, while dynamic reactivity was defined as a calculated change value. The use of different definitions may have obscured a stronger association. Similarly, the greater magnitude of correlations in the Parker et al. (1987) report, compared to those reported by Matthews et al. (1987), may be attributable to methodological differences between investigations or may reflect the different definitions of reactivity (i.e., calculated change values vs. measured values; see "Reliability/Stability," above). Nonetheless, these studies suggest that some children demonstrate substantial similarity in BP reactivity to various procedures; other children may demonstrate responses that are idiosyncratic to particular procedures.

NORMATIVE DATA

If reactivity is associated with later BP, a basis needs to exist for classifying children as hyper-, normo-, or hyporeactors. In comparison with the numbers of children with reported resting BP (e.g., Task Force on Blood Pressure Control in Children, 1987), data on children's reactivity are limited. However, several studies have examined reactivity in large samples (n's > 200) of children. Matthews and Stoney (1988) provided data on responses to serial subtraction, mirror-image tracing, and isometric handgrip from 217 children ranging from 7 to 18 years of age. As described earlier, Hines (1937a) studied cold-pressor responses of 400 children ranging in age from 6 to 18 years. Voors, Webber, and Berenson (1980) reported on the responses to orthostasis, isometric handgrip, and the cold pressor of 278 children from 6 to 13 years of age. Both Alpert and colleagues (Alpert, Dover, Booker, Martin, & Strong, 1981; Alpert et al., 1982; $n = 405$) and Schieken, Clarke, and Lauer (1983; $n = 264$) studied maximal cycle ergometry. Children in the Alpert et al. studies ranged from 6 to 15 years of age, and those studied by Schieken et al. were between 9 and 18 years of age. My colleagues and I, studying children between 6 and 18 years of age, have provided cross-sectional data on video game reactivity of 310 (Murphy, Alpert, Willey, & Somes, 1988) and 481 (Murphy, Alpert, Walker, & Willey, 1988) children. The former report provided percentiles of reactivity (see Figure 3.1; Murphy, Alpert, Willey, & Somes, 1988). Finally, Tell, Prineas, and Gomez-Marin (1988) studied the effects of postural change in 916 children from 14 to 16 years of age. Thus, depending upon the reactivity procedure, data may be available to guide an investigator in evaluating the magnitude of reactivity.

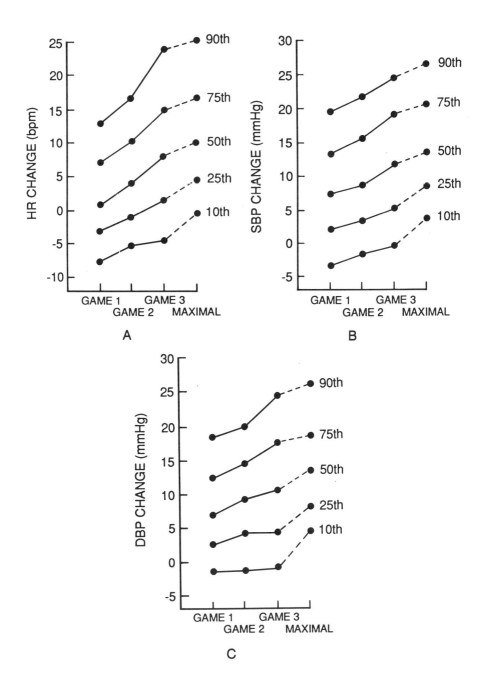

Figure 3.1. Percentiles of reactivity for (A) heart rate, (B) systolic blood pressure, and (C) diastolic blood pressure. From "Cardiovascular Reactivity to Psychological Stress in Healthy Children" by J. K. Murphy, B. S. Alpert, E. S. Willey, and G. W. Somes, 1988, *Psychophysiology*, 25, 144–152. Copyright 1988 by The Society for Psychophysiological Research. Reprinted by permission.

AGE AND GENDER

Although studies of young children (e.g., Lundberg, 1983), infants (e.g., Schwartz, Campos, & Baisel, 1973), and fetuses (e.g., Devoe, McKenzie, Searle, & Sherline, 1985) have been conducted, reactivity studies have generally examined school-age children (i.e., 6–18 years of age) of both genders. Consistent effects of age and gender have not been demonstrated. In the studies of Schieken et al. (1983) and Strong et al. (1978), BP reactivity during exercise was significantly and positively correlated with age; gender differences were not reported. In contrast, James et al. (1980) reported that exercise reactivity was more strongly associated with body size (body surface area) than with age, and that gender differences were mediated by body size. Similarly, Alpert et al. (1981) reported that ethnic differences in exercise reactivity were more consistent with respect to body surface area than to age.

Other studies of physical stressors have provided mixed evidence on the importance of age (Hines, 1937a; Voors et al., 1980). Data from Voors and colleagues indicated that gender (boys > girls) was more closely associated with reactivity than age was, but that association was dependent upon the stressor. Our studies of reactivity to a video game have found both age and gender to be inconsistent correlates of reactivity (Murphy, Alpert, Moes, & Somes, 1986; Murphy, Alpert, Walker, & Willey, 1988; Murphy, Alpert, Willey, & Somes, 1988). Matthews and Stoney (1988) reported that the association of age and gender with reactivity were affected by both the stressor and the hemodynamic parameter; the association of age (younger > older) and HR reactivity was most consistent. Although children and adolescents undergo a substantial number of developmental changes that are both gender-specific (e.g., menstruation and use of birth control pills) and non-gender-specific (e.g., chronological and sexual maturation and increases in height and weight), the contributions of these changes to the reactivity of either boys or girls are incompletely understood.

FAMILIAL REACTIVITY

The data reviewed to this point suggest that reactivity may be associated with later BP. If so, reactivity may be hypothesized to exhibit familial aggregation. In their review, Rose and Chesney (1986) concluded that reactivity demonstrated familial aggregation, and that twin studies (comparisons of monozygotic to dizygotic twins) indicated that aggregation is attributable in part to heritability. Twin studies, in conjunction with studies of parent–child responses (e.g., Hastrup, Kraemer, Hotchkiss, & Johnson, 1986; Matthews et al., 1988), suggest that individual variables are at least as important as genetics in determining the magnitude of reactivity. The study by Matthews et al. exemplifies this research. These investigators were able to study 142 families, comprised of 217 children ages 7–18 years, 141 mothers, and 119 fathers. Reactivity tasks were serial subtraction, mirror-image tracing, and handgrip. Overall, few significant sibling or parent–child associations were reported. The only significant effect with mirror-image tracing was a sister–brother association for HR. Significant handgrip results were (1) a mother–daughter association for both SBP and DBP and (2) a sister–brother association for SBP. Matthews et al. interpreted their results as indicating that extrafamilial influences are most important in determining reactivity.

FAMILIAL HISTORY OF HYPERTENSION

Children of hypertensive parents have been shown to have higher resting BP than offspring of normotensive parents (Munger, Prineas, & Gomez-Marin, 1988). Thus, if hyperreactivity is associated with hypertension, children of hypertensive parents might be expected to exhibit hyperreactivity. Hines (1937b) reported a striking correspondence between parental status and children's responses. If both parents were hypertensive or were hyperreactors, 95% of children were hypertensive or hyperreactors. If only one parent met this definition (hypertensive or hyperreactive), 43.4% of children were categorized similarly. When neither parent met the definition, all children were normoreactive. Unfortunately, the individual contribution of either parental hypertension or parental hyperreactivity cannot be determined. Subsequent evidence for the importance of family history has been mixed, with studies providing both supporting data (e.g., Anderson, Mahoney, Lauer, & Clarke, 1987; Falkner, Onesti, Angelakos, Fernandes, & Langman, 1979; Molineux & Steptoe, 1988) and nonsupporting data (e.g., Hastrup et al., 1986; Matthews, Manuck, & Saab, 1986).

Although even the supporting studies report different distinguishing variables, there does seem to be some consistency in differences in DBP reactivity; that is, children with a positive history demonstrate greater reactivity (Ewart, Harris, Zeger, & Russell, 1986; Falkner, Onesti, Angelakos, Fernandes, & Langman, 1979; Ferrara, Moscato, et al., 1988; Hohn et al., 1983; McCann & Matthews, 1988; Musante, Treiber, Strong, & Levy, 1990; Svensson & Hansson, 1985). Ambulatory monitoring has also indicated increased DBP in children with hypertensive parents (Wilson, Ferencz, Dischinger, Brenner, & Zeger, 1988). Results suggest that the primary effect of a positive family history is an early alteration of peripheral vascular resistance. Ewart et al. (1996) interpreted their results as supporting this conclusion, and Musante et al. (1990), using impedance cardiography, demonstrated that resistance was increased in children with hypertensive parents. Although many factors may influence study outcome (Watt, 1986), regional differences in blood flow may be the most parsimonious explanation for discrepant results (Anderson et al., 1987). Anderson et al. hypothesized that flow differences in one region of the body (e.g., the forearm) may be counteracted by differences in another region (e.g., the splanchnic area). The net result would be an absence of BP differences.

TYPE A BEHAVIOR PATTERN

Another area that has received considerable study is the association between Type A behavior and reactivity. Like the adult literature, the literature on Type A in childhood and adolescence may best be described as equivocal. Studies have reported that Type A was associated with greater reactivity (e.g., Lundberg, 1983; Spiga, 1986); was mediated by another variable, such as parental history of hypertension (McCann & Matthews, 1988); was not associated with greater reactivity (Eagleston et al., 1986; Matthews, Manuck, & Saab, 1986; Murray, Blake, Prineas, & Gillum, 1985); and was dependent upon the Type A measure employed (e.g., Coates et al., 1982; Lawler, Allen, Critcher, & Standard, 1981; Matthews & Jennings, 1984).

Studies indicating different associations for different Type A measures may be particularly pertinent, in view of the multiple measures for assessing children's Type A behavior. Measures include the Matthews Youth Test for Health (Matthews & Angulo, 1980), the Adolescent Structured Interview (Siegel & Leitch, 1981), the Miami Structured Interview (Gerace & Smith, 1985), the Bortner battery (Bortner & Rosenman, 1967), the Hunter-Wolf A-B Rating Scale (Wolf, Sklov, Wenzel, Hunter, & Berenson, 1982), the Butensky Interview (Butensky, Farilli, Heebner, & Waldron, 1976), the Student Type A Behavior Scale (Eagleston et al., 1986), and the Student Structured Interview (Eagleston et al., 1986), as well as various scales and measures assessing attributes or components of the Type A construct. Although no study has utilized all of these instruments, Matthews (1982) has reported on the discordance in Type A instruments. Additional dimensions, such as tasks or gender × task interactions, may further contribute to interstudy differences. Potentially, greater attention to family characteristics, such as positive affiliation or authoritarianism (Woodall & Matthews, 1989), may clarify the importance of children's Type A behavior.

RACE

Despite some limitations in the accuracy of defining individuals as black or white (Cooper, 1984), epidemiological studies have consistently found

Table 3.2. Ethnic Differences in Children's Reactivity

Study	n	Stressor	Results
1. Alpert, Dover, Booker, Martin, & Strong, (1981)	405	Cycle ergometry	HR, B $\approx$ W; SBP, B $>$ W[a]
2. Alpert et al. (1982)	As in study 1	As in study 1	ECG: J point, B $\approx$ W; ST slope, B $>$ W[a]
3. Arensman, Treiber, Gruber, & Strong (1989)	50	Cycle ergometry	HR, B $<$ W; SBP, B $\approx$ W; DBP, B $\approx$ W; RPP, B $\approx$ W; ejection time, B $\approx$ W; time to peak ejection, W $<$ B; velocity change, B $<$ W; flow velocity integral, B $\approx$ W; CI, B $<$ W; SVR, B $>$ W[a,b]
4. Hohn et al. (1983)	141	(1) Postural changes, (2) treadmill	HR, B $\approx$ W; SBP, B $>$ W; DBP, B $>$ W; CO, B $\approx$ W; Na, B $>$ W; K, B $>$ W; Kall, B $>$ W; iPGE, B $\approx$ W; PRA, B $<$ W; NE, B $\approx$ W[a,b]
5. Murphy, Alpert, Moes, & Somes (1986)	213	Video game	HR, B $\approx$ W; SBP, B $>$ W; DBP, B $>$ W[a,b]
6. Murphy, Alpert, Willey, & Somes (1988)	310	Expansion of study 5	HR, B $>$ W; SBP, B $\approx$ W; DBP, B $>$ W[b]
7. Murphy, Alpert, Walker, & Willey (1988)	481	Video game	HR, B $>$ W; SBP, B $>$ W; DBP, B $>$ W
8. Murphy, Alpert, Walker, & Willey (in press)	434	1-year follow-up of study 7	HR, B $>$ W; SBP, B $>$ W; DBP, B $>$ W

9. Murphy, Alpert, Walker, & Niaura (1991)	395	2-year follow up of study 7	HR, B > W; SBP, B > W; SBP, B > W
10. Remington, Lambarth, Moser, & Hoobler (1960)	131	(1) Standing, (2) cold pressor, (3) breath holding, (4) knee bends	No B-W statistical comparisons
11. Tell, Prineas, & Gomez-Martin (1988)	916	Standing	HR, B ≈ W; SBP, B > W; DBP, B ≈ W[a,b]
12. Thomas et al. (1984)	52	Reading aloud	HR, B ≈ W; SBP, B ≈ W; DBP, B ≈ W; MAP, B ≈ W[b]
13. Treiber et al. (1990)	40	Forehead cold	HR, B ≈ W; SBP, B ≈ W; DBP, B > W; CI, B ≈ W; TPR, B > W
14. Treiber, Musante, Strong, & Levy (1989)	75	Treadmill	HR, B < W; SBP, B > W; DBP, B ≈ W[a]
15. Voors, Webber, & Berenson (1980)	278	(1) Standing, (2) handgrip, (3) cold pressor	HR, B < W; SBP, B > W; DBP, B > W[a,b]

Note. B, black; W, white; HR, heart rate; SBP, systolic blood pressure; DBP, diastolic blood pressure; ECG, electrocardiogram; RPP, rate pressure product; CI, cardiac index; SVR, systemic vascular resistance; CO, cardiac output; Na, urinary sodium; K, urinary potassium; Kall, urinary kallikrein; iPGE, urinary immunoreactive prostaglandin E-like material; PRA, plasma renin activity; NE, plasma norepinephrine; MAP, mean arterial pressure; TPR, total peripheral resistance.

[a]Prestressor (baseline) values not incorporated in reactivity analyses (e.g., repeated measures, analysis of covariance, or residuals).
[b]Some B-W differences influenced by another independent variable (e.g., significant interaction between race and gender).

black Americans to have a greater prevalence of hypertension than white Americans (Falkner, 1987). Consequently, a number of investigations have studied reactivity in black children and white children (see Table 3.2). Examination of Table 3.2 indicates that, as in the research areas discussed earlier, ethnic differences are not entirely consistent (e.g., HR). However, more often than not, differences in BP reactivity do seem to occur, and differences do not seem to be a function of task novelty. A recent report (Murphy, Alpert, & Walker, 1991b; see Figure 3.2) demonstrated that the hyperreactivity of blacks was maintained over three annual examinations. In addition, studies by Treiber and colleagues (Arensman, Treiber, Gruber, & Strong, 1989; Musante et al., 1990; Treiber et al., 1990) suggest that black children may exhibit increased vascular resistance.

Finally, ambulatory BP studies indicate that ethnic differences extend beyond the laboratory (Harshfield et al., 1989; Harshfield, Dupaul, et al., 1990). In the first of these reports, blacks and whites were shown to have comparable BP while awake; during sleep, blacks had greater BP (Harshfield et al., 1989). The second report expanded upon the first and suggested that aerobic fitness played a greater role in blacks' than in whites' BP. The lack of ethnic differences in the Southard et al. (1986) report may represent results discrepant with those of Harshfield and colleagues, or may be attributable to either a small sample (9 white boys and 19 black boys) or analysis of the entire 24-hour period.

LEVEL OF BLOOD PRESSURE

An alternative to studying healthy children is to study children who have elevated resting BP (i.e., borderline or essential hypertension). Differences between hypertensive and normotensive children may thereby elucidate childhood hypertension. Although investigators have rather uniformly indicated that elevated BP is associated with altered hemodynamics (Hansen, Hyldebrandt, Nielsen, & Froberg, 1989; Kushner & Falkner, 1981; McCrory, Klein, & Rosenthal, 1982; Santangelo, Falkner, & Kushner, 1989; Wilson, Gaffney, Laird, & Fixler, 1985), the importance of the reactivity measurements (as opposed to the resting measurements) has not been consistently demonstrated (e.g., Hansen et al., 1989).

Because hypertension has clear risks, invasive studies may be justified. For example, McCrory et al. (1982) collected plasma samples before and after standing. Analysis indicated that the hypertensive groups— borderline ($n = 19$) and established ($n = 9$)—had higher resting levels of norepinephrine than normotensives; levels of epinephrine were comparable. Hypertensives exhibited a blunted norepinephrine response to standing. In the borderline group and siblings of hypertensives, SBP was

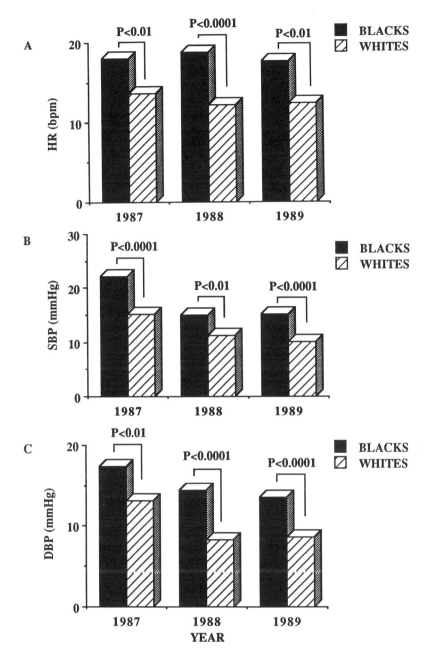

Figure 3.2. Maximal pressor reactivity by ethnicity and year for (A) heart rate, (B) systolic blood pressure, and (C) diastolic blood pressure. From "Stability of Ethnic Differences in Children's Pressor Responses during 3 Annual Examinations" by J. K. Murphy, B. S. Alpert, and S. S. Walker, 1991, *American Journal of Hypertension*, 4, 630–634. Copyright by the American Journal of Hypertension, Inc. Reprinted by permission.

correlated positively with norepinephrine levels, both while at rest and while standing. Santangelo et al. (1989) also interpreted their results as reflecting alterations in the sympathetic nervous system. Treatment data suggest that the magnitude of reactivity, both hemodynamic and catecholaminergic, may be reduced pharmacologically (Falkner, Onesti, Affrime, & Lowenthal, 1982). Finally, ambulatory studies have indicated that hemodynamic irregularities are present throughout the day (Fixler, Wallace, Thornton, & Dimmitt, 1990; Mehta, Bahler, Hanson, Walsh, & Rakita, 1986), but may be most pronounced during school hours (Fixler et al., 1990).

AEROBIC FITNESS

The scant attention given to the effects of children's fitness upon reactivity is probably attributable to equipment and personnel requirements for maximal exercise testing and measurement of oxygen uptake. The ambulatory BP study of Harshfield, Dupaul, et al. (1990) reported that less fit children had higher BP than more fit children. Among black children the effects of fitness were significant; among white children effects were nonsignificant. In contrast, a laboratory study (Murphy et al., 1989) suggested that the salutary effects of fitness might be less consistent among blacks than among whites (fit blacks had greater SBP than unfit blacks). An earlier report (Alpert, Murphy, & Christman, 1986) indicated that maximal oxygen uptake was inversely and significantly associated with video game HR reactivity only among white children. Finally, a study of hypertensive adolescents indicated that an 8-month exercise training program reduced the SBP response to standing (Hagberg et al., 1984). In addition, BP and HR during submaximal exercise testing were reduced after training.

CATECHOLAMINES AND REACTIVITY

As noted in the discussion of BP level and reactivity, the sympathetic nervous system is hypothesized to play a central role in reactivity. A number of studies have examined catecholamine reactivity during stressful situations (e.g., Bergman & Magnusson, 1979; Elwood, Ferguson, & Thakar, 1986; Ferrara, Moscato, et al., 1988; Ferraro, Soro, et al., 1988; Falkner, Onesti, & Angelakos, 1979; Johansson, Frankenhauser, & Magnusson, 1973; Lundberg, Chateau, Winberg, & Frankenhauser, 1981; Tennes & Kreye, 1985; Tennes, Kreye, Avitable, & Wells, 1986). An example of this research is the study of Falkner, Onesti, and Angelakos (1979) of adolescents varying in risk for hypertension. A blood sample was drawn 5 minutes after a 10-minute period of mental arithmetic. Compared to controls (normotensive and a negative family history), "genetic" (normotensive and at least one hypertensive parent) and "labile" (DBP sometimes above the 95th percentile and at least one hypertensive parent) groups demonstrated higher catecholamine levels and greater numbers of individuals with elevated ($>$ 1 ng/ml) levels. Although the higher-risk groups also demonstrated greater BP and HR reactivity, the association between hemodynamic and catecholamine reactivity was not examined. The McCrory et al. (1982) investigation (see "Level of Blood Pressure," above) may provide the most direct evidence that reactivity may be mediated by catecholamines.

ADDITIONAL VARIABLES

Additional variables that have received preliminary study include electrolyte and mineral intake (Alpert et al., 1988; Falkner, Onesti, & Angelakos, 1981), experimenter effects (Murphy et al., 1986, Murphy, Alpert, Willey, & Somes, 1988; Murphy, Alpert, & Walker, 1990), and weight (Ferrara, Soro, et al., 1988). The study by Falkner, Onesti, and Angelakos (1981) suggested that a high salt intake and a family history of hypertension interacted to result in greater reactivity. Cardiovascular reactivity of adolescents with a negative family history was unaffected by 2 weeks of salt loading. Alpert et al. (1988) reported that usual intake of calcium was negatively associated with HR reactivity, whereas usual sodium intake was positively associated with DBP reactivity. More recently, a report by Harshfield et al. (1991) indicated that the pattern of ambulatory BP may be affected by sodium intake in association with plasma renin activity.

In addition to our interest in the interaction between children's ethnicity and reactivity, my colleagues and I have reported on the effects of experimenter race (Murphy et al., 1986; Murphy, Alpert, Willey, & Somes, 1988; Murphy et al., 1990). In the first two reports, which were laboratory studies, an experimenter of the same race as the child increased reactivity. The latest naturalistic study suggested that race-of-experimenter effects were inconsistent and secondary to race-of-subject effects. The full import of experimenter race and other experimental variables remains to be established.

The report by Ferrara, Soro, et al. (1988) indicated a nonsignificant trend for reactivity (as well as urinary catecholamine excretion) to increase with increasing weight (body mass index). Finally, a number of variables studied in adults and potentially important in childhood studies have yet to be examined—for example, caffeine intake (Lovallo et al., 1989), menstrual phase (Kaplan, Whitsett, & Robinson, 1990), and the environmental stress of residing in proximity to commercial (as opposed to residential) development (Fleming, Baum, Davidson, Rectanus, & McArdle, 1987).

TREATMENT OF REACTIVITY

Studies evaluating childhood interventions for reactivity may be premature. The two studies that did evaluate interventions both studied hypertensive adolescents (Falkner et al., 1982; Hagberg et al., 1984). As noted earlier in the discussion of these reports, intensive interventions (medication and exercise training) may reduce reactivity.

SUMMARY

This chapter has provided an admittedly brief overview of research in children's cardiovascular reactivity. Many of the investigations provide conflicting results. However, the evidence also provide some consistency; for instance, the majority of studies indicate an association between reactivity and future BP. Furthermore, the inconsistencies between studies should not be too surprising in view of the mosaic of risk factors for cardiovascular diseases. Future research needs to determine the importance of reactivity within this mosaic.

Acknowledgments

Preparation of this chapter was supported in part by Grant No. HL-44847, National Heart, Lung, and Blood Institute. The secretarial assistance of Linda Moreau is gratefully acknowledged.

REFERENCES

Alpert, B. S., Dover, E. V., Booker, D. L., Martin, A. M., & Strong, W. B. (1981). Blood pressure response to dynamic exercise in healthy children—black vs. white. *Journal of Pediatrics, 99,* 556-560.

Alpert, B. S., Flood, N. L., Strong, W. B., Dover, E. V., DuRant, R. H., Martin, A. M., & Booker, D. L. (1982). Responses to ergometer exercise in a healthy biracial population of children. *Journal of Pediatrics, 101,* 538-545.

Alpert, B. S., Murphy, J. K., & Christman, J. V. (1986). Does fitness protect against excessive heart rate reactivity to psychologic stress? *Pediatric Research, 20,* 167A. (Abstract)

Alpert, B. S., Murphy, J. K., Willey, E. S., Somes, G. W., Stapleton, F. B., & Bittle, J. B. (1988). Sodium, calcium, and cardiovascular reactivity in children. *Pediatric Research, 23*, 214A. (Abstract)

Anderson, E. A., Mahoney, L. T., Lauer, R. M., & Clarke, W. R. (1987). Enhanced forearm blood flow during mental stress in children of hypertensive parents. *Hypertension, 10*, 544-549.

Arensman, F. W., Treiber, F. A., Gruber, M. P., & Strong, W. B. (1989). Exercise-induced differences in cardiac output, blood pressure, and systemic vascular resistance in a healthy biracial population of 10-year-old boys. *American Journal of Diseases of Children, 143*, 212-216.

Barnett, P. H., Hines, E. A., Schirger, A., & Gage, R. P. (1963). Blood pressure and vascular reactivity to the cold pressor test. *Journal of the American Medical Association, 183*, 845-848.

Beidel, D. C. (1989). Assessing anxious emotion: A review of psychophysiological assessment in children. *Clinical Psychology Review, 9*, 717-736.

Bergman, L. R., & Magnusson, D. (1979). Overachievement and catecholamine excretion in an achievement-demanding situation. *Psychosomatic Medicine, 41*, 181-188.

Bortner, R. W., & Rosenman, R. H. (1967). The measurement of pattern A behavior. *Journal of Chronic Diseases, 20*, 525-533.

Butensky, A., Farilli, V., Heebner, D., & Waldron, I. (1976). Elements of the coronary prone behavior pattern in children and teenagers. *Journal of Psychosomatic Research, 20*, 439-444.

Chesney, M. A., & Rosenman, R. H. (Eds.). (1985). *Anger and hostility in cardiovascular and behavioral disorders*. Washington, DC: Hemisphere.

Coates, T. J., Parker, F. C., & Kolodner, K. (1982). Stress and heart disease: Does blood pressure reactivity offer a link? In T. J. Coates, A. C. Peterson & C. Perry (Eds.), *Promoting adolescent health* (pp. 305-321). New York: Academic Press.

Cooper, R. (1984). A note of the biologic concept of race and its application in epidemiologic research. *American Heart Journal, 108*, 715-723.

Daniels, S. R., Loggie, J. M., Burton, T., & Kaplan, S. (1987). Difficulties with ambulatory blood pressure monitoring in children and adolescents. *Journal of Pediatrics, 111*, 397-400.

Devereux, R. B. (1989). Importance of left ventricular mass as a predictor of cardiovascular morbidity in hypertension. *American Journal of Hypertension, 2*, 650-654.

Devoe, L. D., McKenzie, J., Searle, N., & Sherline, D. M. (1985). Nonstress test: Dimensions of normal reactivity. *Obstetrics and Gynecology, 66*, 617-620.

Eagleston, J. R., Kirmil-Gray, K., Thoresen, C. E., Wiedenfield, S. A., Bracke, P., Heft, L., & Arnow, B. (1986). Physical health correlates of Type A behavior in children and adolescents. *Journal of Behavioral Medicine, 9*, 341-362.

Eiff, A. W., Gogolin, E., Jacobs, V., & Neus, H. (1985). Heart rate reactivity under mental stress as a predictor of blood pressure development in children. *Journal of Hypertension, 3*(Suppl. 4), S89-S91.

Elwood, S. W., Ferguson, H. B., & Thakar, J. (1986). Catecholamine response of children in a naturally occurring stressor situation. *Journal of Human Stress, 12,* 154–161.

Ewart, C. K., Harris, W. L., Zeger, S., & Russell, G. A. (1986). Diminished pulse pressure under mental stress characterizes normotensive adolescents with parental high blood pressure. *Psychosomatic Medicine, 48,* 489–501.

Falkner, B. (1987). Is there a black hypertension? *Hypertension, 10,* 551–554.

Falkner, B., Kushner, H., Onesti, G., & Angelakos, E. T. (1981). Cardiovascular characteristics in adolescents who develop essential hypertension. *Hypertension, 3,* 521–527.

Falkner, B., Onesti, G., Affrime, N. B., & Lowenthal, D. T. (1982). Effects of clonidine and hydrochlorthiazide on the cardiovascular response to mental stress in adolescent hypertension. *Clinical Science, 63,* 455s–458s.

Falkner, B., Onesti, G., & Angelakos, E. T. (1979). Hemodynamic response to mental stress in normal adolescents with varying degrees of genetic risk for essential hypertension. In Y. Yamori, W. Lovenberg, & E. D. Freis (Eds.) *Prophylactic approach to hypertensive diseases* (pp. 149–155). New York: Raven Press.

Falkner, B., Onesti, G., & Angelakos, E. T. (1981). Effect of salt loading on the cardiovascular response to stress in adolescents. *Hypertension, 3*(Suppl. II), II-195–II-199.

Falkner, B., Onesti, G., Angelakos, E. T., Fernandes, M., & Langman, D. (1979). Cardiovascular response to mental stress in normal adolescents with hypertensive parents. *Hypertension, 1,* 23–30.

Falkner, B., Onesti, G., & Hamstra, B. (1981). Stress response characteristics of adolescents with high genetic risk for essential hypertension: A five year follow-up. *Clinical and Experimental Hypertension, 3,* 583–591.

Ferrara, L. A., Moscato, T. S., Pisanti, N., Marotta, T., Krogh, V., Capone, D., & Mancini, M. (1988). Is the sympathetic nervous system altered in children with familial history of arterial hypertension? *Cardiology, 75,* 200–205.

Ferrara, L. A., Soro, S., Mainenti, G., Mancini, M., Pisanti, N., Borrelli, R., Moscato, T., & Mancini, M. (1988). Body weight and cardiovascular response to sympathetic stimulation in childhood. *International Journal of Obesity, 13,* 271–277.

Fixler, D. E., Wallace, J. M., Thornton, W. E., Dimmitt, P. (1990). Ambulatory blood pressure monitoring in hypertensive adolescents. *American Journal of Hypertension, 3,* 288–292.

Fleming, I., Baum, A., Davidson, L. M., Rectanus, E., & McArdle, S. (1987). Chronic stress as a factor in physiologic reactivity to challenge. *Health Psychology, 6,* 221–237.

Gerace, T. A., & Smith, G. C. (1985). Children's Type A interview: Interrater, test-retest reliability, and interviewer effect. *Journal of Chronic Diseases, 38,* 781–791.

Gillum, R. F., Taylor, H. L., Anderson, J., & Blackburn, H. (1981). Longitudinal study (32 years) of exercise tolerance, breathing response, blood pressure, and blood lipids in young men. *Arteriosclerosis, 1,* 455–462.

Hagberg, J. M., Goldring, D., Heath, G. W., Ehsani, A. A., Hernandez, A., & Holloszy, J. O. (1984). Effect of exercise training on plasma catecholamines and haemodynamics of adolescent hypertensives during rest, submaximal exercise and orthostatic stress. *Clinical Physiology, 4,* 117–124.

Hansen, H. S., Hyldebrandt, N., Nielson, J. R., & Froberg, K. (1989). Exercise testing in children as a diagnostic tool of future hypertension: The Odense Schoolchild Study. *Journal of Hypertension, 7*(Suppl. 1), S41–S42.

Harlan, W. R., Oberman, A., Mitchell, R. E., & Graybiel, A. (1973). A 30-year study of blood pressure in a white male cohort. In G. Onesti, K. E. Kim, & J. H. Moyer (Eds.), *Hypertension: Mechanisms and management* (pp. 85–91). New York: Grune & Stratton.

Harshfield, G. A., Alpert, B. S., Murphy, J. K., Willey, E. S., & Somes, G. W. (1990). Blood pressure and heart rate of young hyporeactive and hyperreactive black and white subjects in the natural environment. *Proceedings of the 11th Annual Meeting of the Society of Behavioral Medicine, 11,* 22. (Abstract)

Harshfield, G. A., Alpert, B. S., Willey, E. S., Somes, G. W., Murphy, J. K., & Dupaul, L. M. (1989). Race and gender influence ambulatory blood pressure patterns of adolescents. *Hypertension, 14,* 598–603.

Harshfield, G. A., Dupaul, L. M., Alpert, B. S., Christman, J. V., Willey, E. S., Murphy, J. K., & Somes, G. W. (1990). Aerobic fitness and the diurnal rhythm of blood pressure in adolescents. *Hypertension, 15,* 810–814.

Harshfield, G. A., Pulliam, D. A., Alpert, B. S., Stapleton, F. B., Willey, E. S., & Somes, G. W. (1991). Ambulatory blood pressure patterns in children and adolescents: Influence of renin–sodium profiles. *Pediatrics, 87,* 94–100.

Hastrup, J. L., Kraemer, D. L., Hotchkiss, A. P., & Johnson, C. A. (1986). Cardiovascular responsivity to stress: Family patterns and the effects of instructions. *Journal of Psychosomatic Research, 30,* 233–241.

Hines, E. A. (1937a). Reaction of the blood pressure of 400 school children to a standard stimulus. *Journal of the American Medical Association, 108,* 1249–1250.

Hines, E. A. (1937b). The hereditary factor in essential hypertension. *Annals of Internal Medicine, 11,* 593–601.

Hines, E. A., & Brown, G. E. (1932). A standard stimulus for measuring vasomotor reactions: Its application in the study of hypertension. *Proceedings of the Staff Meeting of the Mayo Clinic, 7,* 332–335.

Hines, E. A., & Brown, G. E. (1933). A standard test for measuring the variability of blood pressure. Its significance as an index of the prehypertensive state. *Annals of Internal Medicine, 7,* 209–217.

Hines, E. A., & Brown, G. E. (1936). The cold pressor test for measuring the reactibility of the blood pressure: Data concerning 571 normal and hypertensive subjects. *American Heart Journal, 11*, 1-9.

Hofman, A., & Valkenburg, H. A. (1983). Determinants of change in blood pressure during childhood. *American Journal of Epidemiology, 117*, 735-743.

Hohn, A. R., Riopel, D. A., Keil, J. E., Loadholt, C. B., Margolius, H. S., Halushka, P. V., Privitera, P. J., Webb, J. G., Medley, E. S., Schuman, S. H., Rubin, M. I., Pantell, R. H., & Braunstein, M. L. (1983). Childhood familial and racial differences in physiologic and biochemical factors related to hypertension. *Hypertension, 5*, 56-70.

Holmes, O. W., Jr. (1919). *Abrams v. United States*, 250 U. S. 616, 630.

Horwitz, R. I. (1984). Methodologic standards and the clinical usefulness of the cold pressor test. *Hypertension, 6*, 1295-1296.

Houston, B. K., & Snyder, C. R. (Eds.). (1988). *Type A behavior pattern: Research, theory and intervention*. New York: Wiley.

James, F. W., Kaplan, S., Glueck, C. J., Tsay, J., Knight, M. S., & Sarwar, C. J. (1980). Responses of normal children and young adults to controlled bicycle exercise. *Circulation, 61*, 902-12.

Johansson, G., Frankenhauser, M., & Magnusson, D. (1973). Catecholamine output in school children as related to performance and adjustment. *Scandinavian Journal of Psychology, 14*, 20-28.

Kaplan, B. J., Whitsett, S. F., & Robinson, J. W. (1990). Menstrual cycle phase is a potential confound in psychophysiology research. *Psychophysiology, 27*, 445-450.

Kushner, H., & Falkner, B. (1981). A harmonic analysis of cardiac response of normotensive and hypertensive adolescents during stress. *Journal of Human Stress, 7*(1), 21-27.

Langewitz, W., Eiff, A. W., Gogolin, E., Neus, H., Ruddel, H., & Schmeider, R. (1985). Reliability and validity of ambulatory blood pressure recording in children. *Clinical and Experimental Hypertension, A7*, 217-225.

Lauer, R. M., Clarke, W. R., & Beaglehole, R. (1984). Level, trend, and variability of blood pressure during childhood: The Muscatine Study. *Circulation, 69*, 242-249.

Lawler, K. A., Allen, M. T., Critcher, E. C., & Standard, B. A. (1981). The relationship of physiological responses to the coronary-prone behavior pattern in children. *Journal of Behavioral Medicine, 4*, 203-216.

Lovallo, W. R., Pincomb, G. A., Sung, B. H., Passey, R. B., Sausen, K. P., & Wilson, M. F. (1989). Caffeine may potentiate adrenocortical stress in hypertension-prone men. *Hypertension, 14*, 170-176.

Lundberg, U. (1983). Note on Type A behavior and cardiovascular responses to challenge in 3-6 year old children. *Journal of Psychosomatic Research, 27*, 39-42.

Lundberg, U., Chateau, P., Winberg, J., & Frankenhauser, M. (1981). Catecholamine and cortisol excretion patterns in three-year-old children and their parents. *Journal of Human Stress, 7*, 3-11.

Mahoney, L. T., Schieken, R. M., Clarke, W. R., & Lauer, R. M. (1988). Left ventricular mass and exercise responses predict future blood pressure: The Muscatine Study. *Hypertension, 12,* 206–213.

Matthews, K. A. (1982). Psychological perspectives on the Type A behavior pattern. *Psychological Bulletin, 91,* 293–323.

Matthews, K. A., & Angulo, J. (1980). Measurement of the Type A behavior pattern in children: Assessment of children's competitiveness, impatience-anger, and aggression. *Child Development, 51,* 466–475.

Matthews, K. A., & Jennings, J. R. (1984). Cardiovascular responses of boys exhibiting the Type A behavior pattern. *Psychosomatic Medicine, 46,* 484–497.

Matthews, K. A., Manuck, S. B., & Saab, P. G. (1986). Cardiovascular responses of adolescents during a naturally occurring stressor and their behavioral and psychophysiological predictors. *Psychophysiology, 23,* 198–209.

Matthews, K. A., Manuck, S. B., Stoney, C. M., Rakaczky, C. J., McCann, B. S., Saab, P. G., Woodall, K. L., Block, D. R., Visintainer, P. F., & Engebretson, T. O. (1988). Familial aggregation of blood pressure and heart rate responses during behavioral stress. *Psychosomatic Medicine, 50,* 341–352.

Matthews, K. A., Rakaczky, C. J., Stoney, C. M., & Manuck, S. B. (1987). Are cardiovascular responses to behavioral stressors a stable individual difference variable in childhood? *Psychophysiology, 24,* 464–473.

Matthews, K. A., & Stoney, C. M. (1988). Influences of sex and age on cardiovascular responses during stress. *Psychosomatic Medicine, 50,* 46–56.

Matthews, K. A., Weiss, S. M., Detre, T., Dembroski, T. M., Falkner, B., Manuck, S. B., & Williams, R. B. (Eds.). (1986). *Handbook of stress, reactivity and cardiovascular disease.* New York: Wiley.

Matthews, K. A., Woodall, K. A., & Stoney, C. M. (1990). Changes in and stability of cardiovascular responses to behavioral stress: Results from a four-year longitudinal study of children. *Child Development, 61,* 1134–1144.

McCann, B. S., & Matthews, K. A. (1988). Influences of potential for hostility, Type A behavior, and parental history of hypertension on adolescents' cardiovascular responses during stress. *Psychophysiology, 25,* 503–511.

McCrory, W. W., Klein, A. A., & Rosenthal, R. A., (1982). Blood pressure, heart rate, and plasma catecholamines in normal and hypertensive children and their siblings at rest and after standing. *Hypertension, 4,* 507–513.

Mehta, S. K., Bahler, R. C., Hanson, R., Walsh, J. T., & Rakita, L. (1986). Relative tachycardia in ambulant children with borderline hypertension. *American Heart Journal, 112,* 1257–1263.

Menkes, M. S., Mathews, K. A., Krantz, D. S., Lundberg, V., Mead, L. A., Qaqish, B., Liang, K., Thomas, C. B., & Pearson, T. A. (1989). Cardiovascular reactivity to the cold pressor as a predictor of hypertension. *Hypertension, 14,* 524–530.

Molineux, D., & Steptoe, A. (1988). Exaggerated blood pressure responses to submaximal exercise in normotensive adolescents with a family history of hypertension. *Journal of Hypertension, 6,* 361–365.

Munger, R. G., Prineas, R. J., & Gomez-Marin, O. (1988). Persistent elevation of blood pressure among children with a family history of hypertension: The Minneapolis Children's Blood Pressure Study. *Journal of Hypertension, 6,* 647–653.

Murphy, J. K., Alpert, B. S., Moes, D. M., & Somes, G. W. (1986). Race and cardiovascular reactivity: A neglected relationship. *Hypertension, 8,* 1075–1083.

Murphy, J. K., Alpert, B. S., & Walker, S. S. (1990). Importance of race (subject vs. experimenter) in children's cardiovascular reactivity. *Psychophysiology, 27,* S52. (Abstract)

Murphy, J. K., Alpert, B. S., & Walker, S. S. (1991a). *A longitudinal comparison of hyper- and hyporeactive children.* Manuscript in preparation.

Murphy, J. K., Alpert, B. S. & Walker, S. S. (1991b). Stability of ethnic differences in children's pressor responses during 3 annual examinations. *American Journal of Hypertension, 4,* 630–634.

Murphy, J. K., Alpert, B. S., & Walker, S. S. (1991c). Whether to measure change from baseline or actual level in studies of children's cardiovascular reactivity: A two-year follow-up. *Journal of Behavioral Medicine, 14,* 409–419.

Murphy, J. K., Alpert, B. S., Walker, S. S., & Niaura, R. (1991). Ethnicity, cardiovascular reactivity and the prediction of subsequent blood pressure: A 2 year follow-up. *Psychosomatic Medicine, 53,* 240. (Abstract)

Murphy, J. K., Alpert, B. S., Walker, S. S., & Willey, E. S. (1988). Race and cardiovascular reactivity: A replication. *Hypertension, 11,* 308–311.

Murphy, J. K., Alpert, B. S., Walker, S. S., & Willey, E. S. (in press). Children's cardiovascular reactivity: Stability of racial differences and relation to subsequent blood pressure over a one-year period. *Psychophysiology.*

Murphy, J. K., Alpert, B. S., Willey, E. S., Christman, J. V., Sexton, J. E., & Harshfield, G. A. (1989). Modulation of pressor responses by fitness: Racial differences among children. *American Journal of Hypertension, 2,* 25A. (Abstract)

Murphy, J. K., Alpert, B. S., Willey, E. S., & Somes, G. W. (1988). Cardiovascular reactivity to psychological stress in healthy children. *Psychophysiology, 25,* 144–152.

Murray, D. M., Blake, S. M., Prineas, R., & Gillum, R. F. (1985). Cardiovascular responses in Type A children during a cognitive challenge. *Journal of Behavioral Medicine, 8,* 377–395.

Musante, L., Treiber, F. A., Strong, W. B., & Levy, M. (1990). Family history of hypertension and cardiovascular reactivity in black male children. *Journal of Psychosomatic Research, 34,* 111–116.

Parker, F. C., Croft, J. B., Cresanta, J. L., Freedman, D. S., Burke, G. L., Webber, L. S., & Berenson, G. S. (1987). The association between cardiovascular response tasks and future blood pressure levels in children: Bogalusa Heart Study. *American Heart Journal, 113*, 1174–1179.

Portaluppi, F., Bagni, B., Uberti, D., Montanari, L., Cavallini, R., Trasforini, G., Margutti, A., Ferlini, M., Zanella, M., & Parti, M. (1990). Circadian rhythms of atrial natriuretic peptide, renin, aldosterone, cortisol, blood pressure, and heart rate in normal and hypertensive subjects. *Journal of Hypertension, 6*, 85–95.

Remington, R. D., Lambarth, B., Moser, M., & Hoobler, S. W. (1960). Circulatory reactions of normotensive and hypertensive subjects and of the children of normal and hypertensive parents. *American Heart Journal, 59*, 58–70.

Rose, R. J., & Chesney, M. A. (1986). Cardiovascular stress reactivity: A behavior genetic perspective. *Behavior Therapy, 17*, 314–323.

Sallis, J. F., Patterson, T. L., McKenzie, T. L., Buono, M. J., Atkins, C. J., & Nader, P. R. (1989). Stability of systolic blood pressure reactivity to exercise in young children. *Journal of Developmental and Behavioral Pediatrics, 10*, 38–43.

Santangelo, K. L., Falkner, B., & Kushner, H. (1989). Forearm hemodynamics at rest and stress in borderline hypertensive adolescents. *American Journal of Hypertension, 2*, 52–56.

Schieken, R. M., Clarke, W. R., & Lauer, R. M. (1983). The cardiovascular responses to exercise in children across the blood pressure distribution: The Muscatine Study. *Hypertension, 5*, 71–78.

Schmidt, T. H., Dembroski, T. M., & Blumchen, G. (Eds.). (1986). *Biological and psychological factors in cardiovascular disease.* New York: Springer-Verlag.

Schneiderman, N., Weiss, S. M., & Kaufman, P. G. (Eds.). (1989). *Handbook of research methods in cardiovascular behavioral medicine.* New York: Plenum.

Schwartz, A. N., Campos, J. J., & Baisel, E. J. (1973). The visual cliff: Cardiac and behavioral responses on the deep and shallow sides at five and nine months of age. *Journal of Experimental Child Psychology, 35*, 239–243.

Siegel, J. M., & Leitch, C. J. (1981). Assessment of the Type A behavior pattern in adolescents. *Psychosomatic Medicine, 43*, 45–56.

Southard, D. R., Coates, T. J., Kolodner, K., Parker, F. C., Padgett, N. E., & Kennedy, H. L. (1986). Relationship between mood and blood pressure in the natural environment: An adolescent population. *Health Psychology, 5*, 469–480.

Spiga, R. (1986). Social interaction and cardiovascular response of boys exhibiting the coronary-prone behavior pattern. *Journal of Pediatric Psychology, 11*, 59–69.

Strong, W. B., Miller, M. D., Striplin, M., Salehbhai, M. (1978). Blood pressure responses to isometric and dynamic exercise in healthy black children. *American Journal of Diseases in Children, 132*, 587–591.

Svensson, A., & Hansson, L. (1985). Blood pressure and response to "stress" in 11–16 year old children. *Acta Medica Scandinavica*, (Suppl. 693), 51–55.

Task Force on Blood Pressure Control in Children. (1987). Report of the Second Task Force on Blood Pressure Control in Children—1987. *Pediatrics, 79,* 1–25.

Tell, G. S., Prineas, R. J., & Gomez-Marin, O. (1988). Postural changes in blood pressure and pulse rate among black adolescents and white adolescents: The Minneapolis Children's Blood Pressure Study. *American Journal of Epidemiology, 128,* 360–369.

Tennes, K., & Kreye, M. (1985). Children's adrenocortical responses to classroom activities and tests in elementary school. *Psychosomatic Medicine, 47,* 451–460.

Tennes, K., Kreye, M., Avitable, N., & Wells, R. (1986). Behavioral correlates of excreted catecholamines and cortisol in second grade children. *Journal of the American Academy of Child Psychiatry, 25,* 764–770.

Thomas, J., Semenya, K. A., Neser, W. B., Thomas, D. J., Green, D. R., & Gillum, R. F. (1985). Risk factors and the incidence of hypertension in black physicians: The Meharry Cohort Study. *American Heart Journal, 110,* 637–645.

Thomas, S. A., Lynch, J. J., Friedmann, E., Suginohara, M., Hall, P. S., & Peteron, C. (1984). Blood pressure and heart rate changes in children when they read aloud in school. *Public Health Reports, 99,* 77–84.

Treiber, F. A., Musante, L., Braden, D., Arensman, F., Strong, W. B., Levy, M., & Leverett, S. (1990). Racial differences in hemodynamic responses to the cold face stimulus in children and adults. *Psychosomatic Medicine, 52,* 286–296.

Treiber, F. A., Musante, L., Strong, W. B., & Levy, M. (1989). Racial differences in young children's blood pressure responses to dynamic exercise. *American Journal of Diseases of Children, 143,* 720–723.

Visser, M. C., Grobbee, D. E., & Hofman, A. (1987). Determinants of rise in blood pressure in normotensive children. *Journal of Hypertension, 5,* 367–370.

Voors, A. W., Webber, L. S., & Berenson, G. S. (1980). Racial contrasts in cardiovascular response tests for children from a total community. *Hypertension, 2,* 686–694.

Watt, G. (1986). Design and interpretation of studies comparing individuals with and without a family history of high blood pressure. *Journal of Hypertension, 4,* 1–7.

Wilson, P. D., Ferencz, C., Dischinger, P. C., Brenner, J. I., & Zeger, S.L. (1988). Twenty-four hour ambulatory blood pressure in normotensive adolescent children of hypertensive and normotensive parents. *American Journal of Epidemiology, 127,* 946–954.

Wilson, S. L., Gaffney, F. A., Laird, W. P., & Fixler, D. E. (1985). Body size, composition, and fitness in adolescents with elevated blood pressures. *Hypertension, 7,* 417–422.

Wolf, T. M., Sklov, M. C., Wenzel, P. A., Hunter, S. M., & Berenson, G. S. (1982).

Validation of a measure of Type A behavior pattern in children: Bogalusa Heart Study. *Child Development, 53,* 126–135.

Wood, D. L., Sheps, S. G., Elveback, L. R., & Schirger, R. (1984). Cold pressor test as a predictor of hypertension. *Hypertension, 6,* 301–306.

Woodall, K. L., & Matthews, K. A. (1989). Familial environment associated with Type A behaviors and psychophysiological responses to stress in children. *Health Psychology, 8,* 403–426.

CHAPTER 4

The Conceptual Utility of the Temperament Construct in Understanding Coping with Pediatric Conditions

WILLIAM T. GARRISON
Children's National Medical Center, Washington, D.C.

The specific purpose of this chapter is to explore and illustrate the primary conceptual value of the temperament construct in research and clinical work with pediatric populations. In the broadly defined field of child health and development, it has been suggested that important relationships exist between children's individual differences, as conceived and measured through the temperament approach, and their responses to stress associated with physical disease, handicapping conditions, or life trauma (Garrison & McQuiston, 1989; Johnson, 1987; Rutter, 1981; Wertlieb, Wiegel, Springer, & Feldstern, 1987). In recent years, several empirical studies have lent support to the view that there are significant associations between the construct of temperament and outcomes in pediatric conditions.

This chapter also provides a brief overview of the major issues and problems associated with use of the temperament construct as it may relate to the nature of coping and adjustment in pediatric conditions. More comprehensive reviews of the larger literature on temperament are available elsewhere, and should be consulted for more comprehensive discussion of the theories, methods, and critical issues in this burgeoning area of child developmental research (Garrison & Earls, 1987; Goldsmith et al., 1987; Plomin & Dunn, 1986).

OVERVIEW OF THE CONSTRUCT

Historically, there has been much interest in the concept of "temperament," or constitutionally based individual differences, as such differences may relate to human behavior, development, and health. We do know, for example, that the ancient Greeks and Romans considered the possibility that individual qualities were closely associated to health and disease outcomes, as did Eastern civilizations such as the Hindu and Chinese before them. More contemporary approaches to temperament have tended to emphasize the range and types of behavioral manifestations of individual differences that can be observed and measured very early in human development. In addition, there has been much more attention to the continuities and discontinuities of temperament across the life span. In this way, the construct of temperament has evolved from being viewed as an amalgam of biology and experience, or as "personality," to being perceived as constituting the basic organismic building blocks for human behavior and development.

Most child temperament researchers consider their phenomena of interest as factors inherent to the organism, and as traits or qualities that are constitutional in origin. Temperament is presumed to be directly or indirectly related to a broad array of behavioral, social, and physiological characteristics. Plomin (1982) has argued that a temperament characteristic, in order to be thought of as constitutional in its origin and therefore as distinct from a broader concept such as personality, should meet at least two basic criteria: (1) It should show evidence for *heritability* or a genetic basis; and (2) it should demonstrate moderate *stability* across time and context. If we accept this conservative view, as many have, then the model of temperament Plomin has offered in collaboration with Buss and others is of special interest. Later in this chapter, I use Buss and Plomin's (1984) model of temperament as an illustrative example of how this construct may be especially applicable to the study of psychological coping with pediatric conditions.

A few researchers who have sought to identify constitutionally based temperament qualities have argued that temperament as a *pure* construct may not be easily studied once environmental factors begin to shape and influence child behavior (Goldsmith et al., 1987). They contend that biologically based differences in the newborn infant are rapidly obscured by subsequent, ongoing interactions with caretakers, and by transactions with the broader environment. As a result of this possibility, many temperament researchers have tended to begin their studies with infants or very young children as subjects.

Some investigators have taken a more quantitative, behavioral-genetics approach to the question of temperament differences, employing twin, family pedigree, and adoption research designs. Others have relied heavily upon laboratory-based observations of children in structured situations, which are then compared to parental reports about temperament. Much of the work on temperament to date, however, has primarily used parent- or teacher-generated reports and descriptions of children's behavioral characteristics.

One major approach to temperament that relies upon parental reports has focused on individual differences in what has been called "behavioral style" (Carey & McDevitt, 1978; Thomas & Chess, 1984). The measures that have been developed to describe child temperament from this vantage point have been designed to be sensitive to the *interactional* qualities of individual differences, and to what Thomas and Chess call the "goodness of fit" between the environment and children's inborn individual differences. At this point, however, it seems that a behavioral style approach is not simply an examination of the organismic traits or qualities of children, but is also an attempt to capture transactional processes mediated by a host of child or environmental factors, as well as by the passage of time. As such, it is not clear whether this approach is wholly consistent with the dominant view of temperament in developmental psychology today.

POTENTIAL PROBLEMS IN TEMPERAMENT RESEARCH

Because there are several competing theoretical and methodological approaches to the definition and measurement of the temperament construct, considerable care must be taken to identify the basic differences that exist among them. I have argued elsewhere that it may be misleading to include *all* versions of temperament under the same rubric (Garrison & Earls, 1987), since different methods will often imply very different phenomena. Therefore, those researchers or clinicians who choose a particular temperament approach must be familiar with the theoretical underpinnings of that method, as well as the specific dimensions purported to be measured by the various tools that have been derived. They cannot readily or safely assume that they are examining the same phenomena as those being studied by colleagues who are conducting studies of temperament at another research site and employing different methods.

Perhaps due to a certain amount of confusion in definition, and broad differences in method, there now exist almost as many temperament dimensions as there are researchers in that field of inquiry. I now briefly review some of the findings from the growing literature on temperament and pediatric conditions, as a way to pare the task down in size. It is not my goal to review this growing body of work exhaustively; rather, it is to examine some of the ways in which these studies suggest that a greater sensitivity to individual differences will be important to our attempts to understand children's coping with pediatric conditions.

RESEARCH IN PEDIATRIC SAMPLES

From the outset, it may be useful to stop and consider two overriding questions. First, what are the potential uses or applications of the temperament construct within theoretical and research attempts to understand coping with pediatric conditions? And second, how might persons interested in applying this construct to pediatric samples avoid some of the more serious pitfalls encountered by temperament researchers in other fields? Attention to these two questions will ultimately save precious time and resources as we explore the usefulness of the temperament construct in pediatric conditions.

A number of recent studies have attempted to include attention to temperament differences in children with chronic diseases or handicapping conditions. In samples of such children, there are at least two good reasons for adopting a temperament or behavioral style approach to the measurement of individual differences, as compared with traditional methods that focus on the presence of psychological symptoms or child psychiatric disorders. First, the temperament approach allows a much broader range of behavior to be considered than a view oriented toward psychopathology alone. And second, it can alleviate the stigma associated with a search for child psychiatric disorders amid the normal range of reactions and responses to abnormally stressful conditions and life events (Garrison & McQuiston, 1989).

The studies that are emerging suggest that researchers are becoming more interested in both within-group and between-group temperament comparisons in samples of children affected by pediatric conditions. A quick overview of the field of pediatric psychology indicates certain topics with special relevance to the question of individual differences in temperament. These include broadly defined child coping with chronic diseases or conditions; the range of response to stressful and painful medical procedures; and temperament as an outcome of or covariate to certain forms of pediatric conditions, trauma, or environmental insult.

A few researchers have attempted to relate temperament to clinical outcomes in diabetes mellitus (Garrison, Biggs, & Williams, 1990; Rovet & Ehrlich, 1988). Other studies have sought to distinguish between children with and children without a specific pediatric condition, such as chronic abdominal pain syndrome (Davison, Faull, & Nicol, 1986) or a physical handicap (Wallander, Hubert, & Varni, 1988). More recently, researchers have examined the utility and validity of temperament in the prediction of eventual health outcomes in children at risk for developing disease, such as wheezy babies who subsequently become asthmatic (Priel, Henik, Dekel, & Tal, 1990) or infants with nonorganic failure to thrive (Wolke, Skuse, & Mathisen, 1990).

And we should not forget that clinical work by one of the long-time stalwarts of the behavioral style approach to temperament, William Carey, has repeatedly indicated that it can be a useful construct in understanding and responding to a wide array of common pediatric problems (Carey, 1985; Carey & McDevitt, 1989). These include sleep and feeding patterns, children's responses to illness, and various broadly defined behavioral and developmental problems.

Many associations that have been reported among temperament dimensions and medical outcomes, such as disease control or regimen adherence, have been reasonable and thought-provoking. For example, consider Rovet and Ehrlich's (1988) finding that the temperament dimensions of regularity in biological functioning, reactivity to external stimuli, and activity level, among others, have utility in understanding good versus poor control of diabetes. Similarly, my colleagues and I (Garrison et al., 1990) have found that certain *combinations* of child and parent temperament characteristics are valuable in identifying younger children in very poor control and compliance with diabetes, and that they appear more useful than traditional measures of child behavior disorders.

One of the lessons from this latter study lies in its emphasis on the fact that different temperament dimensions vary in their conceptual and practical utility, largely as a function of the nature of the specific outcome or condition to be assessed. For example, attention span may be related to compliance with a medical regimen, whereas predominant mood (positive or negative) may be associated with certain physiological or treatment parameters of a particular disease or chronic condition. In other words, certain individual differences may be more or less relevant to specific clinical outcomes in pediatric conditions, and thought should be given to this likelihood in the design and implementation of research.

Another important point is that the temperament or behavioral style characteristics of parents, and even of children's health care providers, is an interesting but neglected area of research. Such an emphasis is especially relevant to the study of children's responses to physical conditions and diseases, since understanding the role of the family in shaping child coping is an essential task.

It is also important to point out that a few of these studies suffer from a basic confusion that has characterized the larger literature on temperament and child psychopathology (Garrison & Earls, 1987)—namely, the issue of overlap between measures of temperament and measures of outcome. Sometimes this confounding is subtle, but it can also be rather blatant. For example, one study that examined the relationship between temperament and child behavior problems reported that young children described by mothers as high in activity level, low in attention-span, and high in impulsivity also tended to meet criteria for attention deficit disorder with hyperactivity. A comparison of the items on two purportedly distinct measures would reveal many more similarities than might be first suspected.

Similarly, in the study of outcomes associated with pediatric conditions, it may be tautological to suggest that children who display extremes in such temperamental dimensions as impulsivity, activity level, or distractibility will also have problems with behavioral adherence to their medical regimen. Especially when ratings or measures of adherence or compliance contain items similar to those on the temperament questionnaires (e.g., "Child doesn't pay attention to instructions," "Child acts impulsively," etc.). Likewise, it should not be surprising to find that children with cancer described as displaying predominantly negative mood also happen to be on a current course of chemotherapy.

These studies as a group indicate, at least when within-group comparisons are made, that individual differences in temperament or behavioral style can have both logical and sensible relationships with outcomes in certain pediatric conditions. But few studies have specifically hypothesized how temperament may be more or less valuable in differentiating affected children from matched controls, or in distinguishing between children who cope well and those who do not. Researchers have not always made their basis for such comparisons explicit. Why, for example, might we be led to believe that certain pediatric conditions somehow lead to systematic variations in individual differences? And which temperament dimensions, on an *a priori* basis, are hypothesized to have a functional relationship with the pediatric condition or outcome under study? If these sorts of questions are asked *before* studies are designed, there is a better chance that researchers will choose the temperament approach best suited to their topic of interest.

TEMPERAMENT, STRESS, AND COPING

Let us reflect for a moment on the ways in which attention to individual differences may be important in the study of the relationships among stress, illness, and psychological coping. After all, much of the interest in temperament has been based upon its ability to explain variations across different children or adults in terms of pathology or stress outcomes. To date, though, most of the work concerned with psychological coping in children affected by disease or chronic conditions has emphasized the *cognitive* processes that influence such variability. Successful versus unsuccessful adaptation to painful or stressful medical procedures, for example, has been linked with a child's particular cognitive perspective or approach (Siegel & Smith, 1989; Worchel, Copeland, & Barker, 1987). It appears that the way in which a child seeks out and manages information in the medical environment is associated with the child's overall ability to cope. A variation on this approach has been the emphasis on children's overall capacity to make meaning of stress, given important age and ability differences in their cognitive-developmental level (Brown, O'Keeffe, Sanders, & Baker, 1986; Garrison & McQuiston, 1989).

For example, consider the child who successfully manages information in low- as opposed to high-stress situations. In such a case, attention to temperament differences in emotional arousal and self-regulation may be useful and revealing in understanding observed variation for that child across contexts. Similarly, the child who is described temperamentally as low in social approach may also display a related pattern of avoiding health care workers, instead of actively gathering information about the disease or the stressful procedures the child must endure.

Even a cursory analysis of the relationships among child cognition, temperament characteristics, and psychological coping suggests difficult conceptual and methodological issues. But let us consider how a few researchers have approached this topic. Wertlieb et al. (1987), for example, conducted a study in which they examined the mediating effects of child temperament in coping with stressful experiences. They concluded that certain temperament characteristics do show relationships with differences in behavioral symptom outcomes as a function of life stress, but that these associations are very complex. The study serves to portray the possible associations among different types of life stress, temperament, and behavioral disorder outcomes.

In a very different vein, Boyce and Jemerin (1990; Jemerin & Boyce, 1990) have recently provided a useful conceptual overview of the stress and illness literature as it pertains to children, using the example of cardiovascular markers of vulnerability. They describe recent research suggesting that physiological and temperament or behavioral style measures are intercorrelated. Vagal tone and exaggerated cardiovascular reactivity, for example, are two physiological indices thought to be directly related to children's overt manifestations of behavioral reactions to external stimuli in both laboratory and field settings. Among the other points they make is that attention to temperament, as conceived only in behavioral terms, should be attempted along with the measurement of physiological processes wherever possible. To date, studies that have examined temperament and coping with pediatric conditions have not generally done this.

It is important to be aware that several temperament researchers are employing physiological measures in their work, and readers interested in applications to pediatric conditions might be wise to explore their methods first (Kagan, Reznick, & Snidman, 1987; Rothbart & Posner, 1985). The potential of research on the physiological and psychological parameters of the stress response in various pediatric conditions and procedures should be fairly obvious.

There is at least one important point to keep in mind as we attempt to consider how exactly temperament may fit into conceptual models of psychological coping with pediatric conditions. These models will include attention to factors such as differences in cognitive appraisal, variation in biophysiological parameters, and the availability of and access to environmental supports. The concept of temperament will have relevance to and even overlap with each of these three main variable classes. What the temperament approach (and the literature that provides its basis) may have to offer that is unique is an emphasis on identifying the constitutional *origins* of individual differences in these factors, through a central focus on describing the very earliest manifestations of such differences in human development.

For example, attempts to measure cognitive processes in coping with pediatric conditions have largely involved older, more verbal children. Temperament approaches may offer important links back to earlier development, and to developmental levels not amenable to current measures of cognitive appraisal. Similarly, biological markers of vulnerability to illness conditions, or to successful versus unsuccessful coping with life stress, will have covariates with the behavioral phenomena captured via the temperament approach. Indeed, the psychophysiological parameters of temperament now constitute a major focus within whole approaches to the temperament construct. Also, temperament as it relates to sociability and emotionality may have direct and indirect correspondence to the child's attitudes and behavior related to use of external social supports which are thought to mediate stressful experiences.

CORE TEMPERAMENT DIMENSIONS

Much as in the field of temperament per se, it is wise in the study of temperament as it relates to stress and coping with pediatric conditions to begin by considering two fundamental questions. First, are there core dimensions of temperament or individual differences that appear to overlap the many studies and approaches, thereby offering some degree of confidence as to their replicability and validity? And, if so, do any of these core temperament dimensions have some special applicability to a better understanding of children's coping with pediatric conditions? An overview of the competing approaches to temperament does provide some answers to these questions.

As mentioned previously, one of the major approaches to temperament has been developed by Buss and Plomin (1984). Their approach happens to capture three of the more general temperament dimensions that have repeatedly appeared, in one form or another, throughout the research literature on this construct. Thus, their approach provides an especially useful example for illustrating the major points to be made in the remainder of this chapter. The following sections describe the three dimensions that Buss and Plomin have found to meet the two basic criteria of moderate heritability and stability in individual differences: "emotionality," "activity level," and "sociability."

Emotionality

It has been observed that emotionality, or some trait or quality closely related to it, has appeared consistently in nearly all approaches to the temperament construct (Strelau, 1987). Indeed, several theorists have suggested that emotional arousal and its behavioral expression represent a core concept within temperament research. Although there are variations in how this dimension is operationalized and measured, and in how importantly it figures within a particular theoretical model, it is still clearly one of the most robust and central dimensions discussed in the professional literature on human temperament.

If we use Plomin's model as a working example, we find that he posits three types of emotion captured within ratings of emotionality: distress, fear, and anger. Much debate arises as to whether these are the only important, discrete emotions within the broader dimension of emotionality, but their applicability should be most apparent to anyone familiar with the study of children's coping with pediatric conditions or medical procedures. On the face of it, distress, fear, and anger are three behavioral manifestations in which pediatric researchers are particularly interested as indicators of children's psychological coping. Although investigators must be careful to ensure that measures of emotionality sample widely across situations for a particular child, it is potentially valuable to have an index of individual differences in those children affected by pediatric conditions or medical procedures. In this way, it may be possible to separate behavior peculiar to the medical setting from behavior more typical across situations for a child with a certain pattern of emotionality in temperament.

Activity Level

The second dimension that has been replicated across most studies of temperament, and that meets criteria pertinent to constitutionality, is behavioral activity level. This dimension has often been included and/or correlated with another one, typically referred to as attention span or cognitive distractibility. Some approaches to temperament have separated these two dimensions into more distinct characteristics, but typically they are moderately to highly intercorrelated.

The dimension of activity level, while apparently robust in the temperament research, also offers potential value in applications to practice and research in pediatric conditions. One particular outcome variable that has garnered much attention in research on the chronically or acutely ill has been the quality of life, as reflected in such things as self-care capacities, overall levels of energy, the patient's ability to ambulate, and so on. Each of these has direct relevance to activity level. Also, it is conceivable that this core temperament dimension may be associated with more basic physiological parameters of both coping behavior and disease outcomes. It may even have differential effects, depending upon the outcome under study. For example, high activity level may be a positive trait in relation to metabolic control of diabetes mellitus (Rovet & Ehrlich, 1988), but may have a negative association with good compliance (Garrison et al., 1990).

Sociability

There is clear overlap between the temperament dimension of sociability and with what Eysenck has called the "introversion–extraversion" continuum in human personality—a notion that has received a great deal of support across numerous studies of adult and child personality differences. However, there is controversy in the child temperament literature as to whether this third dimension is more likely to be affected by and to be a manifestation of accrued experience than are the other two core dimensions (emotionality and activity level). Aside from this debate, attention to the sociability dimension of temperament may be very useful in studies of pediatric conditions, especially if they are focused on things such as the child's or parent's use of social supports, successful versus unsuccessful interactions with health care providers, or the ongoing socialization of a recovering or physically incapacitated child.

One particular series of studies relevant to the sociability construct is the work on behavioral inhibition in young children. Kagan, Resnick, and Snidman (1988) have argued that this pattern of behavioral style has distinct covariates in physiology. For example, children who conform to this behavioral pattern appear also to show diminished variability in heart rate, as well as in their approach behavior in novel or familiar situations. And it is of interest that this general pattern of behavior was one of the few thought to have appreciable longitudinal continuity across several decades of development in Kagan's earlier analyses of data from a large longitudinal study.

Whether this pattern should be considered as a manifestation of a core temperament construct known as sociability, or as an amalgam of temperament and early experience, it is still an example of a fascinating body of work that has direct applicability to the study of psychological coping with pediatric conditions.

Applications of the Temperament Dimensions

At this point in the development of temperament, in terms of both theory and methods, it may be wise to approach applications of this idea in the study of pediatric conditions by emphasizing what appear to be its core dimensions. Thus, investigators should pay special attention to the potential value of emotionality, activity level, and sociability. Most major approaches to temperament contain either these core dimensions themselves or ones very similar to them.

Reliance upon more specific temperament dimensions is certainly warranted, but there should be some reasoned basis for it. For example, methods that emphasize a dimension of temperament such as rhythmicity of biological functioning or persistence on task may have special appeal to a researcher examining a particular pediatric condition or outcome. In such a situation, the researcher should take care to map out reasonable hypothesized connections, and should not attempt simply to employ a convenient temperament method within a sample. And again, we must continue to ensure that the domains of what we intend to measure, whether dimensions of temperament or clinical outcomes, are sufficiently distinct to protect against tautological and overlapping results. By and large, however, investigators should be aware that applications with these more specific temperament dimensions are more likely to be fraught with problems of definition and measurement.

The laboratory-based methods for the measurement of temperament have not been used very much at all within pediatric applications. Once again, those techniques that attempt to elicit and rate emotionality, activity level, and sociability appear most robust and stable over time, according to the larger temperament literature. Of course, parent-generated questionnaires are easier and cheaper to administer, but they carry with them certain risks in terms of validity and reliability. Most temperament researchers today use laboratory-based and parent questionnaire methods in tandem—an approach that is wise.

SUMMARY

On a final and positive note, it is important to remember that we stand to profit by heeding an important lesson from the long and controversial history of the temperament concept. That is, we will inevitably need to acknowledge that individual differences, or a construct very similar to temperament, will be important in our ultimate models of human behavior and development. This is likely to be as true in the study of coping with pediatric conditions as in other areas of psychology. Although the theoretical and methodological problems can seem herculean, it is likely that temperament or a concept similar to it is destined to inform our explanations for the observed variation in psychological coping with life stress, as well as our attempts to account for the vagaries of human development.

REFERENCES

Boyce, W. T., & Jemerin, J. M. (1990). Psychobiological differences in childhood stress response: I. Patterns of illness and susceptibility. *Journal of Developmental and Behavioral Pediatrics, 11,* 86–94.

Brown, J. M., O'Keeffe, J., Sanders, S. H., & Baker, B. (1986). Developmental changes in children's cognition to stressful and painful situations. *Journal of Pediatric Psychology, 11,* 343–357.

Buss, A. H., & Plomin, R. (1984). *Early developing personality traits.* Hillsdale, NJ: Erlbaum.

Carey, W. (1985). Clinical use of temperament in pediatrics. *Journal of Developmental and Behavioral Pediatrics, 6,* 137–142.

Carey, W., & McDevitt, S. (1978). Stability and change in individual temperament diagnoses from infancy to early childhood. *Journal of the American Academy of child Psychiatry, 10,* 331–337.

Carey, W., & McDevitt, S. (1989). *Clinical and educational applications of temperament research.* Amsterdam: Swets & Zeitlinger.

Davison, I. S., Faull, C., & Nicol, A. R. (1986). Temperament and behavior in six-year-olds with recurrent abdominal pain: A follow-up. *Journal of Child Psychology and Psychiatry, 27,* 539–544.

Garrison, W. T., Biggs, D., & Williams, K. (1990). Temperament characteristics and clinical outcomes in young children with diabetes mellitus. *Journal of Child Psychology and Psychiatry, 31,* 1079–1088.

Garrison, W. T., & Earls, F. (1987). *Temperament and child psychopathology.* Newbury Park, CA: Sage.

Garrison, W. T., & McQuiston, S. (1989). *Chronic illness during childhood and adolescence: Psychological aspects.* Newbury Park, CA: Sage.

Goldsmith, H., Buss, A. H., Plomin, R., Rothbart, M., Thomas, A., Chess, S., Hinde, R., & McCall, R. (1987). Roundtable: What is temperament? *Child Development, 58,* 505–529.

Jemerin, J., & Boyce, W. T. (1990). Psychobiological differences in childhood stress response: II. Cardiovascular markers of vulnerability. *Journal of Developmental and Behavioral Pediatrics, 11,* 140–150.

Johnson, J. (1987). *Life events as stressors in childhood and adolescence.* Newbury Park, CA: Sage.

Kagan, J., Resnick, J. S., & Snidman, N. (1987). The physiology and psychology of behavioral inhibition in young children. *Child Development, 58,* 1459–1473.

Kagan, J., Resnick, J. S., & Snidman, N. (1988). Biological bases of childhood shyness. *Science, 240,* 176–171.

Plomin, R. (1982). Childhood temperament. In B. Lahey & A. Kazdin (Eds.), *Advances in clinical child psychology* (Vol. 6, pp. 2–80). New York: Plenum.

Plomin, R., & Dunn, J. (1986). *The study of early temperament: Changes, continuities and challenges.* Hillsdale, NJ: Erlbaum.

Priel, B., Henik, A., Dekel, A. & Tal, A. (1990). Perceived temperamental characteristics and regulation of physiological stress: A study of wheezy babies. *Journal of Pediatric Psychology, 15,* 197–210.

Rothbart, M. K., & Posner, M. I. (1985). Temperament and the development of self regulation. In C. Hartlage & C. Telzrow (Eds.), *The neurophysiology of individual differences* (pp. 93–123). New York: Plenum.

Rovet, J. F., & Ehrlich, R. M. (1988). Effect of temperament on metabolic control in children with diabetes mellitus. *Diabetes Care, 11,* 77–82.

Rutter, M. (1981). Stress, coping and development: Some issues and questions. *Journal of Child Psychology and Psychiatry, 22,* 323–356.

Siegel, J. L., & Smith, K. E. (1989). Children's strategies for coping with pain. *Pediatrician, 16,* 110–118.

Strelau, J. (1987). Emotion as a key concept in temperament research. *Journal of Research in Personality, 21,* 510–528.

Thomas, A., & Chess, S. (1984). Genesis and evolution of behavioral disorder: From infancy to early adult life. *American Journal of Psychiatry, 141,* 1–9.

Wallander, J. L., Hubert, N. C., & Varni, J. W. (1988). Child and maternal temperament characteristics, goodness of fit, and adjustment in physically handicapped children. *Journal of Clinical Child Psychology, 17,* 336–346.

Wertlieb, D., Wiegel, C., Springer, T., & Feldstern, M. (1987). Temperament as a moderator of children's stressful experiences. *American Journal of Orthopsychiatry, 57,* 234–245.

Wolke, D., Skuse, D., & Mathisen, B. (1990). Behavioral style in failure-to-thrive infants: A preliminary communication. *Journal of Pediatric Psychology, 15,* 237–254.

Worchel, F. F., Copeland, D. R., & Barker, D. G. (1987). Control-related coping strategies in pediatric oncology patients. *Pediatric Psychology, 12,* 25–48.

CHAPTER 5

Re-Examining Research on Stress and Social Support: The Importance of Contextual Factors

ALEXANDRA L. QUITTNER
Indiana University

Chronically ill children and their families are faced with a number of ongoing stressors that affect several dimensions of their lives. Depending on the medical condition, a child with a serious illness may encounter alterations in physical, social, and emotional functioning (Drotar, Crawford, & Bush, 1984). Parents may also experience increased demands on their time, energy, and resources, as well as dramatic shifts in the enactment of their primary social roles (e.g., parental, marital). Although there is a growing consensus that chronically ill children and their families do not evidence "psychopathology" per se (Cappelli et al., 1989; Kazak & Marvin, 1984), recent surveys suggest that these children are at increased risk for behavioral and emotional problems (Cadman, Boyle, Szatmari, & Offord, 1987; Wallander, Varni, Babani, Banis, & Wilcox, 1988). Studies combining diverse pediatric conditions indicate that children with chronic illnesses and disabilities are approximately twice as likely as normative samples to evidence behavioral difficulties (Perrin & MacLean, 1988). Similarly, several studies of parental adaptation have found increased levels of stress and depression, particularly among mothers (Kazak & Marvin, 1984; Quittner, 1991).

One factor that may mitigate the relationship between ongoing stressors and psychological symptoms is the availability of social support. A plethora of research on stressful life events and illness has documented the role of social support in protecting and maintaining physical and psychological health (for reviews, see Cohen & Wills, 1985; Wallston, Alagna, DeVellis, & DeVellis, 1983). More recently, pediatric researchers have begun to examine the role of social support in the context of childhood illness (Quittner, Glueckauf, & Jackson, 1990; Varni, Wilcox, & Hanson, 1988). In the general stress–illness literature, increasingly sophisticated concepts and measures of social support have emerged, establishing links between inadequate social support and mortality rates (Berkman & Syme, 1979), the onset of physical illness (Cohen, 1988), and increases in both physical and psychological symptoms (Kessler & McLeod, 1985). However, despite the promising results to date, very little is known about the mechanisms underlying these effects (Heller, Swindle, & Dusenbury, 1986). A number of questions remain: What are the specific psychological and interpersonal processes that account for the mitigating effects of social support? And under what conditions are these effects likely to occur?

A primary reason for confusion about the mechanisms linking stressors, supportive transactions, and outcomes has been a lack of contextual specificity (Heller et al., 1986; Quittner, Glueckauf, & Jackson, 1990). Most studies have focused on the assessment of stressful life events or daily hassles, rather than on measuring stressors and support resources embedded within a specific context. This approach has ignored such important factors as the severity and duration of the stressor, the primary social roles (e.g., parental, marital) affected by the stressful event (Pearlin, Lieberman, Menaghan, & Mullan, 1981; Thoits, 1985), and the individual's stage in the life span (Heller, Price, & Hogg, 1990). These factors have considerable relevance for pediatric researchers, because the most frequently studied childhood illnesses last for long periods (e.g., cancer, diabetes); affect all members of the family system (Kazak, 1989); and lead to different consequences, depending upon the child and family's developmental stage (Morrow, Carpenter, & Hoagland, 1984; Rolland, 1987).

A second major shortcoming of prior research on stress and social support has been an emphasis on tests of main versus "buffering" effects. On a conceptual level, buffering effects specify the conditions under which social support may be effective—in this case, when perceptions of stress are high. Statistically, such tests necessitate cross-sectional rather than longitudinal designs, and thus limit the development of specific causal links among stress, social support, and symptomatology. This research emphasis has led to widely held notions that social support protects individuals from the negative consequences of stress, and to premature recommendations that increased support will be beneficial for those under high levels of stress (Coyne, Wortman, & Lehman, 1988; Lieberman, 1986). More research is needed to specify *how* social support works, what types of support are effective for particular problems, and who benefits from it at what points in time.

Researchers in the field of pediatric psychology may be in a unique position to address many of these inadequacies, because of their opportunity to assess stressors and social support processes within a specific context—defined by the type of illness, the developmental stage of the child and family, and the disruption of normative social roles (Cochran & Brassard, 1979; Rolland, 1984). Unfortunately, few studies examining stress in families with chronically ill children have employed such a contextual approach. Rather, a majority of these investigations have been plagued by the same conceptual and methodological limitations found in the broader stress–illness literature, such as inadequate measurement of the stress construct (Kazak, 1987; Varni et al., 1988).

The purpose of this chapter is to propose an alternative framework for conceptualizing and measuring the functions of social support for children with chronic illnesses and their families. Although an extensive review of the social support literature is beyond the scope of this chapter, key concepts and findings are used to highlight this alternative approach. First, various definitions and models of stress and social support are critically discussed as they apply to pediatric populations. Second, distinctions among life events, hassles, and chronic strains are drawn; particular attention is paid to the implications these differences may have for the provision and receipt of support. Third, the advantages of measuring several dimensions of the situation are discussed, including the task demands of the illness, strains in parental and marital roles, and the impact of developmental and life span factors. Finally, a contextual approach to studying chronic stress is illustrated with data from two studies of parents with chronically ill children.

CONCEPTUALIZATIONS AND MODELS OF SOCIAL SUPPORT

Definitions of Social Support

It is widely agreed that "social support" is a construct consisting of several components, including the provision of direct assistance, information, emotional concern, and affirmation (Gottlieb, 1985; House, 1981). Broad distinctions, however, have been drawn between the structural properties of the social network (e.g., size, density) and the functions the network provides (e.g., self-esteem, tangible aid). For example, although the size of an individual's network may be positively associated with the perceived availability of supportive contacts, a large social network may also bring with it increased demands and conflicts (Hirsch, 1980). In general, subjects' perceptions of available support, rather than their number of social contacts, have been most strongly associated with psychological benefits (Wethington & Kessler, 1986). However, given that supportive relationships are embedded within important social structures (e.g., extended family, schools) that may be altered by ongoing stress, it may be premature to eliminate consideration of structural measures (Cutrona, 1986; Heller et al., 1990). For parents of a child recently diagnosed with cancer, it may be critically important to add health care professionals to the support network.

Social network analysis provides a framework for testing long-held notions that families with handicapped or chronically ill children are socially isolated (Fewell & Gelb, 1983). Kazak and colleagues conducted a series of studies examining the network characteristics of families of children with spina bifida, phenylketonuria (PKU), and severe mental retardation (Kazak & Marvin, 1984; Kazak, Reber, & Carter, 1988). Compared to matched comparison families, mothers of children with spina bifida had *smaller* social networks, particularly with respect to number of friends. These families also had *denser* networks (i.e., network members knew one another to a greater extent), and higher density was associated with greater parental distress (Kazak & Wilcox, 1984). Unfortunately, measures of perceived support were not obtained, so the relationship between network structure and perceptions of the quality of support could not be determined. In contrast, no differences in network characteristics were found among parents of children with PKU or families of adolescents institutionalized with mental retardation. Thus, network structure differed among the three disability groups.

Smaller networks were also found among mothers of hearing-impaired children (Quittner, 1991), who reported significantly fewer family members, relatives, and friends in their network than mothers of matched hearing children. However, no significant differences between the groups were found on measures of perceived support. In order to clarify this potential discrepancy, analyses of the providers of support were conducted, revealing dramatic differences in the two groups. Mothers of deaf children listed health care professionals (e.g., home-visiting teachers) more frequently in their networks, and attributed a substantially larger percentage of functional (e.g., tangible aid) and emotional support to these sources (12%), as compared to mothers of hearing children (3%). The notion that certain types of support providers may compensate for decreased support from other members of the network has only recently been raised, and few studies have addressed this issue empirically (Coyne, Ellard, & Smith, 1990).

Both Kazak and colleagues' and my own results suggest that smaller networks may be found in some samples of mothers of handicapped children, but not in others. One possible interpretation of these results is that structural differences vary with the visibility of the child's handicap.

Both spina bifida and profound deafness are publicly observable (e.g., use of a wheelchair, communication deficits), and network members may be reluctant to offer help or may feel anxious in unfamiliar and stigmatizing situations (Chesler & Barbarin, 1984; Wortman & Lehman, 1985). In contrast, PKU does not produce visible differences in children, and the institutionalized adolescents with mental retardation lacked any direct contact with mothers' networks. Other research has indicated that the visibility of a handicap has a significant influence on how others communicate and interact with persons with disabilities (Strohmer, Grand, & Purcell, 1984).

It should be noted that studies combining medically diverse samples may not detect important differences in social support processes as a function of these contextual variations; they may thus lead to premature and potentially inaccurate generalizations. Together, the results of these studies (Kazak & Marvin, 1984; Quittner, 1991) also highlight the importance of measuring *perceptions* of support, since they may not be linked to network size, but rather to the availability of specific support providers (e.g., teachers familiar with childhood deafness) who can provide the most beneficial types of support (Cutrona & Russell, 1990).

Turning now to functional rather than structural types of support, five basic dimensions have appeared in most models of social support: (1) emotional support, (2) social integration (sense of belonging), (3) esteem support (sense of competence and value), (4) tangible aid, and (5) informational support (see Cutrona & Russell, 1990). Social support measures typically assess most of the supportive functions listed above, with varying measurement formats and degrees of psychometric validity (see Barrera, 1986, and Tardy, 1985, for reviews of support measurement).

Studies examining the effects of perceived support for families of chronically ill children have generally found positive associations between perceptions of available support and psychological functioning for parents of children with cancer (Frydman, 1981; Kupst & Schulman, 1988), children with developmental delays (McKinney & Peterson, 1987), and premature infants (Crnic, Greenberg, Ragozin, Robinson, & Basham, 1983). Interestingly, the beneficial effects of social support seem to be related primarily to perceptions of availability rather than actual receipt (Kessler, 1991). Although a majority of studies have found main effects for social support (Frydman, 1981), interaction (i.e., buffering) effects have been found only for selected support measures (Crnic et al., 1983; McKinney & Peterson, 1987). Methodological problems, such as inadequate support measures (McKinney & Peterson, 1987), differing definitions of stress (i.e., stressful life events vs. parenting stress), and confusion over the statistical differences between mediators and moderators (Frydman, 1981) may account for the discrepant results.

One emerging trend in this literature is noteworthy: Studies examining specific *sources* of support have reported stronger effects for spousal support than any other type. Spousal or intimate support was positively related to parental adjustment to children's cancer (Barbarin, Hughes, & Chesler, 1985; Kupst & Schulman, 1988), and seizure disorders (Quittner, 1989), as well as to maternal attitudes and interactive behavior with at-risk infants (Crnic et al., 1983). Furthermore, marital satisfaction was the single best predictor of parents' problems with developmentally delayed children over an 8-month period (Friedrich, Wilturner, & Cohen, 1985). Several social support researchers have argued that relationships with family members (in particular, a spouse) largely account for the positive association between social support and adaptation to stress, and that this relationship is less clear for other support providers (Coyne et al., 1988; House, 1981). For parents of chronically ill children, spousal support may represent increased involvement in the child's care and a greater sense of shared responsibility for performing medical routines, traveling to clinics, and caring for healthy siblings (Barbarin et al., 1985; Bristol, Gallagher, & Schopler, 1988). There is also some evidence that as stressors related to parenting an ill child increase (e.g., more frequent hospitalizations), perceptions of spousal support and marital satisfaction decrease (Barbarin et al., 1985; Quittner, 1989). A greater understanding of how parents of chronically ill children divide child care and household responsibilities is needed, with a particular focus on how these role issues affect levels of marital intimacy and satisfaction (Quittner & Eigen, 1990).

Models of Social Support

In assessing the mechanisms by which social support modifies the negative consequences of stress, two competing models have been tested: the "main effects" and "buffer" models. According to the main effects model, social support has beneficial effects on physical and psychological outcomes, regardless of the person's level of stress (Cohen & Wills, 1985). Thus, in general, parents who report satisfaction with their support resources will be less likely to develop psychological or physical symptoms. In contrast, the moderator or buffer model specifies an interaction between levels of stress and social support: Parents who report high levels of stress, but who also have satisfying social relationships, will be protected from the negative impact of stress. Several explanations for these buffering effects have been proposed, including (1) altered appraisals of the stressor, and (2) the maintenance of self-esteem during stressful periods, which may facilitate the use of adaptive coping strategies (Cohen & McKay, 1984; Cutrona & Troutman, 1986).

In addition to the main effects and buffer models, a third possibility may be considered—a "mediating" model. In this model, social support functions as an intervening variable between the stressor and outcome. Lin and Ensel's (1984) "support deterioration model" illustrates the role of social support as a mediator. According to this model, some stressful events elicit withdrawal or avoidance responses from members of the social network (Barrera, 1988). Traumatic or stigmatizing events, such as serious illness or death of a child, may lead network members to avoid contact or to respond in ways that are unhelpful (Wortman & Lehman, 1985). Researchers have recently discussed processes whereby support efforts may "miscarry" (e.g., undermine independence), potentially leading to more negative perceptions of the availability of support by the receiver, and in turn to increased symptoms of depression and anxiety (Anderson & Coyne, 1991). Alternatively, those who are experiencing chronic stress conditions and are in need of frequent assistance may exhaust their resources, or they may perceive the support provided by others as less helpful because it highlights their own inadequacy (Coyne et al., 1990; Hobfoll & Lerman, 1988).

Support for the mediating role of social support was obtained in a recent study of mothers of hearing-impaired and matched hearing children (Quittner, Glueckauf, & Jackson, 1990). Child stressors (e.g., behavior problems, moodiness) and maternal stressors (e.g., competence, attachment) were associated with lower perceptions of support, which in turn were related to increases in symptoms of depression, anxiety, and hostility. Although the cross-sectional design of this study precluded tests of causal associations, mediational models tested within a longitudinal framework may increase our understanding of how social support exerts its influence on the stress process.

STRESSFUL LIFE EVENTS, HASSLES, AND CHRONIC STRAINS

Although considerable attention has been given to identifying potential moderators of stress, such as social support and coping behaviors, relatively little attention has been paid to defining, measuring, and understanding the origins of stress itself (Pearlin & Turner, 1987). Clearly, the measurement of stressors and that of intervening variables are inextricably bound, and progress in understanding how social and behavioral factors modify the negative effects of stress is unlikely to occur without a clear delineation of the nature and manifestations of the stressor being studied. Several dimensions of the stressor warrant further attention, including its temporal nature (acute vs. chronic) and the extent to which it is anticipated (normative vs. non-normative). To date, the majority of studies in this field have assessed the effects of stressful life events as antecedents of stress (Cohen & Wills, 1985), without consideration of temporal or contextual factors.

Stressful life events are typically measured by summing the total number or severity of events over the past year (Holmes & Rahe, 1967). This approach to stress measurement has several major disadvantages. First, different kinds of stressful events are likely to lead to very different challenges and adjustments (e.g., loss of a job vs. death of a spouse). Simply adding a number of disparate events tells us little about the daily experience of stress for that individual. Not surprisingly, tests of the association between life stress, measured as an amalgam of events, and psychological and health outcomes have proven disappointing, accounting for minimal amounts of variance (Rabkin & Struening, 1976; Quittner, Glueckauf, & Jackson, 1990).

Second, measuring stress in terms of a heterogeneous list of life events obscures the relationship between the *type* of stress and the specific helping behaviors that may be needed (Cohen & Wills, 1985). Several researchers have suggested that a match between the demands of the stressor and the types of support provided will lead to the strongest mediating effects (Cutrona & Russell, 1990; Pearlin et al., 1981). Thus, identifying these matches would also have the greatest implications for intervention. Third, processes of adjustment to discrete events may differ greatly from those occurring in response to more enduring chronic strains (Pearlin & Schooler, 1978; Quittner, Glueckauf, & Jackson, 1990). For example, the provision of instrumental support may be beneficial for someone relocating to a new city who is in need of basic information and social contact. However, that same boost of support may be viewed negatively under chronic circumstances, such as parenting an ill or disabled child. Within this context, such support efforts may be viewed as intrusive or suggestive of incompetence (Hobfoll & Lerman, 1988).

Finally, research on major life events has virtually ignored the extent to which the stressor is a normally occurring event (such as marriage or birth of a child) as opposed to an unexpected or non-normative event (such as serious childhood illness) (Pearlin & Turner, 1987; Schulz & Rau, 1985). Although normative events may precipitate temporary difficulties, they have not been shown to be major sources of stress (Menaghan, 1983). Two explanations may account for this finding. First, normative events are expected, allowing individuals a chance to anticipate the changes that may occur and attempt to prepare for them. For example, although the birth of a first child may be initially stressful, leading to readjustments in sleeping schedules and the development of new parental roles, couples have had nearly a year to anticipate the difficulties that may arise and have established supportive contacts to assist them in making the transition (e.g., having grandparents visit and help out). Second, normative events are more likely to be associated with traditions that elicit support from informal network members (e.g., baby showers), as well as more formal organized resources (e.g., postnatal exercise classes); both types of resources naturally provide many of the supportive functions that may be needed, such as information, emotional support, and a sense of belonging.

In contrast, non-normative events, such as the birth of a disabled child, are typically unexpected, leaving those affected with no opportunity to prepare for the event or its sequelae (e.g., greater time demands, changes in parenting roles). These events by definition occur to relatively few people, and so are less likely to elicit effective indigenous support, because network members may have little experience with this type of event and may not know how to respond (Chesler & Barbarin, 1984; Heller, 1990; Schulz & Rau, 1985). Furthermore, although the need may be greatest, there are likely to be fewer community support resources available for relatively rare events. In sum, normative events that occur as part of the developmental life cycle may be differentiated from non-normative events with respect to both the levels of stress that may result and the availability of social support.

Researchers have also begun to assess "small events" or daily hassles for their effects on physical and psychological well-being (Kanner, Coyne, Schaefer, & Lazarus, 1981). However, this line of research may be vulnerable to the same criticisms leveled at the literature on stressful life events—namely, a lack of attention to the context in which these events occur, and therefore few clear links between the frequency of daily hassles and processes of support provision and receipt (Dohrenwend & Shrout, 1985). In an effort to go beyond this limitation, recent studies have looked for linkages between major life events and daily, ongoing stressors (Felner, Farber, & Primavera, 1983). Felner and colleagues, for example, have provided some evidence that major life events exert their greatest impact on psychological outcomes through the day-to-day changes and adaptations required by the initial event (e.g., adjusting to the birth of a baby). As noted above, these *scheduled* transitions are less likely to produce potent stress effects, and are usually associated with naturally occurring social support.

Although examining hassles and daily stressors may facilitate an understanding of the sequelae of major life events, the generalizability of this theoretical and measurement framework to more severe, chronic types of stress is questionable. Hassles and chronic strains are likely to differ in several ways. First, the effects of severe chronic stressors (e.g., a child with cystic fibrosis) are likely to be more pervasive, leading to alterations in several domains—for example, marital and work roles, interactions among siblings (Breslau & Prabucki, 1987; Opipari, Quittner, & Winslow, 1991), and relationships with larger community institutions (e.g., hospitals, schools) (Pearlin et al., 1981). Second, the chronicity of this type of stress implies its continuation into the future, potentially altering expectations for the accomplishment of normal milestones (e.g., independent functioning as a young adult), and requiring new shifts and adaptations in response to the stressor throughout the developmental life cycle. Thus, in terms of both its scope and its enduring impact, chronic stress as described above may be distinguished from both major life events and daily hassles.

A CONTEXTUAL APPROACH TO CHRONIC STRESS

In addition to considering the temporal and normative aspects of the stressor, the inclusion of relevant situational factors may increase our understanding of how and under what conditions social support influences adaptation to stress. Given that supportive transactions are likely to be effective within a specific situation or domain, researchers must begin to define the contexts in which these transactions occur (Heller et al., 1990; Menaghan, 1983). In this regard, stressful life events may be considered a *global* rather than a *specific* type of stress, providing little information about the context in which such events take place or the ways in which they influence current roles or daily circumstances (e.g., time demands).

An alternative to the life stress approach is to study stressors embedded within a particular context, such as chronic childhood illness (Cutrona & Russell, 1990; Quittner, Glueckauf, & Jackson, 1990; Quittner, Steck, & Rouiller, 1991). This approach to stress measurement has several advantages: (1) It provides a framework for assessing stressors tied directly to the task demands imposed by the illness as well as normal development; (2) it embeds the stress process within the developmental and life span goals of the family; and (3) it points to the relevant life roles that may be altered (e.g., parental). This framework should allow for the matching of types of support (e.g., information) and support providers (e.g., health care professionals) to the specific needs of patients and family members, and subsequently to more effective interventions.

Tasks and Demands of Childhood Illness

In discussing adaptation to chronic illness, several investigators have argued that we should assess the specific tasks and demands that must be mastered for successful functioning (Meyerowitz, Heinrich, & Schag, 1983). For childhood illness, in particular, Melamed, Siegel, and Ridley-Johnson (1988) have advocated the assessment of one set of illness-related tasks (e.g., treatment regimens), and a second set of tasks developmentally relevant for all children (e.g., peer relations, school attendance). In my own research, I used a similar approach to assess the chronic stressors associated with parenting children with seizure disorders and hearing impairments, and was able to account for substantial proportions of the variance in parental outcomes (Quittner, 1989, 1991).

It is important to note that this approach requires the assessment of stressors related to a *specific disease*, rather than the sampling of heterogeneous chronically ill populations—a practice common in much of the research published to date (Jessop, Riessman, & Stein, 1988). Although commonalities among medical conditions may be found, such as performance of a treatment regimen, the specific challenges and demands required by each disease may vary greatly (e.g., chest physiotherapy for cystic fibrosis vs. insulin regulation for diabetes).

Rolland (1984) has recently developed a typology of illness that includes the following characteristics: onset (gradual, acute), course (episodic, progressive), outcome (shortened life span, terminal), and level of incapacitation. To the extent that diseases vary on these dimensions, they are likely to make different demands on children and families, and to require different types of social support. For example, the demands faced by parents caring for a child with an episodic condition such as epilepsy (e.g., monitoring medications, worrying about physical injury) are different from those faced by parents caring for a child with cystic fibrosis (e.g., time demands related to the medical regimen, long hospitalizations) (Quittner, 1989; Quittner, DiGirolamo, & Rouiller, 1990).

Developmental and Life Span Factors

Another important aspect of the context of disability is the child's and family's stage in the life cycle. Most studies of adaptation to childhood illness have examined children ranging in age from 2 to 18 (Phillips, Bohannon, Gayton, & Friedman, 1985; Varni et al., 1988). This approach ignores both the meaning and demands of the illness as they vary with the child's developmental age and the family's life span goals (Glueckauf & Quittner, 1984; Rolland, 1987). For example, adherence to a medical regimen may pose no difficulties for parents of a school-age child; however, greater stress may occur during adolescence, when responsibility for management of the condition shifts to the child (Johnson, 1988). Similarly, the illness may affect the family's accomplishment of life goals, leading to feelings of frustration and depression (Quittner, Glueckauf, & Jackson, 1990; Rolland, 1987). Parents looking forward to more free time and independence as their children mature may feel ambivalent about a young adult's continued need to live at home because of a medical condition. Thus, the areas of stress for both the child with the illness and the child's family may be directly related to developmental and life span issues (Pearlin & Turner, 1987), with greatest stress associated with those limitations that preclude the accomplishment of normative transitions and goals.

Furthermore, the types of social support that may mediate these difficulties are also likely to vary with the child's and parents' age and stage of development. For example, compliance with a medical regimen may be strongly influenced by the supportive statements and reactions of the adolescent's peer network, but peer support may have little impact on a younger school-age child, who may look to the teacher for support. A failure to measure both the stressors and the support resources relevant for the family's stage in the life cycle may lead to weak relationships between stress and indices of adjustment, and little specific information about which supportive functions are most beneficial.

Social Roles

Instead of focusing on life events and the amount of readjustment they require, a shift toward examining the impact of events on social roles may prove more informative. "Social roles" have been defined as a set of behaviors expected of, or assigned to, a person occupying a particular place in the family system (Efron & Glueckauf, 1989). Alterations or difficulties in these roles have been termed "role strains" (Pearlin & Turner, 1987).

Social roles may serve as important contexts for examining stress processes for several reasons. First, focusing on role strains allows us to identify specific stressors that arise from an event, whereas merely counting global events over the past year does not. A major stressful event, such as the diagnosis of illness in a family member, is likely to alter the performance of primary social roles. Moreover, these alterations are likely to be observable in the daily tasks and routines in which families engage (Quittner, DiGirolamo, & Rouiller, 1990). For example, at the outset of a disabling childhood illness, parents may focus their efforts on providing emotional and instrumental support to the ill child, leaving them less time to spend together in social and recreational activities. Strains in their marital relationship may emerge, which can be measured in terms of these alterations in daily activities. Thus, role strains may be examined as antecedents or correlates of distress, providing a gauge for monitoring how individuals or subsystems (e.g., husband–wife) adapt to chronic stress.

Second, roles, such as those of spouse or parent, are usually highly valued by both the individual and the larger society. Considerable amounts of time and importance are associated with the enactment of these roles, and thus perceptions of inadequate role performance are likely to lead to decreases in self-esteem (Pearlin et al., 1981; Thoits, 1985). Childhood illness, for example, has the potential for dramatically altering both expectations and performance of parental roles, varying as a function of the child's need for physical care and level of independence

(Rolland, 1987). Consider the parents of a profoundly deaf child who must drastically alter expectations for normal communication with that child, as well as decisions regarding when the child may safely cross the street or play alone (Quittner, 1991; Quittner et al., 1991). Parents faced with these challenges may perceive themselves as less effective in their parenting role, which may lead to feelings of depression and low self-esteem. Support for the impact of role strain on parental depression and anxiety was recently obtained in two studies of maternal adaptation to childhood deafness and seizure disorders (Quittner, 1989, 1991).

Finally, social roles provide a link between the individual and the larger family system. Because roles by definition represent the emotional and behavioral interconnections among family members (e.g., mother-daughter), they provide us with an opportunity to operationalize and measure family-level problems. For example, parents of children with chronic illnesses may find themselves struggling for the time and energy to perform several roles (e.g., wife, mother, caregiver). How families set priorities among these competing roles may be a potent source of stress, measurable at both the individual level (e.g., less time for healthy siblings) and the systemic level (e.g., postponing family vacations).

Despite the recent emphasis on assessing the effects of stress on the *family* (Kazak, 1989; McCubbin & Patterson, 1982), much of the family research to date assesses the *individual's* perception of family functioning via questionnaire measures of such constructs as "cohesion" and "expressiveness" (Olson, Russell, & Sprenkle, 1983; Moos & Moos, 1981), rather than interactions among members of the system. Two problems with this approach may be identified. First, without a referent in terms of specific interactions or relevant problems, it is unclear what these terms mean behaviorally. What dimensions or behaviors underlie the notion of "cohesion," and what specific aspects of family functioning are relevant for assessing this? Second, if these items are not embedded within a specific context, the subject is forced to define the situation in which these behaviors occur. Therefore, each subject may respond to the item idiosyncratically, based on his or her own interpretation of what is meant. This may lead to decreases in the reliability and construct validity of the measure. For example, using a scale such as the Family Adaptibility and Cohesion Evaluation Scales (FACES) (Olson et al., 1983) to compare levels of cohesion in families with a chronically ill child versus families with a healthy child may be problematic, because it is unclear whether or not parents in these two groups use similar referents when responding to these items. In contrast, assessing role functioning and role strain may be advantageous in this regard because of the potential for operationalizing role issues in specific behavioral terms (e.g., less time for healthy siblings).

In sum, employing a contextual approach to measuring family stressors is more likely than questionnaire data to focus us on the behaviors and interactions relevant to family functioning. This should lead to a more process-oriented assessment of the impact of chronic stress on the family, and to the development of interventions matched to the specific problems that families identify. Social support, for example, may have beneficial effects to the extent that it facilitates the performance of key social roles (Crnic et al., 1983; Thoits, 1985). Parents caring for a child with cystic fibrosis may have few opportunities to engage in social and recreational activities as a couple, leading to reports of greater marital distress (Quittner, DiGirolamo, & Rouiller, 1990). Social support in the form of babysitting assistance may mediate the relationship between marital role strains and satisfaction, thus functioning to preserve a vital family role.

APPLYING A CONTEXTUAL MODEL OF STRESS TO PARENTS OF CHRONICALLY ILL CHILDREN

In applying a contextual framework to research on stress and social support, two studies of maternal adaptation to childhood illness were conducted (Quittner, 1989, 1991; Quittner, Glueckauf, & Jackson, 1990). In both of these investigations, several contextual factors were controlled, including the duration of the stressor, the developmental stage of the child, and the specific demands of the medical condition. Three samples of children were included in this research: severely to profoundly deaf children, children with a seizure disorder, and children matched on relevant demographic variables who served as healthy controls. All children in the deaf and seizure groups had been diagnosed for a minimum of 1 year; at the time of the study, dealing with a child's disability thus represented a familiar, ongoing stressor for parents, rather than an unfamiliar, acute event. In addition, the samples were confined to children 2 to 5 years of age, in order to facilitate the measurement of stressors related to the normal tasks of parenting a preschool-age child (e.g., toilet training, bedtime routines), as well as those imposed by the medical condition (e.g., compliance with the use of hearing aids and seizure medications). Finally, we focused on the role of parenting because of its central importance at this stage in the life span. Although only results on mothers' adaptation to parenting stress are considered here, data on fathers in the seizure and comparison groups were also obtained (Quittner, 1989).

The specific objectives of the studies were (1) to assess the extent of parenting stress, social support, and psychological distress among mothers of hearing-impaired, seizure-disordered, and matched comparison children; (2) to identify the specific stressors associated with each group's parenting role, as well as their relative contributions to measures of emotional distress; and (3) to test the moderating versus mediating effects of social support on psychological adjustment. A thorough review of both studies is beyond the scope of this chapter; therefore, only the measurement procedures and results relevant to employing a contextual approach to stress research are discussed.

Procedure

Subjects

The samples consisted of 96 mothers of severely to profoundly deaf children (i.e., 70-dB loss or greater across the speaking range); 106 mothers of children referred to a neurologist because of recurrent seizures; and 118 mothers of healthy children matched on maternal age, marital status, years of education, family income, and child's age. No significant differences were found among the groups on any of the demographic variables.

Measures

The major variables in the model were parenting stress, perceived social support, and psychological distress. Multiple indicators of each variable were obtained through interview and questionnaire procedures. A 100-item structured interview was conducted in each mother's home to collect demographic and medical information, as well as to identify and measure child-rearing and disability-specific stressors.

Measuring Contextual Stressors. Three parenting stress scales were derived from the structured interview. First, a list of generic tasks related to parenting a preschool-age child was generated from the developmental and parenting literature, and through problem situations elicited from mothers during the pilot phase. Parenting responsibilities were sampled across several domains (e.g., bedtime and mealtime routines, sibling concerns), facilitating the measurement of ongoing role-related strains The average number of problems reported across these domains was then calculated to form the Parenting Routines Inventory—Problem scale (PRI-P). Tasks specific to each medical condition were also generated. For mothers of hearing-impaired children, the problems and tasks included those related to communication (e.g., choice of oral or total communication methods); language training; use of hearing aids; and reactions of family, friends, and community members. For mothers of children with seizure conditions, problems were sampled in the areas of medications, obtaining medical care, and education (see Figure 5.1 for examples).

A measure assessing perceptions of parenting stress, titled the Parenting Routines Inventory—Stress scale (PRI-S), was also derived from the

BEDTIME ROUTINES

I'm going to read you a list of things you may have encountered while getting _____ ready for bed. Please tell me whether any of these problems have occurred in the last month.

TYPE OF PROBLEM	NO	YES
1. Tantrums	0	1
2. Dawdling	0	1
3. Feeling frightened of the dark	0	1
4. Uncooperative	0	1
5. Staying awake	0	1
6. Sleeping in places other than own bed	0	1
7. Getting up several times	0	1
8. Nightmares	0	1
9. Not having time for yourself	0	1
10. Other _____		

TOTAL SCORE _____

MEDICATIONS

I'm going to read you a list of difficulties you might be having with medications. Please tell me whether any of these things have happened in the past month.

TYPE OF PROBLEM	NO	YES
1. Finding the best drug to control them [symptoms]	0	1
2. Finding the right dosage	0	1
3. Remembering to give it to the child	0	1
4. Resisting/refusing to take medication	0	1
5. Expense	0	1
6. Side effects	0	1
7. Fluctuations in seizure control	0	1
8. Other _____		

TOTAL SCORE _____

Figure 5.1. Measuring stressors related to bedtime routines and medications.

interview. Stress ratings on a 5-point scale ranging from "not at all stressful" (1) to "extremely stressful" (5) were obtained for each domain (e.g., routines, medications). Finally, a more general measure of stress, the Family Stress Scale (FSS), was developed to sample relevant *family* issues that might be problematic for parents with young children (e.g., finances, outings in the community). The FSS consisted of 14 items rated on a similar 5-point scale.[1]

Standardized Measures. In addition to the interview-based measures of parenting stress described above, two other indices of stress were administered: the Parenting Stress Index (PSI; Abidin, 1983) and the Eyberg Child Behavior Inventory (ECBI; Eyberg & Ross, 1978). The PSI is designed to identify sources of stress in parent–child subsystems, and yields a total stress score, three domain scores (Child, Parent, and Life Stress), and 15 subscale scores reflecting both child characteristics (e.g., demandingness) and maternal role strain (e.g., competence).[2] The ECBI was administered to identify the frequency and types of behavior problems observed by parents.

Two measures of social support were given: the Norbeck Social Support Questionnaire (NSSQ; Norbeck, Lindsey, & Carrieri, 1983) and the Arizona Social Support Interview Schedule (ASSIS; Barrera, 1981). The NSSQ measures the extent of perceived emotional support (e.g., affirmation, aid) and network structure (e.g., size). The NSSQ is unique in providing information about the *sources* of support (e.g., friends, health care professionals), as well as the relative contribution of network members to the provision of these supportive functions.[3] The ASSIS assesses perceived satisfaction with six categories of support: material aid, physical assistance, intimate interaction, guidance, feedback, and positive social interaction. Finally, psychological distress was assessed using the Center for Epidemiological Studies—Depression Scale (CES-D; Radloff, 1977) and subscales from the Symptom Checklist 90—Revised (SCL-90-R; Derogatis & Cleary, 1977).

Relevant Findings

Extent of Parenting Stress Among the Three Groups

It was hypothesized that mothers of children with chronic medical conditions would report higher levels of parenting stress than mothers of healthy children. Furthermore, because childhood deafness involves deficits in communication between children and parents, leading to potentially pervasive difficulties in parenting, mothers in this group were expected to report greater stress in their role than mothers of children with seizure disorders. Significant group differences were obtained on the overall multivariate analysis of variance (Hotellings $T^2 = 2.07$), $F(2, 313) = 10.56$, $p < .001$. Follow-up univariate analyses of variance revealed significant differences on 13 of the 15 parenting stress measures. Mothers of children in both the deaf and seizure groups rated their children as more demanding, moody, and distractible and as less adaptable than mothers in the control group rated their children. They also reported more frequent behavior problems, and had more difficulty with family routines and activities. Not surprisingly, mothers in these groups also reported significantly lower perceptions of competence in fulfilling their role than did mothers of healthy children. As hypothesized, mothers of deaf children had higher parenting stress scores across nearly all of the measures than did mothers in the seizure group, with significant differences found on measures of family and parenting routines, role restriction, and child distractibility and demandingness.

It was also hypothesized that tasks related directly to the child's medical condition or disability would receive higher stress ratings than tasks related to normal parenting. In general, this hypothesis was supported. Other than stress related to behavior problems, which received high rankings across the groups, mothers tended to rank disability-specific problems as most stressful (see Table 5.1). For mothers of deaf children, these stressors were related to language training, communication, and finding an appropriate educational placement. In contrast, mothers of children with seizure disorders ranked safety issues, medications, and controlling seizures as most stressful. Having a comparison group was important for determining the specific areas of parenting that were most stressful, because it was clear from the data that parents of preschoolers generally find controlling their children's behavior fairly stressful.

A final hypothesis was that relationships between stressors measured contextually and outcome variables would be stronger than relationships between stressors and outcomes measured more generally. The patterns of correlations between the interview-based measures of stress (i.e., the PRI-S and FSS) and the PSI Child domain score (the PSI represents an improvement over measuring general life stress because it embeds problems within the parenting role) were contrasted. This hypothesis received moderate support. An average correlation of .40 across the groups was obtained between the interview measures of stress and the two psychological distress measures (i.e., CES-D and SCL-90-R subscales). In contrast, the average correlation between the PSI Child domain score and the psychological distress measures was .29. Correlations between a life events measure and distress scores were even lower ($r = .11$), accounting for little of the variance in the dependent measures.

Comparisons of Network and Perceived Support Across the Three Groups

Network Support. Significant differences in network support were found among the three groups. Mothers of hearing-impaired children had substantially *smaller* networks than mothers of children with seizure disorders or healthy controls. An examination of specific types of network members indicated that mothers of deaf children listed fewer family members and friends, but more health care professionals, than mothers in either the seizure or comparison groups. Mothers of children with seizure disorders reported a slightly different pattern of network providers, listing more family members and fewer friends in their networks than comparison mothers. Significant group differences in the average duration of

Table 5.1. Rankings of Parenting Stressors

Rank	Parents of deaf children	Parents of seizure-disordered children	Parents of control children
1	Behavior problems during language training	Safety	Behavior problems at home
2	Behavior problems at home	Behavior problems away from home	Sibling rivalry
3	Communication	Medications	Toilet training
4	Dual role as mother and teacher	Behavior problems at home	Mealtimes
5	Finding a school program	Mealtimes	Behavior problems away from home
6	Crossing the street	Controlling seizures	Bedtimes

relationships were also found among the three groups: Mothers of children with seizure problems had known members of their networks longer than mothers of healthy or hearing-impaired children, with mothers in the deaf group reporting the shortest relationships across types of network members.

Perceived Support. In contrast to the structural support characteristics reported above, mothers of deaf children did not differ significantly from mothers of healthy children in their perceptions of available support. Mothers in both groups reported similar levels of affirmation, affection, and material aid. However, significant differences in perceived support were found between mothers in the deaf and seizure groups, in that mothers of children with seizure disorders reported *less* support in the areas of affirmation and affection. Mothers in the seizure group also reported significantly less emotional support than controls. An inspection of support providers suggested that mothers of deaf children perceived family members and friends as more emotionally supportive than did mothers in either of the other groups. Thus, although mothers of hearing-impaired children had the smallest number of family members and friends in their networks, their perceptions of support equaled or surpassed those of the other mothers. This discrepancy between network characteristics and perceived emotional support highlights the multidimensional nature of the social support construct and the need to identify both the positive and negative aspects of support transactions.

Comparisons of the Moderating versus Mediating Effects of Social Support

In order to increase the reliability and validity of the variables used to test the buffering versus mediating effects of social support, multiple indicators of each construct were employed. These measures were then subjected to a principal-components factor analysis, followed when appropriate by a varimax rotation. Factor scores based on the rotated factor loadings were employed in the subsequent tests of the models (Quittner, Glueckauf, & Jackson, 1990).

A factor analysis of the parenting stress measures yielded a two-factor solution accounting for 61% of the variance. Factor 1 was labeled Child Stressors and was defined by high loadings on measures of stress in daily routines and negative characteristics of the child (e.g., demanding, hyperactive). Factor 2, labeled Maternal Stressors, was characterized by high loadings on attachment to the child, perceptions that the child was rewarding, and maternal sense of competence. Three factors were extracted from the social support measures (i.e., Network Support, Perceived Support, and Need for Support), accounting for 70% of the variance. Finally, one large unrotated Psychological Distress factor was extracted from the various psychological distress measures, accounting for 68% of the variance.

Prior to testing the two competing models, multiple-regression analyses were conducted to assess the effects of group membership. The results suggested that group membership (e.g., mothers in the deaf vs. control group) had no influence on the relationships between the variables. Therefore, the groups were collapsed for tests of the models. In the interests of simplicity, the analyses relating only to the deaf and control groups are presented here, although similar results were obtained for the seizure group.

Buffering Effects of Social Support. According to the buffer model, perceived social support was expected to moderate psychological adjustment at high levels of stress. In order to test this hypothesis, four multiple-regression equations were generated to test for interactions between the Support and Stress factors. None of the interaction terms contributed significantly to the prediction of distress. In contrast, significant direct effects were found for Perceived Support and Stress factors. Perceived Support, in particular, explained a large proportion of the variance in Distress scores, controlling for the effects of Child and Maternal Stressors (i.e., 13% and 18.5% of the variance, respectively). In sum, little support was obtained for the buffer model of social support.

Mediating Effects of Social Support. In contrast to the results just described, a mediating model predicted that social support would intervene between parenting stress and psychological adjustment. Parenting stress was expected to lower perceptions of support, leading to increases in symptoms of distress. Although path-analytic techniques could not rule out alternative causal explanations or reciprocal effects, mediating effects might provide important information about links between model variables.

To test the mediating effects of Perceived Support, a series of regression analyses was conducted, and the strengths of the paths were estimated (Baron & Kenny, 1986). A strong direct effect was found between Child Stressors and Psychological Distress ($r = .54$), accounting for 29% of the variance in distress scores. However, as can be seen in Figure 5.2, a significant mediating relationship was also obtained. Child Stressors were associated with lower Perceived Support, which in turn was related to increased symptoms of depression, anxiety, and hostility. In contrast, Network Support did not mediate the relationship between Child Stressors and Psychological Distress.

Mediating effects were also found for Maternal Stressors using *both* Perceived and Network Support, although the direct effect of this type of stress accounted for less of the variance in distress scores ($r = .17$).

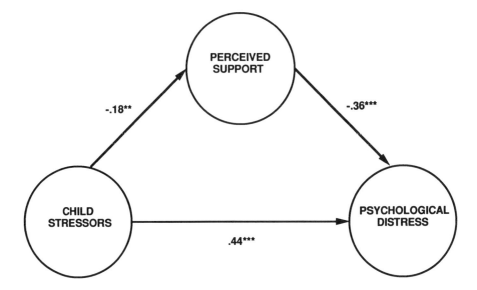

Figure 5.2. Mediating effects of perceived support. (Direct effects of Child Stressors on Psychological Distress = .54*** [**p < .01; ***p < .001].) From "Chronic Parenting Stress: Moderating versus Mediating Effects of Social Support" A. L. Quittner, R. L. Glueckauf, and D. N. Jackson, 1990, *Journal of Personality and Social Psychology, 59*, p. 1275. Copyright 1990 by the American Psychological Association, Inc. Reprinted by permission.

Mothers who perceived themselves as less competent, less attached to their children, and less rewarded in their parenting role had smaller networks, fewer social contacts, and lowered perceptions of being loved, respected, and aided (e.g., money). This in turn was associated with higher symptom scores. It should be noted that although the direct effect of Maternal Stressors on Psychological Distress was less dramatic, almost perfect mediation of this relationship was achieved with the addition of Perceived and Network Support (see Figure 5.3), suggesting that social support may be critically affected by this type of role strain.

Conclusions

The results of these investigations provided strong evidence that mothers of children with severe hearing losses and seizure disorders experienced greater stress in their parenting role and poorer emotional adjustment than mothers of nonimpaired children. Substantial group differences were found on nearly all parenting stress measures. In addition, substantial support for the importance of role strain was obtained in both studies. Although prior research on family adaptation to a variety of childhood disorders has focused on the incidence of *child* behaviors and deficits, the current results suggest that role-related stressors (e.g., perceptions of maternal competence) should be considered as well. Furthermore, by comparing stressors related to typical parenting tasks and the problems associated with the child's medical condition, these studies indicated that mothers had greatest difficulty managing disability-specific stressors, and thus point us toward specific areas in which parents may need greater support.

In terms of social support, mothers of hearing-impaired children had significantly smaller networks than mothers in either of the other groups, particularly in the domains of family and friends. This may not be surprising, given the large number of problems related to relatives, friends, and community members endorsed by mothers of deaf children (including misconceptions about their child's condition, advice giving,

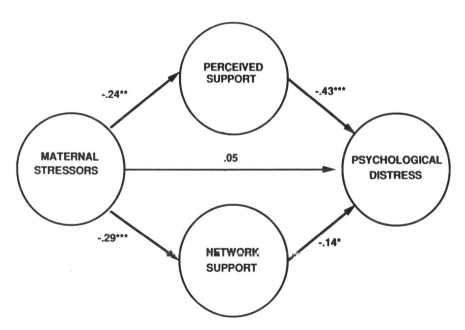

Figure 5.3. Mediating effects of network and perceived support. (Direct effects of Maternal Stressors on Psychological Distress = .173*** [*p < .05; **p < .01; ***p < .001].) From "Chronic Parenting Stress: Moderating versus Mediating Effects of Social Support" A. L. Quittner, R. L. Glueckauf, and D. N. Jackson, 1990, *Journal of Personality and Social Psychology,* 59, p. 1275. Copyright 1990 by the American Psychological Association, Inc. Reprinted by permission.

and underestimates of the child's ability). These reactions may have led mothers of hearing-impaired children to withdraw from network members who were critical, poorly informed, or overly intrusive. On measures of functional and emotional support, mothers of deaf children did not differ from mothers of healthy children, but reported more emotional support than mothers of children with seizure disorders. Thus, although mothers of deaf children had fewer network members on whom they could rely, they were satisfied with the availability of help. As other studies have noted, network size may not be related to perceptions of the availability of support or to the receipt of actual helping behaviors.

To turn to tests of the models, little evidence of buffering effects was found for social support across the three groups. Although main effects for both network and perceived support were observed, high-stress/high-support mothers did not report better psychological adjustment than high-stress/low-support mothers. In contrast, significant mediating effects for social support were obtained. Although causal conclusions cannot be drawn because of the cross-sectional nature of the design, chronic parenting stress was associated with decreases in perceived support and increases in symptoms of distress. Several explanations may account for these results, including the measurement of chronic strain rather than life stress, the assessment of stressors embedded within highly valued social roles, and the use of multiple indicators of each variable. A replication of these findings using longitudinal data is needed to confirm the causal ordering employed in these investigations. In addition, the causal links proposed by this mediating model represent a unidirectional pattern that may not fully describe what is most likely a reciprocal process (e.g., perceptions of support may also influence reports of child and maternal stressors).

FINAL NOTE

In order to advance our understanding of the stress process, including the role of potential mediators such as social support, we must begin to carefully define the contexts in which stressors and supportive transactions occur. Several temporal and contextual factors have been put forward in this chapter as worthy of consideration, such as the severity and chronicity of the stressor, and the extent to which it represents a normative or non-normative event. Once the situation has been more narrowly defined, a framework for measuring specific stressors tied to important roles and life span factors naturally emerges. This framework facilitates a similar level of specificity in measuring support processes. Identifying matches between and among types of support, support providers, and specific needs should yield the greatest benefits for physical and psychological health. Furthermore, this approach should increase our understanding of the situations in which supportive transactions are considered intrusive or unhelpful.

As pediatric researchers, we are in a unique position to contribute conceptually and empirically to knowledge of these processes. Chronic childhood illness provides a vehicle for examining the specific demands of an ongoing stressor, as well as the role social support may play (both positive and negative) in altering its impact on developmental processes and family roles. This approach also poses greater challenges, because it necessitates the study of homogeneous populations with respect to medical condition and stage in the life span. Moreover, in order to more closely capture the behaviors and transactions underlying the adaptation process, we will have to move beyond questionnaire data toward more innovative measurement approaches (e.g., diary methods). Despite these difficulties, we are likely to reap substantial benefits in terms of our understanding of the process, as well as our ability to translate this knowledge into effective interventions.

Acknowledgments

This research was supported by Grant No. 949-86-88 from the Ontario Mental Health Foundation and Grant No. 12-174 from the March of Dimes Birth Defects Foundation. I would like to thank Robert L. Glueckauf, Emily B. Winslow, Ann M. DiGirolamo, and Lisa C. Opipari for their helpful comments on an earlier version of this chapter.

NOTES

1. The psychometric properties of these scales have been described elsewhere (Quittner, Glueckauf, & Jackson, 1990).
2. Only three subscales from the Parent domain were used in this research because of potential confounding between stressors measured in the Parent domain (e.g., social isolation, depression) and the mediating (i.e., social support) and dependent (i.e., emotional distress) variables in the model (Thoits, 1982).
3. The NSSQ confounds network size and ratings of perceived support. This confound was eliminated by dividing the perceived support ratings by the number in the network.

REFERENCES

Abidin, R. R. (1983). *Parenting Stress Index (PSI): Manual and administration booklet.* Charlottesville, VA: Pediatric Psychology Press.

Anderson, B. J., & Coyne, J. C. (1991). "Miscarried helping" in families of children and adolescents with chronic diseases. In J. H. Johnson & S. B. Johnson (Eds.), *Advances in child health psychology* (pp. 167–177). Gainesville: University of Florida Press.

Barbarin, O., Hughes, D., & Chesler, M. (1985). Stress, coping, and marital functioning among parents of children with cancer. *Journal of Marriage and the Family, 47*, 473–480.

Baron, R. M., & Kenny, D. A. (1986). The moderator–mediator variable distinction in social psychological research: Conceptual, strategic, and statistical considerations. *Journal of Personality and Social Psychology, 51*, 1173–1182.

Barrera, M. (1981). social support in the adjustment of pregnant adolescents: Assessment issues. In B. H. Gottlieb (Ed.), *Social networks and social support* (pp. 69–96). Beverly Hills, CA: Sage.

Barrera, M. (1986). Distinctions between social support concepts, measures, and models.. *American Journal of community Psychology, 14*, 413–445.

Barrera, M. (1988). Models of social support and life stress: Beyond the buffering hypothesis. In L. H. Cohen (Ed.), *Life events and psychological functioning: Theoretical and methodological issues* (pp. 211–236). Newbury Park, CA: Sage.

Berkman, L. F., & Syme, S. L. (1979). Social networks, host resistance, and mortality: A nine-year follow-up study of Alameda County residents. *American Journal of Epidemiology, 109*, 186–204.

Breslau, N., & Prabucki, K. (1987). Siblings of disabled children: Effects of chronic stress in the family. *Archives of General Psychiatry, 44*, 1040–1046.

Bristol, M. M., Gallagher, J. J., & Schopler, E. (1988). Mothers and fathers of young developmentally disabled and nondisabled boys: Adaptation and spousal support. *Developmental Psychology, 24*, 441–451.

Cadman, D., Boyle, M., Szatmari, P., & Offord, D. R. (1987). Chronic illness, disability, and mental and social well-being: Findings of the Ontario Child Health Study. *Pediatrics, 79*, 805–813.

Cappelli, M. A., McGrath, P. J., Heick, C. E., MacDonald, N. E., Feldman, W., & Rowe, P. (1989). Chronic disease and its impact: The adolescent's perspective. *Journal of Adolescent Health Care, 10*, 283–288.

Chesler, M. A., & Barbarin, O. A. (1984). Difficulties of providing help in a crisis: Relationships between parents of children with cancer and their friends. *Journal of Social Issues, 40*, 113–134.

Cochran, M., & Brassard, J. (1979). Child development and personal social networks. *Child Development, 50*, 601–616.

Cohen, S. (1988). Psychosocial models of the role of social support in the etiology of physical disease. *Health Psychology, 7*, 269–297.

Cohen, S., & McKay, G. (1984). Social support, stress and the buffering hypothesis: A theoretical analysis. In A. Baum, S. E. Taylor, & J. E. Singer (Eds.), *Handbook of psychology and health* (pp. 253–267). Hillsdale, NJ: Erlbaum.

Cohen, S., & Wills, T. A. (1985). Stress, social support, and the buffering hypothesis. *Psychological Bulletin, 98*, 310–357.

Coyne, J. C., Ellard, J. H., & Smith D. A. (1990). Social support, interdependence, and the dilemmas of helping. In B. R. Sarason, I. G. Sarason, & G. R. Pierce (Eds.), *Social support: An interactional view* (pp. 129–149). New York: Wiley.

Coyne, J. C., Wortman, C. B., & Lehman, D. R. (1988). The other side of support: Emotional overinvolvement and miscarried helping. In B. H. Gottlieb (Ed.), *Marshaling social support: Formats, processes and effects* (pp. 305–330). Newbury Park, CA: Sage.

Crnic, K. A., Greenberg, M. T., Ragozin, A. S., Robinson, N. M., & Basham, R. B. (1983). Effects of stress and social support on mothers of premature and full-term infants. *Child Development, 54,* 209–217.

Cutrona, C. E. (1986). Objective determinants of perceived social support. *Journal of Personality and Social Psychology, 50,* 349–355.

Cutrona, C. E., & Russell, D. (1990). Type of social support and specific stress: Toward a theory of optimal matching. In B. R. Sarason, I. G. Sarason, & G. R. Pierce (Eds.), *Social support: An interactional view* (pp. 319–366). New York: Wiley.

Cutrona, C. E., & Troutman, B. R. (1986). Social support, infant temperament, and parenting self-efficacy: A mediational model of postpartum depression. *Child Development, 57,* 1507–1518.

Derogatis, L., & Cleary, P. (1977). Confirmation of the dimensional structure of the SCL-90: A study in construct validation. *Journal of Clinical Psychology, 33,* 981–989.

Dohrenwend, B. P., & Shrout, P. E. (198‾). "Hassles" in the conceptualization and measurement of life stress. *American Psychologist, 40,* 780–785.

Drotar, D., Crawford, P., & Bush, M. (1984). The family context of childhood chronic illness: Implications for psychosocial intervention. In M. G. Eisenberg, L. C. Sutkin, & M. A. Jansen (Eds.), *Chronic illness and disability throughout the life span: Effects on self and family* (pp. 103–129). New York: Springer.

Efron, D. E., & Glueckauf, R. L. (1989). Pragmatics of the tiger–shark integrative model of family therapy. *Journal of Strategic and Systemic Therapies, 8,* 1–17.

Eyberg, S. M., & Ross, A. W. (1978). Assessment of child behavior problems: The validation of a new inventory. *Journal of Clinical Child Psychology, 7,* 113–116.

Felner, R. D., Farber, S., & Primavera, J. (1983). Transitions and stressful life events: A model for primary prevention. In R. D. Felner, L. Jason, J. Moritsugu, & S. Farber (Eds.), *Preventive psychology: Theory, research, and practice* (pp. 199–215). Elmsford, NY: Pergamon Press.

Fewell, R.R., & Gelb, S.A. (1983). Parenting moderately handicapped persons. In M. Seligman (Ed.), *The family with a handicapped child: Understanding and treatment* (pp. 175–202). New York: Grune & Stratton.

Friedrich, W. N., Wilturner, L., & Cohen, D. S. (1985). Coping resources and parenting mentally retarded children. *American Journal of Mental Deficiency, 90,* 130–139.

Frydman, M. I. (1981). Social support, life events and psychiatric symptoms: A study of direct, conditional and interaction effects. *Social Psychiatry, 16,* 69–78.

Glueckauf, R. L., & Quittner, A. L. (1984). Facing physical disability as a young adult: Psychological issues and approaches. In M. Eisenberg, L. Sutkin, & M. Jansen (Eds.), *Chronic illness and disability through the life span: Effects on self and family* (pp. 167–183). New York: Springer.

Gottlieb, B. H. (1985). Social support and the study of personal relationships. *Journal of Social and Personal Relationships, 2,* 351–375.

Heller, K. (1990). Social and community intervention. *Annual Review of Psychology, 41,* 141–168.

Heller, K., Price, R. H., & Hogg, J. R. (1990). The role of social support in community and clinical interventions. In B. R. Sarason, I. G. Sarason, & G. R. Pierce (Eds.), *Social support: An interactional view* (pp. 483–507). New York: Wiley.

Heller, K., Swindle, R., & Dusenbury, L. (1986). Component social support processes: Comments and integration. *Journal of Consulting and Clinical Psychology, 54,* 466–470.

Hirsch, B. J. (1980). Natural support systems and coping with major life change. *American Journal of Community Psychology, 8,* 159–172.

Hobfoll, S., & Lerman, M. (1988). Personal relationships, personal attributes, and stress resistance: Mothers' reactions to their child's illness. *American Journal of Community Psychology, 16,* 565–589.

Holmes, T., & Rahe, R. (1967). The Social Readjustment Rating Scale. *Journal of Psychosomatic Research, 11,* 213–218.

House, J. S. (1981). *Work stress and social support.* Reading, MA: Addison-Wesley.

Jessop, D. J., Riessman, C. K., & Stein, R. E. K. (1988). Chronic childhood illness and maternal mental health. *Journal of Developmental and Behavioral Pediatrics, 9,* 147–156.

Johnson, S. B. (1988). Diabetes mellitus in childhood. In D. K. Routh (Ed.), *Handbook of pediatric psychology* (pp. 9–31). New York: Guilford Press.

Kanner, A. D., Coyne, J. C., Schaefer, C., & Lazarus, R. S. (1981). Comparisons of two models of stress management: Daily hassles and uplifts versus major life events. *Journal of Behavioral Medicine, 4,* 1–39.

Kazak, A. E. (1987). Families with disabled children: Stress and social networks in three samples. *Journal of Abnormal Child Psychology, 15,* 137–146.

Kazak, A. E. (1989). Families of chronically ill children: A systems and social-ecological model of adaptation and challenge. *Journal of Consulting and Clinical Psychology, 57,* 25–30.

Kazak, A. E., & Marvin, R. S. (1984). Differences, difficulties and adaptation: Stress and social networks in families with a handicapped child. *Family Relations, 33,* 66–77.

Kazak, A. E., Reber, M., & Carter, A. (1988). Structural and qualitative aspects of social networks in families with young chronically ill children. *Journal of Pediatric Psychology, 13,* 171–182.

Kazak, A. E., & Wilcox, B. (1984). The structure and function of social support networks in families with a handicapped child. *American Journal of Community Psychology, 12,* 645-661.

Kessler, R. (1991). Perceived support and adjustment to stress: Methodological considerations. In H. O. F. Veiel & U. Baumann (Eds.), *The meaning and measurement of social support.* Washington, DC: Hemisphere.

Kessler, R., & McLeod, J. (1985). Social support and mental health in community samples. In S. Cohen & S. Syme (Eds.), *Social support and health* (pp. 219-240). New York: Academic Press.

Kupst, M., & Schulman, J. (1988). Longterm coping with pediatric leukemia: A six year follow-up study. *Journal of Pediatric Psychology, 13*(1), 7-22.

Lieberman, M. A. (1986). Social supports—the consequences of psychologizing: A commentary. *Journal of Consulting and Clinical Psychology, 54,* 461-465.

Lin, N., & Ensel, W. (1984). Depression-mobility and its social etiology: The role of life events and social support. *Journal of Health and Social Behavior, 25,* 176-188.

McCubbin, H. I., & Patterson, J. M. (1982). Family adaptation to crises. In H. McCubbin, A. Cauble, & J. Patterson (Eds.), *Family stress, coping and social support* (pp. 26-47). Springfield, IL: Charles C Thomas.

McKinney, B., & Peterson, R. (1987). Prediction of stress in parents of developmentally delayed children. *Journal of Pediatric Psychology, 12,* 133-150.

Melamed, B. G., Siegel, L. J., & Ridley-Johnson, R. (1988). Coping behaviors in children facing medical stress. In T. M. Field, P. M. McCabe, & N. Schneiderman (Eds.), *Stress and coping across development* (pp. 109-137). Hillsdale, NJ: Erlbaum.

Menaghan, E. G. (1983). Individual coping efforts and family studies: Conceptual and methodological issues. *Marriage and Family Review, 6,* 113-135.

Meyerowitz, B. E., Heinrich, R. L., & Schag, C. C. (1983). A competency-based approach to coping with cancer. In T. G. Burish & L. A. Bradley (Eds.), *Coping with chronic disease: Research and applications* (pp. 137-158). New York: Academic Press.

Moos, R. H., & Moos, B. S. (1981). *Family Environment Scale manual.* Palo Alto, CA: Consulting Psychologists Press.

Morrow, G. R., Carpenter, P. J., & Hoagland, A. C. (1984). The role of social support in parental adjustment to pediatric cancer. *Journal of Pediatric Psychology, 9,* 317-329.

Norbeck, J., Lindsey, A., & Carrieri, V. (1983). Further development of the Norbeck Social Support Questionnaire: Normative data and validity testing. *Nursing Research, 32,* 4-9.

Olson, D., Russell, C., & Sprenkle, D. (1983). Circumplex model of marital and family systems: VI. Theoretical update. *Family Process, 22,* 69-83.

Opipari, L. C., Quittner, A. L., Winslow, E. B. (1991, April). *Diary analyses of differential treatment of siblings in ill versus healthy families.* Paper presented at the Third Florida Conference of Child Health Psychology, Gainesville.

Pearlin, L. I., Lieberman, M. A., Menaghan, E. G., & Mullan, J. T. (1981). The stress process. *Journal of Health and Social Behavior, 22,* 337-356.

Pearlin, L. I., & Schooler, C. (1978). The structure of coping. *Journal of Health and Social Behavior, 19,* 2-21.

Pearlin, L. I., & Turner, H. A. (1987). The family as a context of the stress process. In S. V. Kasl & C. L. Cooper (Eds.), *Stress and health: Issues in research methodology* (pp. 143-165). New York: Wiley.

Perrin, J. M., & MacLean, W. E. (1988). Children with chronic illness: The prevention of dysfunction. *Pediatric Clinics of North America, 35,* 1325-1337.

Phillips, S., Bohannon, W. E., Gayton, W. F., & Friedman, S. B. (1985). Parent interview findings regarding the impact of cystic fibrosis on families. *Journal of Developmental and Behavioral Pediatrics, 6,* 122-127.

Quittner, A. L. (1989, August). *Coping with childhood seizures: A comparison of maternal and paternal perceptions of stress and adjustment.* Paper presented at the 97th Annual Meeting of the American Psychological Association, New Orleans.

Quittner, A. L. (1991). Coping with a hearing impaired child: A model of adjustment to chronic stress. In J. H. Johnson & S. B. Johnson (Eds.), *Advances in child health psychology* (pp. 206-223). Gainesville: University of Florida Press.

Quittner, A. L., DiGirolamo, A. M., & Rouiller, R. L. (1990, August). *Parental adjustment to childhood illness during the diagnosis phase.* Paper presented at the 98th Annual Meeting of the American Psychological Association, Boston.

Quittner, A. L., & Eigen, H. (1990). *Coping with cystic fibrosis: The longitudinal impact of role strain and activities on marital adjustment* (Funded grant proposal, March of Dimes Birth Defects Foundation). Bloomington: Indiana University.

Quittner, A. L., Glueckauf, R. L., & Jackson, D. N. (1990). Chronic parenting stress: Moderating versus mediating effects of social support. *Journal of Personality and Social Psychology, 59,* 1266-1278.

Quittner, A. L., Steck, J. T., & Rouiller, R. L. (1991). Cochlear implants in children: A study of parental stress and adjustment. *The American Journal of Otolaryngology, 12*(5), 95-104.

Rabkin, J. G., & Struening, E. L. (1976). Life events, stress, and illness. *Science, 194,* 1013-1020.

Radloff, L. S. (1977). The CES-D Scale: A self-report depression scale for research in the general population. *Applied Psychological Measurement, 1*(3), 385-401.

Rolland, J. (1984). Toward a psychosocial topology of chronic and life threatening illness. *Family Systems Medicine, 2,* 245-262.

Rolland, J. (1987). Chronic illness and the life cycle: A conceptual framework. *Family Process, 26,* 203-221.

Schulz, R., & Rau, M. T. (1985). Social support through the life course. In

S. Cohen & S. L. Syme (Eds.), *Social support and health* (pp. 129-149). New York: Academic Press.

Strohmer, D. C., Grand, S. A., & Purcell, M. J. (1984). Attitudes toward persons with a disability: An examination of demographic factors, social context, and specific disability. *Rehabilitation Psychology, 29,* 131-145.

Tardy, C. H. (1985). Social support measurement. *American Journal of Community Pscyhology, 13,* 187-202.

Thoits, P. A. (1982). Conceptual, methodological and theoretical problems in studying social support as a buffer against life stress. *Journal of Health and Social Behavior, 23,* 145-159.

Thoits, P. A. (1985). Social support and psychological well-being: Theoretical possibilities. In I. G. Sarason & B. R. Sarason (Eds.), *Social support: Theory, research, and applications* (pp. 51-72). Dordrecht, The Netherlands: Martinus Nijhoff.

Varni, J. W., Wilcox, K. T., & Hanson, V. (1988). Mediating effects of family social support on child psychological adjustment in juvenile rheumatoid arthritis. *Health Psychology, 7*(5), 421-431.

Wallander, J. L., Varni, J. W., Babani, L., Banis, H. T., & Wilcox, K. T. (1988). Children with chronic physical disorders: Maternal reports of their psychological adjustment. *Journal of Pediatric Psychology, 13,* 197-212.

Wallston, B. S., Alagna, S. W., DeVellis, B. M., & DeVellis, R. F. (1983). Social support and physical health. *Health Psychology, 2,* 367-391.

Wethington, E., & Kessler, R. C. (1986). Perceived support, received support, and adjustment to stressful events. *Journal of Health and Social Behavior, 27,* 78-89.

Wortman, C. B., & Lehman, D. R. (1985). Reactions to victims of life crises: Support attempts that fail. In I. G. Sarason & B. R. Sarason (Eds.), *Social support: Theory, research, and applications* (pp. 463-489). Dordrecht, The Netherlands: Martinus Nijhoff.

CURRENT RESEARCH PERSPECTIVES

Overview

ANNETTE M. LA GRECA
University of Miami
JAN L. WALLANDER
University of Alabama at Birmingham

Within the realm of pediatrics, medical conditions differ markedly in terms of management requirements and demands placed on the child and family. Pediatric conditions vary along a continuum from very acute, short-term problems requiring a brief course of treatment, to chronic conditions that demand lifelong management. Disease chronicity has been linked with poor adherence; in general, treatment difficulties abound with chronic, long-term regimens (Litt & Cuskey, 1980; Varni, 1983). Pediatric treatments also vary with respect to their complexity and the degree to which they involve unpleasant or aversive procedures. Treatments that are complex, entail activity restrictions, or require changes in personal habits and lifestyle are difficult for children and families to manage (La Greca, 1988). Furthermore, medical procedures that are painful, unpleasant, or aversive, such as chemotherapy or steroid medication, will be avoided by some individuals, even in the face of life-threatening consequences for nonparticipation. At the very least, they put further stress on children and families whose coping resources may already be taxed. For children and families who must endure aversive procedures, efforts to minimize discomfort and maximize quality of life become important considerations.

In order to appreciate the stressful nature of certain pediatric conditions, and to identify the processes involved in successful coping, we must first consider the nature of the challenge posed by the specific pediatric condition. The chapters in this section of the text recognize the varied challenges posed by different medical problems. Several focus on youngsters' and families' coping responses in the face of specific unpleasant medical stressors (e.g., invasive medical procedures, anesthesia induction, dental procedures), which may be characterized as acute but aversive (Chapters 6-8). Others consider chronic diseases, such as diabetes or cancer, to represent long-standing stressors that involve numerous adaptations and coping responses from children and families across time and development (Chapters 9-13). Not surprisingly, coping strategies that may be effective in acute, unpleasant circumstances, such as distraction and disengagement from the situation, contrast sharply with those that are adaptive for chronic conditions; in fact, avoidant behaviors may be counterproductive for coping with chronic diseases (see Chapters 9 and 10).

Several themes underlie the material presented herein. First of all, across all the chapters, it is apparent that children's coping must be viewed in the context of the broader social systems within which children function (e.g., see Chapters 7 and 12). Although research on children's coping strategies is certainly important, we recognize that parents, siblings, friends, school personnel, and health care professionals exert significant and diverse influences on youngsters' adaptation. Most of the research on stress and coping to date has emphasized the youngster in a family context (e.g., see Chapters 6-9). Within the family unit, mothers have been the most common focus of study. This emphasis is understandable, in that mothers are often the primary family members involved in youngsters' medical (and emotional) care. Yet we need more research on fathers and other caregivers.

We are also beginning to encounter investigations that extend beyond these traditional boundaries. For instance, Hanson (Chapter 10) articulates a systems approach, which incorporates diverse social systems and sources of influence, to understanding coping with childhood diabetes. In her model of adaptation for youths with diabetes, the family, peer, school, and health care systems are viewed as diverse, independent, and yet integrated influences on youngsters' adaptation and course of medical management. This emerging, multivariate model has guided the thinking and direction of Hanson's research in this area. Consistent with this contextual perspective, work by Kazak (Chapter 12) and Wallander and Varni (Chapter 13) also illustrates the utility of developing comprehensive, multivariate models to conceptualize children's coping and adaptation within broad social-ecological systems.

Future research might extend our understanding of children's social systems even further. For instance, fruitful areas for further investigation include the role of children's friendships and peer relationships in children's coping; the interdependent nature of youngsters' and families' interactions with the health care system; community influences on adaptation and health; and the effects of medical stressors on diverse aspects of family functioning (e.g., family members other than the ill child). Some of these areas are considered briefly herein, but represent a small fraction of current research on children's coping.

Another well-demonstrated theme in this section of the text is that programmatic efforts are necessary for learning about stress and coping with pediatric conditions. The concepts of stress and coping are sufficiently complex and multifaceted that single studies will not yield much useful information. Most of the chapters describe programmatic research, in which multiple studies build upon one another. Programmatic investigation typically requires a conceptual basis, as exemplified in several of the chapters (e.g., Chapters 10, 12, and 13).

A third theme evident throughout this section is the importance of adopting a developmental framework for understanding stress and coping. "Development" can be viewed from the perspective of the child, the disease, or the medical procedure. In terms of the developing child, Achenbach (1978) aptly notes that "even small differences in developmental level can have a large impact on [children's] capabilities, the ways in which they construe situations, the kinds of experiences they have, and the behavior they elicit from others" (p. 761). Thus, effective coping is inextricably linked with youngsters' developmental stage, at least within the broad age groupings of infancy, preschool/early childhood, middle childhood, and adolescence. Accordingly, the chapters in this section present material that covers the age range from infancy through adolescence. Field (Chapter 6), for example, describes strategies that have been effective for diminishing stress associated with the invasive and painful procedures that are a necessary part of medical management of the preterm newborn, such as massaging the infant and providing pacifiers for sucking. In contrast, more assertive and self-initiated behaviors, such as information seeking (e.g., asking questions) and distraction, are common strategies invoked by preadolescents in the face of unplea. int medical procedures (Chapters 6, 7, and 8). Developmental themes are also apparent throughout the chapters on chronic illness (Chapters 9–13). In particular, Hanson (Chapter 10) articulates a developmental sequence of stress and coping young youths with diabetes; this has clear application to other chronic pediatric conditions.

The developmental stage of the disease or its treatment is also an important part of the overall picture of adaptation. The chapter by Miller, Sherman, Combs, and Kruus (Chapter 8) notes that children's coping responses were observed to fluctuate as a function of the phase of the dental stressor (e.g., anticipatory, during the procedure, after the procedure). Melamed (Chapter 7) describes similar findings regarding anesthesia induction. In contrast, with a chronic illness such as diabetes, greater social support and family involvement may be apparent following onset or during the early course of the disease, and may become less salient as disease duration increases. Moreover, as Delamater (Chapter 9) and Hanson (Chapter 10) note, maladaptive coping strategies such as avoidance and wishful thinking become more common as disease duration increases. Developmental study of disease benefits from longitudinal research designs, which, unfortunately, are rare. An exception to this appears in the chapter by Kupst (Chapter 11), who carefully describes long-term coping with pediatric cancer.

A final theme that can be observed within this section is the necessity of obtaining multiple measures and multiple perspectives when studying stress and coping. Most investigators have obtained reports from children and family members; others have included the perspectives of medical personnel (e.g., see Chapters 6-8). Observational assessment adds yet another dimension to our understanding of children's coping behaviors; not surprisingly, observational data do not necessarily correspond directly with self-reports. Moreover, work by Delamater (Chapter 9) and Field (Chapter 6) clearly illustrates the value of obtaining hormonal, metabolic, and/or cardiovascular indices of stress, to document the presence of a stressor as well as the effects of various coping and intervention strategies.

In summary, the chapters in this section provide a sampling of significant and state-of-the-art research on stress and coping with pediatric conditions. Most especially, the material herein reveals considerable breadth and scope of research in pediatric psychology.

REFERENCES

Achenbach, T. M. (1978). Psychopathology of childhood: Research problems and issues. *Journal of Consulting and Clinical Psychology, 46*, 759-776.

La Greca, A. M. (1988). Adherence to prescribed medical regimens. In D. K. Routh (Ed.), *Handbook of pediatric psychology* (pp. 299-320). New York: Guilford Press.

Litt, I. F., & Cuskey, W. R. (1980). Compliance with medical regimens during adolescence. *Pediatric Clinical of North America, 27*, 3-15.

Varni, J. W. (1983). *Clinical behavioral pediatrics: An interdisciplinary approach.* Elmsford, NY: Pergamon Press.

Infants' and Children's Responses to Invasive Procedures

TIFFANY FIELD
University of Miami School of Medicine

Until very recently, people believed that infants and children did not experience pain because they could not verbally describe or remember the painful experience. More recently, several behaviors have been interpreted as responses to painful procedures, including facial and vocal distress behaviors, elevated respiration and heart rate, diminished oxygen tension (TcPO$_2$), and plasma/saliva cortisol levels. Thus, with the development of our measurement technology, we have been able to document stressful responses to painful procedures in a number of different systems. As in almost any study on groups of individuals, repeated investigations reveal large individual differences in responsivity. This phenomenon also applies to the experience of pain following invasive procedures. Some children show significant changes in their biochemistry but exhibit very little distressed behavior, whereas others show rigorous vocal protest and facial grimacing but exhibit little change in their physiology and neuroendocrine activity.

The purpose of this chapter is to briefly review some of the data from my own and others' laboratories on the behavioral, physiological and neuroendocrine responses to invasive procedures by infants and children. Most of the review focuses on group data, although some material on individual differences are also mentioned. In addition, because coping and soothing techniques are so critical to alleviating these kinds of stress, some coping strategies are described. Because most of the literature has focused on the newborn in intensive care and the hospitalized child, data examples are limited to those samples.

THE HEALTHY NEWBORN'S RESPONSE
TO INVASIVE PROCEDURES

During the newborn period of the healthy neonate, the two most common painful events are the heelstick and circumcision. Because the heelstick is universally administered to all newborns to screen for metabolic disorders, this procedure has been the most frequently studied for the newborn's response to pain. In these studies various measures have been employed, including behavioral state, heart rate, respiration, $TcPO_2$, and cortisol (Anders, Sachar, Kream, Roffwarg, & Hellman, 1970; Field & Goldson, 1984; Franck, 1986; Grunau & Craig, 1987; Gunnar, Connors, Isensee, & Wall, 1988; Tennes & Carter, 1973). Typically, in heelstick studies baseline measures are taken of behavior, physiology, and blood or saliva samples for cortisol levels. These are followed by the pricking of the newborn's heel and squeezing of the foot for the release of a very small amount of blood. Usually the infant cries during this procedure. Yet crying is not a sufficiently convincing demonstration that the infant is experiencing pain. Thus investigators have looked for convergent measures to document the infant's response to pain. For example, in a recent study by Lewis, Worobey, and Thomas (1989), both vocalization and facial expressions were coded prior to, during, and following the heelstick procedure. Vocalizations were rated on a 3-point scale from no vocalization to continuous crying, and facial responses were coded in a similar fashion from no facial response to full distress with the brows, cheeks, and mouth grimacing. Because these vocal and facial responses were highly correlated, they were combined to form one intensity score. Plotting the curve of this intensity response, Lewis et al. (1989) noted an immediate significant increase in the intensity score, indicating a high initial reactivity to the procedure. This was followed by a diminution in the intensity scores and a later reactivation of the distress response.

Considerable individual differences were noted in this sample. For example, some infants had low thresholds but quieted quickly, whereas other infants with low thresholds took longer to quiet down. Some infants with high thresholds remained upset once they started to cry, and continued to be upset over a long period of time. Thus individual differences emerged over both the initial response and the latency-to-quietness variables. Of further interest was the observation that the highly reactive newborns were the healthier infants: The infants who were more reactive at 2 days had less illness at an 18-month follow-up period.

Lewis et al. (1989) also explored the problem of the stability of responsivity over time by making a comparison between the responses to heelsticks at the newborn period and to inoculations at two months of age. The subjects were divided into 2 groups of responders based on their responses to the heelstick—namely, high reactors and moderate to low reactors. At 2 months, these investigators noted that 86% of the high reactors remained high, whereas only 10% of the moderate to low responders remained in this category. They suggested, therefore, that highly reactive infants are more likely to remain reactive independent of their experience over the 2-month period, whereas low reactors may be more responsive to environmental influences. It is possible that in this moderate to low group a responsive environment led to moderate to low reactivity, whereas a less responsive environment led to high reactivity.

It is interesting in this context that Lewis (in press) has also reported on cross-cultural differences in infants' responses to inoculations that may relate to differences in the infants' socialization. For example, in a comparison of Japanese and American infants, the American infants cried and were more upset at 3 to 5 months of age during inoculations, whereas the Japanese infants showed no crying and very little vocal and facial distress. Lewis (in press) suggests that because Japanese infants are constantly carried around they do not have to signal their mothers when distressed, while American infants are often placed at a distance from their caregivers and need to cry loudly to get their mothers' attention. Thus it would appear that newborns are born with different thresholds to pain and different dispositions for reactivity, but that these responses are rapidly complicated by different responses from the environment.

The most commonly accepted measure of the infant's response to stress is the plasma cortisol level change. Much of this work has been conducted in the lab of Megan Gunnar. As can be seen in Table 6.1 (Gunnar, 1989), Gunnar and her colleagues and others have documented elevations in plasma cortisol concentrations following various invasive procedures, including the circumstraint board (Malone, Gunnar, & Fisch, 1985), a discharge examination (Gunnar et al. 1988), weighing and measuring (Gunnar et al., 1988), heelstick sampling (Gunnar et al., 1988), circumcision by experienced physicians (Gunnar, Malone, Vance, & Fisch, 1985) and circumcision by residents (Gunnar, Fisch, Korsvik, & Donhowe, 1981; Gunnar, Fisch, & Malone, 1984). The last-mentioned levels were eight times higher than the levels of plasma cortisol in resting undisturbed newborns.

A number of investigators have noted individual differences in newborns' physiological responses to stress. For example, Porter, Porges, and Marshall (1988) noted that individual differences in vagal tone measured prior to circumcision surgery were predictive of physiological and acoustic (cry acoustic) reactivity to subsequent stress. Individual differences have also been noted by Gunnar and her colleagues (Gunnar et al., 1988). During the newborn period they noted that some babies

Table 6.1. Plasma Cortisol Concentrations under Various Conditions in the Newborn

Condition	n	Cortisol
Resting undisturbed[b]	50	3.0 μg/dl
Resting undisturbed[c]	10	3.6 μg/dl
Resting undisturbed (before circumcision)[d]	80	5.2 μg/dl
Circumstraint board[c]	10	6.1 μg/dl
Vaginal delivery (cord blood)[a,e]	13	8.2 μg/dl
Discharge exam[b]	50	9.2 μg/dl
Weigh and measure[b]	20	10.4 μg/dl
High-risk delivery (cord blood)[a,f]	21	11.0 μg/dl
Heelstick blood sampling[b]	49	11.7 μg/dl
Circumcision by experienced physicians[g]	30	17.0 μg/dl
Circumcision by residents[h]	26	24.4 μg/dl
High-risk delivery (scalp vein blood)[f]	14	25.5 μg/dl

Note: With the exception of delivery, poststimulation samples were obtained at either 20 or 30 minutes following onset of stimulation. "Resting undisturbed" reflects over 1 hour of sleep. Before circumcision, many infants were more than 3 hours postprandial. From "Studies of the Human Infant's Adrenocortical Response to Potentially Stressful Events" by M. Gunnar, 1989, in M. Lewis and J. Worobey (Eds.), *Infant Stress and Coping* (pp. 3–18). San Francisco: Jossey-Bass. Copyright 1989 by Jossey-Bass, Inc. Reprinted by permission.
[a]Because of rapid conversion to cortisone, cord blood may underestimate cortisol response to labor and delivery.
[b]Data from two experiments: Gunnar, Connors, Isensee, and Wall (1988).
[c]Data from Malone, Gunnar, and Fisch (1985), Experiment 2.
[d]Data from Gunnar, Malone, Vance, and Fisch (1985).
[e]Data from Talbert, Pearlman, and Potter (1977).
[f]Data from Sybulski, Goldsmith, and Maughn (1975).
[g]Data from Gunnar, Malone, Vance, and Fisch (1985) and Stang, Gunnar, Snellman, Condon, and Kestenbaum (1988).
[h]Data from two experiments: Gunnar, Fisch, Korsvik, and Donhowe (1981) and Gunnar, Fisch, and Malone (1984). Residents had performed an average of five circumcisions.

showed no responses even to blood sampling, and others showed a dramatic cortisol response even to being undressed, weighed, and measured. Gunnar et al. (1988) also noted that increases in cortisol were not always associated with behavioral distress in infants. In fact, large elevations in cortisol were sometimes observed in quiet babies. Some of the individual variability and discordance in response systems (i.e., the cortisol response's inconsistency with the behavioral reaction) could be accounted for by individual differences in baseline levels, with newborns of low concentrations showing greater increases than newborns with higher basal levels. Thus some of this variability may be governed by the law of initial values. Individual variability may also be affected by differences in the rate at which infants habituate their cortisol response to repeated experiences with the painful stimulus.

THE PRETERM NEWBORN'S RESPONSE
TO INVASIVE PROCEDURES

The preterm newborn typically experiences medical complications that require treatment in an intensive care nursery. There the infant experiences significant numbers of invasive procedures. As Lucey (1985) has noted,

> Almost everything done to or for the infant is painful, and that pain can certainly be felt, although it cannot be communicated. The infant who must have an endotracheal tube cannot cry and is not fed by mouth for weeks. His or her feet are slashed periodically for blood samples. (p. xvii)

The "gold standard" measure in intensive care units for documenting stressful responses is $TcPO_2$. Decreases in $TcPO_2$ are typically noted during invasive procedures and are cause for considerable clinical concern. Several authors have noted diminished $TcPO_2$ levels following heelsticks (Danford, Miske, Headley, & Nelson, 1983; Morrow et al., 1990). For example, in the Morrow et al. (1990) study, the heelstick procedure (in this case, used for assaying bilirubin levels) led to $TcPO_2$ drops that averaged 14 mm. Similar decreases in $TcPO_2$ have been noted during other invasive procedures, such as endotracheal suction (Long, Alistair, Philip, & Lucey, 1980). The latter investigators attempted to alleviate this stress by instructing nurses to monitor the infants' $TcPO_2$ levels as they modified their procedures and to limit those procedures that were considered undesirable (those that reduced the $TcPO_2$ levels) to particular times of day. When the nurses monitored the infants, the amount of "undesirable time" was reduced from 40 minutes to 6 minutes for 24-hour intervals. For example, endotracheal suction in the monitored group essentially did not change, whereas suctioning in the group that was not monitored led to significant decreases in $TcPO_2$. Thus stress can be alleviated by simply monitoring an infant during invasive procedures.

Even procedures that are less obviously stressful or invasive have been associated with physiological changes suggestive of stress. For example, in our neonatal intensive care unit (NICU), my colleagues and I noted that weaning from the incubator was a stressful procedure. This was a serendipitous finding in a study on supplemental stimulation of preterm infants (Field, 1987). In this protocol, plasma was sampled by heelsticks on day 1 and day 5 of the study. The neonates were weaned from their ventilators 1 to 2 days prior to their participation in our study. As can be seen in Table 6.2, their plasma levels for cortisol were significantly higher on day 1 ($M = 61$ ng/ml) than on day 5 ($M = 41$ ng/ml). The average change from day 1 to day 5 was a 25% decrease in cortisol

Table 6.2. Plasma Level of Cortisol (ng/ml) at Day 1 and Day 5 (Days 9 and 10 in Parentheses) Following Weaning from Ventilator

Newborn	Day 1	Day 5	Percentage change from day 1
1	60	39 (41, 37)	−35
2	47	25 (25, 25)	−47
3	90	64 (68, 61)	−29
4	33	32 (29, 35)	−3
5	34	30 (27, 32)	−13
6	123	57 (67, 47)	−54
7	38	42 (42, 41)	+9

Note. Average percentage change from day 1 to day 5 = − 25% (± 7%), $p < .05$. Adapted from Field (1987).

values. This is perhaps not surprising, given that infants who had been dependent on life support systems would then experience adjustment reactions to the weaning.

Another less obviously painful procedure is the neonatal behavioral assessment (in particular, the Brazelton Neonatal Behavioral Assessment Scale). This finding was another serendipitous observation from the study of supplemental stimulation (Field, 1987). The data suggested that preterm neonates were stressed during the Brazelton, as manifested by decreases in growth hormone levels. Although growth hormone levels are typically elevated in children and adults who are stressed, growth hormone levels are typically diminished in stressed infants. As can be seen in Table 6.3, the growth hormone levels prior to the Brazelton (at baseline) were higher than those immediately following the Brazelton. The mean baseline level for plasma growth hormone was 21.5 ng/ml, and the mean value following the Brazelton was 14.4 ng/ml. This 32% decrease in growth hormone following administration of the Brazelton suggests that assessments of this kind can also be stressful for preterm newborns even though they do not appear to be causing pain.

Several investigators have attempted to diminish these stressful experiences, as, for example, in the study by Long et al. (1980), in which nurses carefully monitored their infants' responses and limited invasive procedures to particular times of day. These attempts have generally led many NICUs to adopt a policy of "minimal touch." This policy basically limits the number of stressful procedures as well as their periodicity. In addition, my colleagues and I have tried a number of intervention procedures to minimize the amount of stress experienced during invasive procedures. One of the ways we have alleviated stress is simply giving infants pacifiers to suck on. Although this seems intuitive and basic, most infants are not given pacifiers in newborn nurseries. Because pacifiers appear to calm newborns, we conducted a study in which preterm neonates were given pacifiers during heelsticks. The infants who were allowed to suck on the pacifiers showed significantly less fussing and crying during and after the procedure than those not given pacifiers (Field & Goldson, 1984). As can be seen in Table 6.4, the neonates who were given the pacifiers were also less physiologically aroused (lower heart rate and respiration rate) than those not given pacifiers.

We also gave pacifiers to newborns during gavage or tube feedings, a procedure that was once considered invasive and stressful for the preterm newborn. In this study (Field et al., 1982), we simply gave preterm newborns in the NICU pacifiers to suck on during their tube feedings. As compared to the control group, these infants required fewer tube feedings; they were easier to bottle-feed; their average weight gain per day was greater; they were hospitalized fewer days; and their hospital costs were significantly lower (see Table 6.5).

Another intuitive but rarely used calming procedure is simply placing hands on an infant. For example, in a study by Jay (1982), nurses simply placed their hands on infants' heads and abdomens for 12 minutes four times per day. In this case the nurse provided this treatment at times other than those reserved for invasive procedures, in order that the children would not experience painful stimuli simultaneous with gentle human touch. Of some concern, of course, is the possibility that infants come to associate touch with painful procedures to such an extent that when they are simply touched the stressful reaction is elicited. This simple "placing on of hands" by the nurses was associated with a decreased need for oxygen and with fewer stress behaviors (e.g., startle responses and clenched fists).

Table 6.3. Plasma Level of Growth Hormone (ng/ml) at Baseline and after Brazelton Assessment

Newborn	Baseline	After Brazelton	Percentage change
1	26.0 (27, 25)	19.0	−27
2	20.0 (20, 20)	12.0	−40
3	29.5 (31, 28)	14.0	−53
4	19.5 (18, 21)	9.0	−54
5	19.0 (17, 21)	9.0	−24
6	25.0 (31, 19)	19.0	−4
7	13.5 (12, 15)	13.0	−4
8	19.5 (25, 14)	19.0	−5

Note. Average percentage change $= -32\%$ ($\pm 7\%$), $p < .02$. Adapted from Field (1987).

Table 6.4. Means for Measures Taken during Heelsticks for Treatment (Non-Nutritive Sucking) and Control Groups in Minimal and Intensive Care Nurseries

Measures	Minimal care			Intensive care		
	Treatment	Control	p	Treatment	Control	p
Crying (% time)	25	41	.005	01	19	.001
Heart rate (BPM)	172	187	.05	165	168	n.s.
Respiration rate	81	72	.05	51	54	n.s.

Note. BPM, beats per minute. Adapted from Field and Goldson (1984).

Table 6.5. Means for Clinical Outcome Measures of Treatment Group Receiving Non-Nutritive Sucking Stimulation and Control Group

Measures	Treatment	Control	p
Number of tube feedings	219.0	246.0	.05
Days of tube feeding	26.0	29.0	.01
Daily weight gain (g)	19.3	16.5	.05
Number of hospital days	48.0	56.0	.05
Hospital cost	16,800.0	20,294.0	.01

Note. Adapted from Field et al. (1982).

In a more active touching intervention, we have provided massage for preterm infants during their stressful hospitalization experience (Field et al., 1986; Scafidi et al., 1990). The treatment group received massage for three 15-minute periods during 3 consecutive hours per day for a 10-day period. These massage sessions were comprised of three 5-minute phases, including a first and third phase of massage-like stroking and a middle phase of passive movements of the limbs. In a prone position, the newborn was stroked on the head and face, neck and shoulders, back, legs, and arms for five 1-minute segments. The chest and abdomen were not massaged because of the neonate's apparent aversion to being touched in this area. These preterms may have formed an association between the invasive procedures that are typically performed in these regions and pain. Thus, they preferred not to be massaged in those places. In both of these studies (see Tables 6.6 and 6.7), the massaged infants gained more weight, showed fewer stress behaviors, and were hospitalized for fewer days at significant savings in hospital costs. More recently, providing massage for even more stressed cocaine-exposed preterm newborns has had similar effects (Field, 1990).

Thus, as can be seen in the converging data from these studies, self-comforting stimulation such as sucking on a pacifier, and natural caregiver stimulation such as gentle massage, can alleviate distress behavior and physiology in the preterm newborn during stressful NICU procedures. Because of these effects and the positive side effects (e.g., weight gain and shorter hospital stay) these would appear to be cost-effective interventions.

Table 6.6. Means for Measures Differentiating Tactile/Kinesthetic Stimulation Preterm Neonates from Controls

Measures	Stimulation	Control	*p*
Feedings (number per day)	8.6	9.0	n.s.
Formula (cc/kg/day)	171.0	166.0	n.s.
Calories/kg/day	114.0	112.0	n.s.
Calories/day	169.0	165.0	n.s.
Daily weight gain (g)	25.0	17.0	.0005
% time awake	16.0	7.0	.04
% time movement	32.0	25.0	.04
Brazelton scores			
Habituation	6.1	4.9	.02
Orientation	4.8	4.0	.02
Motor	4.7	4.2	.03
Range of state	4.6	3.9	.03

Note. Adapted from Field et al. (1986).

Table 6.7. Means (and Standard Deviations) for the Formula Intake and Weight Gain Data

Measures	Treatment		Control	
	M	*(SD)*	*M*	*(SD)*
Average daily weight gain prior to study (3 days) (g)	19.6	(10.5)	24.5	(11.1)
Average daily weight gain during study (g)	33.6	(5.4)	28.4	(5.5)[a]
Number of feeds per day	8.6	(0.7)	8.9	(1.4)
Average fluid intake (cc/kg/day)	161.8	(13.2)	163.7	(8.9)
Calories per kg/day	118.9	(11.4)	121.1	(14.5)
Calories per ounce	21.5	(1.71)	21.5	(1.76)

Note. Adapted from Field et al. (1986).
[a]Group difference at *p* = .003.

CHILDREN'S COPING WITH INVASIVE PROCEDURES

In later infancy and early childhood, the pain experience is assumed to occur because of more developed cognitive skills. At this developmental stage, the research focus has been directed more specifically at individual styles in children's coping and ways to facilitate coping with stressful invasive procedures (LaMontagne, 1984; Peterson & Toler, 1986). For example, children have been noted to show considerable variability in their coping behaviors during stressful procedures as a function of whether their mothers are present or absent (Gross, Stern, Levin, Dale, & Wojnilower, 1983; Shaw & Routh, 1982). And the children themselves show different responses to invasive procedures as a function of their coping style—for example, depending on whether they are "sensitizers" or "repressors." A study we conducted on these different coping styles of children is the focus of the remainder of this chapter.

In a number of studies on hospitalized children, some children have appeared to behave like sensitizers and some like repressors. In the literature on adults' coping with stressful hospital procedures, sensitizers tend actively to seek additional information concerning the nature of the stressor. Repressors, in contrast, avoid information about the stressor and appear to use defenses such as denial (Shipley, Butt, & Horwitz, 1979). These kinds of responses have been noted in children prior to surgery. For example in a study by Burstein and Meichenbaum (1979), one group of children behaved in a nondefensive way during play periods prior to hospitalization, whereas another group was defensive and avoided playing with hospital-related toys. The group that behaved in a defensive way showed more distress and anxiety following surgery. In another study by Siegel (1977), children who had been classified as successful copers (those who were cooperative, were low in anxiety, and had high thresholds for visible discovery) requested more information about the nature of their surgery than did children who were unsuccessful copers. In still another study (Knight et al., 1979), children with sensitizing patterns showed significantly lower cortisol levels during hospitalization, suggesting that they were less anxious. These children seemed to want to hear every detail of the procedures, whereas the children who were defensive covered their ears and tried to block out all the information. Thus this literature suggests that children with repressive forms of coping appear to experience more anxiety and distress than children with sensitizing behaviors.

In a study we conducted, 4- to 10-year-old children were observed during their hospitalization for their individual responses to invasive procedures (Field, Alpert, Vega-Lahr, Goldstein, & Perry, 1988). First, an attempt was made to classify the children as sensitizers or repressors, on the basis of a scale given to their mothers. In addition, the mothers were given the adult version of the Sensitizer–Repressor Scale to determine whether there was any similarity in the children's and the mothers' style, and both the mothers and children were given the State-Trait Anxiety Inventory to determine their current levels of anxiety. The mothers and children were then observed in a 10-minute play session with a giant set of Legos (a special set called Hospital Legos, which included building blocks, a Lego hospital, and Legos for an ambulance and an operating room) and a doctor's kit. This observation was conducted to determine whether there was more avoidance of hospital-related toys by either group, as there had been in the earlier study by Burstein and Meichenbaum (1979). Two invasive procedures were then observed for all the children: a blood test and a preoperative injection, both of which were rated by the mothers and the children. Following each of these procedures, each child was given an interview on coping strategies (Siegel, 1981), which asked the child basically which strategies the child would recommend to a friend for coping with the procedures. The child's affect during the procedure was also determined, by asking the child to point to one of a series of faces to indicate how the child felt during the procedure. The mother was asked to rate the child's reactions to medical procedures, including crying, clinging, and aggressive behavior, as well as necessary attempts to restrain the child (based on a questionnaire we developed).

As can be seen in Table 6.8, the repressor and sensitizer children did not differ on baseline measures, demographic measures or the amount of

Table 6.8. Means for Demographic and Baseline Measures for Each Coping Style Group

Measure	Repressor	Sensitizer	p
Child's age (months)	79.6	76.5	n.s.
Mother's age (years)	32.7	31.2	n.s.
Socioeconomic status	3.9	3.7	n.s.
Previous hospitalizations	2.7	3.1	n.s.
Hospital preparation	3.8	3.8	n.s.
Prehospital behavior questionnaire	21.0	19.7	n.s.
Prehospital coping behavior	41.0	43.3	n.s.
Sensitizer–repressor—child	8.4	11.2	.01
Sensitizer–repressor—mother	9.9	12.4	.05
State anxiety—child[a]	44.6	50.2	.10
State anxiety—mother[a]	42.6	47.6	.10

Note. From "Hospitalization Stress in Children: Sensitizer and Repressor Coping Styles" by T. Field, B. Alpert, N. Vega-Lahr, S. Goldstein, and S. Perry, 1988, Health Psychology, 7(5), 433-435. Copyright 1988 by Lawrence Erlbaum Associates. Reprinted by permission.
[a]Lower score indicates greater anxiety.

hospital preparation. Of some interest was the finding that sensitizer mothers tended to have sensitizer children and repressor mothers tended to have repressor children. Also, a trend in the data suggested that repressor children and repressor mothers had higher anxiety scores than the sensitizer children and their mothers prior to their surgery. As Table 6.9 demonstrates, the hospital play observation data suggested that the sensitizer children were more talkative, more affectively expressive (smiling/laughing), and more active than the repressor children. The mothers of the sensitizers were also more involved in their children's play behavior, engaging in more fantasy play, showing more positive affect and being more active; in other words, their behavior was much like their children's behavior. As can be seen in Table 6.10, the sensitizer children experienced more sensitivity and fear during the invasive procedures (the blood test and the preoperative injection). Their coping behavior questionnaire scores suggested that the sensitizer children more often observed the invasive procedures, sought more information about those procedures, and showed more protest behavior during the procedures than the repressor children. Also, the sensitizing children reported feeling more negative affect on the happy–afraid faces following the blood test and the preoperative injection. Although no differences were noted between the two groups on the number of recovery hours or their physiological measures (pulse, respiration, and blood pressure) following surgery,

Table 6.9. Means for Hospital Play Observation Measures

Behavior	Repressor	Sensitizer	p
Observer-coded play[a]			
Child			
Hospital-related fantasy play (.81)	47.8	47.1	n.s.
Talking (.89)	30.4	46.2	.05
Smiling/laughing (.87)	7.2	15.6	.01
Activity level (.82)	2.2	2.8	.05
Mother			
Involved in play (.81)	43.8	57.8	.05
Talking (.95)	46.7	51.4	n.s.
Smiling/laughing (.89)	6.8	11.6	.01
Activity level (.83)	2.3	2.7	.05
Child's drawing of his or her self[b]	4.8	4.0	n.s.

Note. From "Hospitalization Stress in Children: Sensitizer and Repressor Coping Styles" by T. Field, B. Alpert, N. Vega-Lahr, S. Goldstein, and S. Perry, 1988, *Health Psychology, 7*(5), 433–435. Copyright 1988 by Lawrence Erlbaum Associates. Reprinted by permission.
[a]Means are percentages of observation time that behaviors occurred, except for activity level, which is a 3-point rating from low to high. Proportions in parentheses are interobserver reliability coefficients.
[b]Mean scores represent number of depressed/disorganized features.

Table 6.10. Means for Invasive Procedures and Clinical Measures

Measure	Repressor	Sensitizer	p
Coping behavior during blood test[a]	7.5	9.2	.05
Affect during blood test[b]	5.0	6.2	.05
Coping behavior during preoperative injection[a]	7.8	9.3	.05
Affect during preoperative injection[b]	5.3	6.8	.05
Hours in surgery	3.5	3.3	n.s.
Hours in recovery room	0.7	0.5	n.s.
Pulse recovery	107.6	111.9	n.s.
Respiration recovery	20.4	23.2	n.s.
Systolic blood pressure recovery	110.8	106.5	n.s.
Postsurgical adverse effects	8.4	8.5	n.s.
State anxiety—child (postsurgery)	45.5	49.5	n.s.
State anxiety—mother (postsurgery)	38.3	40.1	n.s.
Hours in intensive care	17.4	9.9	.01
Days in hospital	8.0	7.4	n.s.
Posthospital behavior questionnaire	22.4	21.2	n.s.

Note. From "Hospitalization Stress in Children: Sensitizer and Repressor Coping Styles" by T. Field, B. Alpert, N. Vega-Lahr, S. Goldstein, and S. Perry, 1988, *Health Psychology*, 7(5), 433–435. Copyright 1988 by Lawrence Erlbaum Associates. Reprinted by permission.
[a]Higher score reflects greater sensitivity.
[b]Higher score reflects greater fear.

the group of repressor children required significantly more hours in intensive care than the sensitizer children for monitoring purposes.

These data, then, generally suggest that sensitizer children (as rated by their mothers) were more active, talkative, and affectively expressive during their play observations, and were more active, inquisitive, and behaviorally distressed during invasive procedures. In addition, they required fewer hours of intensive care. However, these data may simply reflect the mothers' perceptions of their children's behavior. The mothers of sensitizers (who were typically sensitizers themselves) may have been biased, not unlike the repressor mothers of the repressor children. Despite this potential bias, there were several consistencies between the mothers' ratings and those made by observers. For example, the mothers rated the sensitizer children as being more active during invasive procedures, and the trained observers rated the same children as being more active during play observations. Burstein and Meichenbaum (1979) also reported higher activity levels in sensitizer children. This greater activity level may have also contributed to the mothers' viewing the sensitizer children as needing more restraint during invasive procedures, and to the children's being more readily released from intensive care simply because they were less passive and sedentary. In addition, there was consistency between the mothers' rating of children as seeking more information during the invasive procedures and the observers' rating them as more talkative during the play sessions. This greater talkativeness may have also contributed to both the greater protest behavior and the greater information seeking in the sensitizer children, not unlike the seeking of more information by sensitizer children reported by Knight et al. (1979).

It is not clear over the long run whether it is more adaptive to be a sensitizer (resistive, expressive, active, protesting) or a repressor (cooperative, stoic) during invasive procedures. In this particular study, it was difficult to know whether the positive effects of being sensitizers (e.g., being in recovery for fewer hours) were directly or even indirectly related to the qualities of the sensitizer children. Monitoring physiological indicators of stress, such as cortisol, during invasive procedures of this kind might suggest which form of coping is clinically optimal. In addition, the discrepancy between these data and data reported by others on children's protest behavior during invasive procedures (e.g., Siegel, 1977) suggests that the greater protest behavior observed in the sensitizer children in this study may have been related to the mothers' presence during the procedures. The similarities in sensitization in the mothers and children in this case may have been reinforcing during this invasive procedure. Manipulation of the mothers' presence–absence and ratings of the children by independent observers during invasive procedures would be needed to separate these confounding factors.

These data, combined with those in the literature, suggest that there are highly individualized experiences during invasive procedures that may vary as a function of the child's temperament/personality, the mother's temperament/personality, and other contextual features. Responses to invasive procedures are clearly determined by several factors, including personality variables, the type of situation, and the people in the situation. More complex study designs may be required to sort out the individual and combined effects of these variables. Presumably, the optimal intervention strategies for facilitating coping with painful invasive procedures will depend upon knowing individual differences in coping styles.

Acknowledgments

This research was supported by National Institute of Mental Health (NIMH) Research Scientist Award No. MH00331 and NIMH Research Grant No. MH40779.

REFERENCES

Anders, T. F., Sachar, E. J., Kream, J., Roffwarg, H. P., & Hellman, H. (1970). Behavioral state and plasma cortisol response in the human newborn. *Pediatrics, 46,* 532–537.

Burstein, S., & Meichenbaum, D. (1979). The work of worrying in children undergoing surgery. *Journal of Abnormal Child Psychology, 7,* 121–132.

Danford, D., Miske, S., Headley, J., & Nelson, R. M. (1983). Effects of routine care procedures on transcutaneous oxygen tension in neonates: A quantitative approach. *Archives of Disease in Childhood, 58,* 20–23.

Field, T. (1987). Alleviating stress in the NICU neonate. *Journal of the American Osteopathic Association, 87,* 646–650.

Field, T. (1990). Facilitating growth and development in preterm newborns by massage. Paper presented at the annual meeting of the American Psychological Association. Boston, August 1990.

Field, T., Alpert, B., Vega-Lahr, N., Goldstein, S., & Perry, S. (1988). Hospitalization stress in children: Sensitizer and repressor coping styles. *Health Psychology, 7*(5), 433–445.

Field, T., & Goldson, E. (1984). Pacifying effects of nonnutritive sucking on term and preterm neonates during heelstick procedures. *Pediatrics, 74,* 1012–1015.

Field, T., Ignatoff, E., Stringer, S., Brennan, J., Greenberg, R., Widmayer, S., & Anderson, G. (1982). Nonnutritive sucking during tube feedings: Effects on preterm neonates in an ICU. *Pediatrics, 70,* 381–384.

Field, T., Schanberg, S., Scafidi, F., Bauer, C., Vega-Lahr, N., Garcia, R., Nystrom, J., & Kuhn, C. (1986). Tactile/kinesthetic stimulation effects on preterm neonates. *Pediatrics, 77,* 654–658.

Franck, L. (1986). A new method to quantitatively describe pain behavior in infants. *Nursing Research, 35,* 28–31.

Gross, A. M., Stern, R. M., Levin, R. B., Dale, J., & Wojnilower, D. A. (1983). The effect of mother–child separation on the behavior of children experiencing a diagnostic medical procedure. *Journal of Consulting and Clinical Psychology, 51,* 783–785.

Grunau, R. V. E., & Craig, K. D. (1987). Pain expression in neonates: Facial action and cry. *Pain, 28,* 395–410.

Gunnar, M. (1989). Studies of the human infant's adrenocortical response to potentially stressful events. In M. Lewis & J. Worobey (Eds.), *Infant stress and coping* (pp. 3–18). San Francisco: Jossey-Bass.

Gunnar, M., Connors, J., Isensee, J., & Wall, L. (1988). Adrenocortical activity and behavioral distress in human newborns. *Developmental Psychology, 21,* 297–310.

Gunnar, M., Fisch, R., Korsvik, S., & Donhowe, J. (1981). The effect of circumcision on serum cortisol and behavior. *Psychoneuroendocrinology, 6*(3), 269–276.

Gunnar, M., Fisch, R., & Malone, S. (1984). The effects of pacifying stimulus on behavioral and adrenocortical responses to circumcision. *Journal of the American Academy of Child Psychiatry, 23,* 34–38.

Gunnar, M., Malone, S., Vance, G., & Fisch, R.O. (1985). Coping with aversive stimulation in the neonatal period: Quiet sleep and plasma cortisol levels during recovery from circumcision in newborns. *Child Development, 56,* 824–834.

Jay, S. (1982). The effects of gentle human touch on mechanically ventilated very short gestation infants. *Maternal Child Nursing Journal, 11*, 199-256.

Knight, R. B., Atkins, A., Eagle, C., Evans, M., Finkelstein, J. W., Fukushima, D., Katz, J., & Weiner, H., (1979). Psychological stress ego defenses and cortisol production in children hospitalized for elective surgery. *Psychosomatic Medicine, 1*, 40-90.

LaMontagne, L. L. (1984). Children's locus of control beliefs as predictors of preoperative coping. *Nursing Research, 33*, 76-85.

Lewis, M. (in press). Culture and biology: The role of temperament. In R. Barr & P. Zelazo (Eds.), *Challenges to developmental paradigms*. Hillsdale, NJ: Erlbaum.

Lewis, M., Worobey, J. & Thomas, D. (1989). Behavioral features of early reactivity: Antecedents and consequences. In M. Lewis & J. Worobey (Eds.), *Infant stress and coping* (pp. 33-46). San Francisco: Jossey-Bass.

Long, J., Alistair, G., Philip, A. G. S., & Lucey, J. (1980). Excessive handling as a cause of hypoxemia. *Pediatrics, 65*, 203-207.

Lucey, J. (1985). Foreword. In A. W. Gottfried & J. L. Gaiter (Eds.), *Infant stress under intensive care* (p. xvii). Baltimore: University Park Press.

Malone, S., Gunnar, M., & Fisch, R. O. (1985). Adrenocortical and behavioral responses to physical restraint and blood sampling in human neonates. *Developmental Psychology, 18*, 435-446.

Morrow, C., Field, T., Scafidi, F., Roberts, J., Eisen, L., Larson, S., Hogan, A., & Bandstra, E. (1991). *Massage and heelstick effects on transcutaneous oxygen tension in preterm infants. Infant behavior and development*, in press.

Peterson, L., & Toler, S. M. (1986). An information seeking disposition in child surgery patients. *Health Psychology, 5*, 343-358.

Porter, F. L., Porges, S. W., & Marshall, R. E. (1988). Newborn pain cries and vagal tone: Parallel changes in response to circumcision. *Child Development, 59*, 495-505.

Scafidi, F., Field, T., Schanberg, S., Bauer, C., Tucci, K., Roberts, J., Morrow, C., & Kuhn, C. M. (1990). Massage stimulates growth in preterm infants: A replication. *Infant Behavior and Development, 13*, 167-188.

Shaw, E. G., & Routh, D. K. (1982). Effect of mother presence on children's reaction to aversive procedures. *Journal of Pediatric Psychology, 7*, 33-42.

Shipley, R. H., Butt, J. H., & Horwitz, B. (1979). Preparation to re-experience a stressful medical procedure: Effect of amount of stimulus pre-exposure and coping style. *Journal of Consulting and Clinical Psychology, 47*, 485-492.

Siegel, L. (1977, December). *Therapeutic modeling as a procedure to reduce the stress associated with medical and dental treatment*. Paper presented at the meeting of the Association for Advancement of Behavior Therapy, Atlanta.

Siegel, L. (1981, April). *Naturalistic study of coping strategies in children facing medical procedures*. Paper presented at the meeting of the Southeastern Psychological Association, Atlanta.

Stang, H., Gunnar, M., Snellman, L., Condon, L., & Kestenbaum, R. (1988). Local anesthesia for neonatal circumcision: Effects on distress and cortisol response. *Journal of the American Medical Association, 259*, 1507-1511.

Sybulski, S., Goldsmith, W., & Maughn, G. (1975). Cortisol levels of fetal scalp, maternal and umbilical cord plasma. *Obstetrics and Gynecology, 46,* 268–271.

Talbert, L., Pearlman, W., & Potter, H. D. (1977). Maternal and fetal serum levels of total cortisol and cortisone, unbound cortisol and corticosteroid binding globulin in vaginal delivery and cesarean section. *Obstetrics and Gynecology, 129,* 781–786.

Tennes, K., & Carter, D. (1973). Plasma cortisol levels and behavioral states in early infancy. *Psychosomatic Medicine, 35,* 121–128.

CHAPTER 7

Family Factors Predicting Children's Reaction to Anesthesia Induction

BARBARA G. MELAMED
Yeshiva University

Most children experience medical procedures as significant stressors. The main objective of this chapter is to support the point that an understanding of child behavior within the context of the family system is a prerequisite for enhancing coping responses during acute experiences, such as hospitalization and medical procedures. This notion is based on a program of research that attempts to put into perspective the role of the family in dealing with the medical care system. The mother's role appears critical: Her initial role is in detecting a problem and communicating to the physician the symptoms and history of events that may have led to the need for action; then she must prepare the child for the examinations and, if necessary, hospital procedures; moreover, she interacts with the family in terms of her anxiety and knowledge of the child's coping potentials.

The mother functioning as advocate for the child is a role that has evolved over the past decade, from her being a passive recipient of information to her taking an active role in the process of preparing the child and helping in the adjustment to a brief hospitalization or diagnostic procedure. Many review articles (e.g., Melamed & Ridley-Johnson, 1988; Routh & Sanfilippo, 1991) as well as controlled studies (Manne et al., 1990) demonstrate that the anxiety of the child may be directly or indirectly influenced by the mother's attitudes, behaviors, and autonomic arousal when the dyad is interacting with health care providers.

How to minimize the stressfulness of an unpleasant but unavoidable medical experience is a critical and practical question. The research presented herein addresses the extent to which aspects of particular medical procedures, the mother's parenting behavior, and the individual child's characteristics influence the mother–child dyad's interaction, which in turn affects the child's coping. The data obtained in this research fit a model in which family's and the child's resources, including previous experiences and temperament characteristics, are used to predict the optimal intervention for system integrity. The model is a systems modification of a conception I have presented elsewhere (Melamed, 1990), which views the individual's coping resources as part of the schemas involving interaction of the individual with the transactions of the environmental agencies (including physicians and parents) in order to provide balance.

The studies to be described stem from 10 years of research undertaken at the University of Florida, in which the interactions involved in children's elective surgery are postulated to be an analogue for the transactions between individuals under stress in general. These studies are presented within the context of a growing literature on surgery preparation, which suggests that psychological preparation of the child that also involves the parent reduces stress and enhances coping (Peterson, 1989; Pinto & Hollandsworth, 1989; Zastowny, Kirschenbaum, & Meng, 1986). We have begun with the feeling of helplessness often generated in the main caregiver (i.e., the mother) when a child is ill. (Research by Kaplan-Cohn (1983) suggests that there is also a serious need for research regarding interactions within the practitioner–mother–child triad.) The actual prediction of the child's response during the stressful event is improved by looking at the mother's influence on the child's response during events where she is present and either active or passive in the child's behalf. The data to be presented herein have made the case that a situation in which a child must cope alone (e.g., anesthesia induction) can be better understood by studying the mother's anxiety, prediction of the child's cooperation or upset, and behavior in preparing the child. The influence of the child's own predisposing factors, whether they be temperamental characteristics, coping style preferences or previous negative experiences (Onufrak, 1989), must all be considered in deciding whether a given child needs psychological preparation and whether it is better to exclude or include a parent as a support person.

BACKGROUND FOR THE RESEARCH PROGRAM

The widely held belief that all children will benefit from hospital-presented psychological preparation for surgery has not been borne out. Some children have been shown to be sensitized by receiving information if they are too young to understand what they are being told; if they have had a prior unpleasant experience; if they are told too far in advance of the procedure; or if they are told by the wrong individual (Melamed, Dearborn, & Hermecz, 1983; Melamed, Myers, Gee, & Soule, 1976). The prevalence rates of posthospital behavioral problems of a regressive or more than transient nature after some type of formal preparation have varied widely (from 10% to 90%), which suggests a lack of clarity regarding the role of preventive intervention (Vernon, Foley, & Schulman, 1967). This has suggested that the preparation of a particular child must be based on the nature of the procedure, the age and previous experience of the child, and the parental influence in understanding the child's need. In addition, the presentation of information needs to be tailored to the child's coping style, temperament, anxiety level, and level of understanding.

My colleagues and I (Melamed, Siegel, & Ridley-Johnson, 1988) have pointed out the necessity for understanding the event itself and establishing a taxonomy of what is stressful, depending upon the age of the child, the anxiety of the caregiver, and the future implications of the procedure (i.e., whether it is an ongoing or a single procedure and whether it is likely to minimize future discomfort and enhance well-being). This chapter focuses on those procedures in which hospitalization is required for an overnight or short stay to correct a medical problem and involves anesthesia induction, but is not expected to have long-lasting medical sequelae.

In reviewing the literature, we (Melamed et al., 1988) identified the following taxonomy of stressors: (1) separation from parent during some acute procedures; (2) a fear of loss of control; (3) the need to interact with strangers; (4) expectation of some uncomfortable or painful procedures; (5) separation from peer group and siblings in routine daily events; (6) possibility of being alone overnight for the first time; and (7) fear of anesthesia induction or being unconscious. It is clear that although this list contains common features, not every child will respond to them in a typical manner. The data from the literature on hospitalizations indicate that most children do express concerns about pain, needles, and strangers, but that fewer express concern about dying or general anesthesia per se (Bothe & Goldston, 1972; Melamed & Ridley-Johnson, 1988). The nature of the stress will depend upon the child's previous experience with such procedures, the parent's ability to communicate the impending event and what it will involve, the practitioner's care in imparting instructions in advance of each event that are age-appropriate and geared to the child's level of understanding, and the child's ability to carry out the instructions.

There has been a dramatic change in hospital policies over the past decade, allowing many parents to choose to room in with their children and involving them actively in the children's preparation and hospital care. The need for mothers to support and assist directly in reducing anxiety was identified some years ago (Visintainer & Wolfer, 1975), but until recently, few efforts at including them actively were initiated. This reluctance may originally have been based on notions of limiting spread of infection and not pre-empting nursing responsibilities, but may have been perpetuated by a lack of knowledge about many parents' ability to respond favorably when they receive information on how they can assist. Several articles in the literature (Gross, Stern, Levin, Dale, & Wojinilower, 1983; Shaw & Routh, 1982) may have delayed the inclusion of mothers further by showing that children receiving inoculations or routine venipunctures cried or showed more emotional upset in their mothers' presence than in their absence. It needs to be pointed out that the mothers in both of these studies were allowed to be present, but were not given an active role. The children's fretting may have been an attempt to elicit comforting responses from their mothers in a situation in which this was not allowed. Studies reviewed elsewhere (Melamed & Bush, 1986) indicated that when mothers voluntarily accompanied their children to the operating room or chose to stay overnight, children's cooperation increased and anxiety was reduced.

A focus on individual factors that may interact with the type of preparation provided has been stressed by Peterson (1989). Our own studies have assessed (1) children's previous experience in medical situations (Dahlquist et al., 1986; Melamed et al., 1983); (2) their knowledge about what would occur; and (3) the anxiety and coping behaviors of both the children and the parents accompanying them. Recent studies by other research groups (e.g., Field, Alpert, Vega-Lahr, Goldstein, & Perry, 1988; Peterson & Toler, 1986) have also begun to show the importance of measuring and considering the preference style or temperament of the child.

CURRENT RESEARCH

The studies to be described here were all conducted on children between the ages of 4 and 12 who were facing an impending stressful event. This event was typically either an elective outpatient or inpatient procedure, or, in the case of the last study, videotaped exposure to a peer going through elective surgery. The studies were conducted by graduate students at the University of Florida who were fellows in the National Institute of Dental Research behavioral training program.

Study 1

The investigation by Kaplan-Cohn (1983) is unique because it involved the triadic interaction of the mother, child, and pediatrician in the presurgical evaluation of the child's condition at a tertiary care facility. In many of these cases, nothing more than simple elective procedures involving ear, nose, and throat (ENT) operations were involved. The objectives of the study were (1) to develop an observational coding scale of the triadic interaction of the mother, child, and pediatrician in the communication of information; and (2) to assess how the feeling of self-control influenced the mother's ability to communicate information to the examining physician. Another study has shown that high anxiety can lead a mother to communicate anxiety to her child, verbally or nonverbally (Bush, Melamed, Sheras, & Greenbaum, 1986).

In the Kaplan-Cohen (1983) investigation, 50 mothers and their children were observed during the examination period using a procedure designed specifically to evaluate the process of information transmission. An Observational Rating Scale of Information Seeking was devised that achieved high average interrater reliability when coded for mother, doctor, and child behaviors. The results indicated that certain active information-seeking behaviors by the mothers co-occurred. If a mother actively sought information by asking questions, acknowledging, and providing information, the pediatrician was likely to ask fewer questions and to provide more information. Although these correlations were significant, they did not provide evidence of the directionality of this relationship. More sophisticated analysis is now possible using the Child–Adult Medical Personal Interaction Scale (Blount et al., 1989), which is being further refined.

This research also provided information regarding the nature of mothers' anxiety and their perception of control in this situation. Mothers who rated themselves as internally oriented on the Health Locus of Control Scale (Wallston, Wallston, Kaplan, & Maider, 1978) and whose physicians rated them as high on anxiety, tended to show increasing frequencies of cooperative behavior as their levels of anxiety increased. The contrasting finding of a decrease in maternal cooperation was found in mothers who reported having more of an external health locus of control when they showed increasing levels of anxiety. An additional finding emerged from the mothers' reports on the Billings and Moos (1981) Coping Scale about what they were likely to do to support their children. Those mothers who reported an internal health locus of control reported the use of active coping strategies, whereas those mothers who believed that "powerful others" had control over their health tried to cope with the emotional impact of the stressor rather than to take some direct problem-solving action.

Study 2

The next study, by Lumley (1987), was undertaken specifically (1) to establish the baseline of difficulties that might occur in children who were to undergo a mask procedure for anesthesia induction; and (2) to address whether the actual mother–child interaction prior to surgery, the mother's anxiety and expectations for the child's adjustment and the temperament characteristics of the child could account to a greater extent for a child's coping behaviors than could nonpsychosocial factors (e.g., birth order, age, education of the mother, number of siblings with prior surgeries) (Lumley, Abeles, Melamed, Pistone, & Johnson, 1990).

Lumley (1987) first set out to determine which characteristics of anesthesia induction were most stressful for most children. The prevalence of elevated anxiety in children was evaluated during three phases of the procedure: (1) separation from the parent, (2) placement on the operating table and visual contact with instrumentation and personnel, and (3) the actual induction of anesthesia by mask. A second issue was to determine whether a child's reaction to anesthesia induction could be predicted from the child's age and the quantity and quality of his or her previous medical experience. It was expected that younger children would have more negative stress reactions. As for the role of previous experience, it was predicted that a mother's report of a child's previous reaction to medical situations would correlate directly with the child's behavior during this experience.

The subjects in this study were 50 children ages 4 to 10 years, who underwent elective surgery for ENT dysfunctions. None was admitted to the hospital or sedated prior to surgery, but all were administered the anesthetic by mask induction. The mothers accompanied the children to the waiting area, and no one refused to participate in the study.

All the predictor variables were measured during a preoperative visit to the ENT clinic, and all the dependent measures were obtained the next day during the preparation for surgery. The three independent variables of interest were (1) the child's age; (2) the quantity and quality of the previous medical, dental or surgical/hospital experiences as reported by the mother; and (3) the child's behavior with the mother during the final presurgical examination. Other measures obtained included the child's sex, race, birth order, and history of nonsurgical experiences, and the mother's prediction of her child's cooperation during anesthesia induction.

The dependent variables measured during the anesthesia induction were the child's behavioral distress and cooperation throughout the entire period, and heart rate and blood pressure changes at mask presentation. The anesthesiologist's ratings of behavioral distress were used in addition to those of an independent observer. The Operating Room Cooperation Scale was a 7-point Likert scale, which was modified from a scale by Venham, Gaulin-Kremer, Munster, Bengston, and Cohan (1980). The Observer Rating Scale of Anxiety was modified from Melamed et al. (1983) so that the entire phase 1 period, from separation from the mother to placement upon the table, was rated on a 1-4 scale of intensity, defined as magnitude of the behavior and the proportion of the phase duration that the behavior occurred. A child's distress score for each phase was the sum of the intensity ratings of all present behaviors. Physiological measures of heart rate and blood pressure were obtained after separation, during phase 2 (placement upon the operating table and mask in view) and phase 3 (actual application of mask until first signs of anesthesia effects). These measures were taken every 3 seconds and were recorded for every 10 seconds of the duration of the phase. Mean heart rate during phase 2 was subtracted from the mean heart rate during phase 3, in order to provide difference scores during phase 3. Similar difference scores were calculated for systolic and diastolic blood pressure.

Age was trichotomized as less than 6 years; 6 years to 7 years, 11 months; and 8 years or above. Age differences were revealed in behavioral distress and cooperation during phases 1 and 2, but not during phase 3, with the youngest group being more distressed and less cooperative than the middle age group, but no different from the oldest age group. Diastolic blood pressure and heart rate were significantly elevated in younger children during phase 3 when compared with the oldest children.

The relationship between previous experience and current reaction was analyzed with 24 children who had had previous experience and 26 who had not. There were 34 males, and 40 of the children were white and 10 black. The presence or absence of presurgical experience was not correlated with any of the dependent variables. However, the actual number of prior surgeries was related positively to distress during phases 2 and 3, and negatively to cooperation during phases 1 and 2. Regarding mothers' reports about the quality of their children's previous experience to dental or general medical procedures, results indicated that more negative past surgery experience was related to more distress during phase 2, whereas negative past dental experience was related to less cooperation during all three phases. Diastolic blood pressure was elevated during phase 3 in children with more previous negative dental experience. Heart rate changes were unrelated to quality of prior experience. When Dahlquist et al.'s (1986) classification was used, those children who had had negative past medical experience were more distressed during the first two phases and less cooperative during all phases than were the children who had had neutral or positive experiences. Diastolic blood pressure showed greater increases for the children who had had negative past experience. Heart rate differences were not significant.

Stepwise regressions were completed on data averaged across all three phases for behavioral and physiological outcome measures, using the mean of each as the dependent variable in separate regression analyses. The prediction of children's behavioral distress to anesthesia induction was predicted by being young, having had negative overall medical experience, having had a prior surgery, and showing low presurgical distress. The overall quality of previous experience was the single variable accounting for the greatest proportion of the variance. Twenty-four percent of the variance in behavioral distress and 26% of the variance in cooperation were accounted for by these models. Elevated heart rate changes were predicted by being young and having had a previous surgery, which accounted for 16% of the variance in heart rate change during phase 3.

Lumley's (1987) data showed that only 16% of the children were behaviorally distressed during separation, but that over twice as many, or 36%, were rated as distressed at mask presentation. Also the high relationship between behavioral distress and cooperation indicated that the concept of cooperation and its inverse, anxiety, are measures of the same construct.

This study did define the parameters of the event and the risk factors for children that put them under stress during the induction of anesthesia. Specifically, children become more distressed and uncooperative as anesthesia induction proceeds from the initial separation from the parent, through the period of waiting on the operating table, to the presentation of the mask. Most children are physiologically activated, with an average of 50% of all children showing a heart rate increase of at least five beats per minute prior to the mask induction.

Regarding previous experience, the stepwise regression did show that even when age and quality of previous experience were partialed out, the children who had undergone more frequent surgeries reacted with more distress and less cooperation to the current induction. Therefore, future research should be directed at eliciting whatever memory schemas have been formed during such children's previous medical experiences. Imagery-based therapies in addition to film modeling may be useful in altering these perceptions. Classical conditioning is likely to be responsible for the conditioned fear response. Perhaps through changing prior information or imparting a sense of controllability these children can be helped to cope better with the repeated surgical experiences.

The seemingly paradoxical finding that higher levels of distress behavior during the mother–child interaction at the presurgical examination on the day prior to the operation were related to less behavioral distress during induction can be understood through previous findings. Janis (1958) proposed many years ago that the "work of worrying" is critical to prepare children emotionally for an impending stressor. Knight et al. (1979) also found an inverse relationship between physiological arousal 2 weeks prior to surgery and children's reaction to being hospitalized. The findings of Burstein and Meichenbaum (1979)—namely, that those children who were high on denial and anxiety did not play with hospital related toys to help them prepare—further support this notion. A colleague and I (Melamed & Siegel, 1975) demonstrated an increase in autonomic arousal in children at a preoperative preparation session that included a peer modeling film; however, immediately after surgery these children showed lower anxiety and physiological distress than those children who were shown a neutral film unrelated to the upcoming experience. Therefore, the involvement of parents in instigating readiness responses must be more closely examined. In fact, other investigators (e.g., Zastowny et al., 1986) showed a clear benefit of including parents in the preoperative preparation process and teaching them to coach their children in relaxation and other active coping skills prior to and during stressful procedures.

Study 3

In order to be more direct in the assessment of the mother–child interaction, the next study in our research program (Pistone, 1989) focused on evaluating the use of maternal coping strategies during venipuncture and the surgeon's examination immediately following, to understand the influence of the mother's interaction with the child on the child's distress. The Dyadic Prestressor Interaction Scale (DPIS; Bush et al., 1986), a valid and sensitive measure developed especially for observing mother–child dyads in the waiting room period, was used to define the independent maternal behaviors. The Observation Scale of Behavioral Distress (OSBD; Jay, Ozolins, Elliott, & Caldwell, 1983), which is an independently validated scale of children's distress and discomfort, was used during the venipuncture. This medical procedure is very similar to the ones for which the OSBD was developed and used (Jacobsen et al., 1990).

The predictions made here were based upon the results of two previous studies on a wide range of elective surgeries (Bush et al., 1986; Greenbaum, Melamed, Cook, Abeles, & Bush, 1988). These studies showed that mothers' use of active, problem-focused coping strategies was associated with less distress behavior and more positive coping in children than mothers' use of emotion-focused behaviors of agitation and ignoring. Therefore, Pistone (1989) predicted that mothers' use of emotion-focused behaviors (DPIS codes of Agitation, Ignoring, Reassurance, and Restraint) would be associated with higher distress behaviors in their children during the venipuncture and with greater distress and attachment in the subsequent examination. Mothers who reported higher state anxiety on the State–Trait Anxiety Inventory (Spielberger, Gorusch, & Lushene, 1970) were also predicted to be more likely to use these less effective, emotion-focused coping strategies as they awaited the final presurgical examination with their children. Regarding the role of previous experience, it was also expected (on the basis of Lumley's [1987] study and the research of others) that those children with prior negative experiences would show greater distress during the venipuncture and report greater distress than children with either no prior experience or positive or neutral previous experiences. Some developmental age differences were also expected, based on prior research with younger children between 4 and 6 years of age; it was predicted that younger children's behaviors would show more association with the mothers' behaviors than those of older children.

Forty-six mother–child dyads, in which the children were 4- to 10-year-old pediatric outpatients arriving for venipuncture immediately prior to a preoperative exam for elective surgery in the ENT clinic, were selected. Unfortunately, because of hospital construction, Pistone was only able to follow a reduced sample of 28 dyads during the waiting period observation subsequent to the venipuncture. All subjects were videotaped, and acceptable observer reliability was established for the DPIS and OSBD, which were used to evaluate the hypotheses. The sample contained mostly nonprofessional, white, intact families. The large majority of children had had previous experience with venipunctures, and at least half had had previous surgery or medical experience in the hospital.

The results of this study indicated that mothers who were anxious had children who were anxious in response to a medical procedure. There was support for the hypothesis that mothers who used active, problem-focused behaviors (information provision, distraction), as opposed to reactive, emotion-focused behaviors, had children who were less distressed and displayed positive coping behaviors. Children demonstrated behavior and self-reported distress differences according to age as expected, with the younger children expressing more fear. However, the use of restraint by the mothers with younger children was the main difference in maternal behavior. Those children who had had negative past experience with venipunctures reported more fear and showed greater distress during the venipuncture. In this situation, mothers were (and generally are) not given an active role other than to hold the very youngest children on their laps. Expectations of their influence were examined. Canonical correlations showed strong relationships between maternal and child behavior, with the strongest relationship being found between greater maternal use of restraint and agitation and children's increased distress and decreased exploratory behaviors during the venipuncture.

Stepwise multiple-regression analyses to delineate the specific maternal coping behaviors that predicted child behavior immediately following the venipuncture, while the dyad awaited the surgeon's examination, found some data supportive of the hypothesis that mothers' prediction of distress may lead to anticipatory restraining and agitated behaviors. However, given the small sample size ($n = 28$ dyads), the generalizability of these findings awaits cross-validation. The results indicated that the mothers who ignored their children had children who showed less attachment behavior. However, mothers who used ignoring and distraction had children who demonstrated low child distress as measured by the DPIS. The most powerful predictors of children's exploration of the environment were less maternal ignoring and distraction and greater maternal provision of information. It was also found that mothers who were agitated, had children who showed low social-affiliative behaviors, whereas distraction and ignoring had an opposite effect.

Maternal self-reported trait anxiety during the waiting period related positively to her exhibiting agitation. During the venipuncture procedure, maternal state anxiety was significantly associated with maternal use of distraction and agitation. Maternal state anxiety was also predictive of child distress during the venipuncture on both the DPIS and the OSBD, even when socioeconomic status was controlled for. Child behavioral distress during the venipuncture was positively related to maternal state anxiety after the venipuncture and to maternal trait anxiety. Child-reported fear on both the Hospital Fears (Melamed & Lumley, 1988) and the Fear Faces (Katz, Kellerman, & Siegel, 1982) after the venipuncture showed that behavioral distress as measured by the OSBD was related to childhood anxiety. The influence of previous experience also emerged during the venipuncture: Children who were rated by their mothers as having had past negative experience reported more fear on all the self-report measures and showed greater behavioral distress than those who had had less negative experiences. These children were rated by the phlebotomists as significantly more fearful and less cooperative.

Research reported elsewhere (Lumley et al., 1990) demonstrated a relationship between a mother's perception of her child's temperament and the child's reaction to anesthesia induction. In summary, it was found that mothers who saw their children as more "difficult" or less likely to "approach" in a novel situation were less distressed when they had used distraction rather than information provision in the waiting room period preceding the surgeon's examination. Those mothers who had children who were "easy" or tended to approach novel situations did better if they used ignoring. Studying the cues between individual dyads of mother and children would enhance our knowledge regarding the development of these patterns of communication and might limit the transmission of maladaptive learning experiences.

Study 4

The final study (Onufrak & Melamed, 1991) had as its major goals (1) to investigate the interactive influence of coping style and quality of previous medical experience in determining children's responses to information provision; and (2) to evaluate the utility of the Child Medical

Coping Inventory (CMCI), a new measure designed to assess information-seeking preferences of children. The dependent variables in this research were the children's pre–post anxiety level and the correctness of information obtained on their coping style preferences. The subjects were 144 children ages 7 years, 11 months to 13 years, 1 month, who were attending third- to sixth-grade classes. This population was selected to be similar in age to the child model in the hospitalization film *Ethan Has An Operation*, first used by Melamed and Siegel (1975), as well as to represent a broad range of socioeconomic and racial distribution. Moreover, none of them were expecting to have an operation in the immediate future. In this study, parental consent and a history of each child's previous dental and medical experiences were obtained.

In the interest of obtaining data on coping style preferences in children that could be easily employed by the pediatric psychologist, the CMCI was designed to measure children's self-reported interest in receiving information in advance of a stressful experience such as hospitalization. It consisted of 14 statements, which the child was asked to rate as "true about me" or "not true about me." The statements indicated information-seeking or avoidant attitudes about medical situations and typical behavior in such situations. The parent-rated History of Coping Questionnaire was scored to obtain two items representing "methods of coping" (the child's typical methods of coping with a medical procedure, ranging from concentration to distraction), and four items representing the "degree of distress" (the child's typical levels of upset during medical situations). Parents also completed ratings of their children's reactions in previous medical situations. There was little relationship between the children's reports of information-seeking preferences and the parents' predictions.

In a second part of the Onufrak and Melamed (1991) study, 50 children who had previous experience in a hospital and 50 who did not were surveyed. The CMCI was administered in the classroom on two occasions 2 weeks apart. On the first occasion, the children were administered the CMCI in a group session. Two weeks later, they again completed the CMCI, as well as the Hospital Information Test and Hospital Fears Rating Scale, before viewing the hospitalization film. Immediately after this, the Hospital Fears Rating Scale and the Ethan Information Test (a 16-item multiple-choice questionnaire designed to assess retention of material from the film) were administered. The most interesting result was that those children who reported prior negative hospital experience, and who also reported that they preferred to avoid getting information, were the most anxious. They retained the least correct information following the group viewing of the film *Ethan Has an Operation*. However, this finding held only for the child-rated CMCI and not the parent-rated History of Coping Questionnaire.

DISCUSSION

These studies clearly point out the need for more sophisticated research on the causes of anxiety in, and interventions to be used in preventing anxiety and enhancing coping in, children who require short-term elective surgery. These studies do show that it is possible, within the context of the natural environment, to ask questions that have both theoretical and practical implications. The advantage of using a theoretical model to generate possible pathways of relationships between children's characteristics and parents' and physicians' support–nonsupport behaviors has been demonstrated.

The strongest conclusion that can be drawn is that the reciprocal interactions between the mother and child are critical in establishing the child's abilities to cope effectively with the stressor. The conclusions drawn from these studies are generally supportive of both the "emotional contagion" hypothesis (Escalona, 1953)—namely, that maternal anxiety is communicated both verbally and nonverbally to the child—and the "crisis-parenting" hypothesis (Melamed & Bush, 1986). The latter specifically emphasizes that some parents may display disorganized behavior at times of great stress, which leads their children to develop anxiety rather than adequate coping skills (Kaplan, Smith, Grobstein, & Fischman, 1973). Thus, regarding practical suggestions for training of parents, one might attempt to encourage mothers to use active coping methods (e.g., distracting their children, or providing information) in helping to promote more adaptive child behaviors. Emotion-focused coping (e.g., ignoring the children, providing reassurance or restraint, or exhibiting agitation) should be discouraged.

The studies described herein have limitations in terms of the sizes of the samples and the representation of the subject populations. Subjects came largely from intact families and were primarily white, and the sample sizes in some comparisons were small. More research on physician interactions, such as those studied by Kaplan-Cohn (1983), would add to our understanding of how their role might preclude the development of transmission of anxiety. Already, Blount et al. (1989) have demonstrated that the use of audiotape recording and lag analyses can be helpful in determining conditional probabilities in the interactions between adults and children. They have demonstrated that a child's behavior depends upon the procedure and the present adult's responses immediately preceding and following the procedure. The tools for more productive research methodology exist, including path analyses, which could test models and illuminate the direction of influences.

The continued efforts of clinical researchers in this area will make it much more likely that individual preventive packages will be developed for practitioners to provide better health care to family units. These will be more successful and cost-effective if they are applied only to those who are at risk if no preventive package is provided. Then we can encourage health care policy decisions that are not only empirically based, but cost-effective as well.

Acknowledgments

The ideas and efforts of my research fellows and the colleagues involved in the National Institute of Dental Research Training Grant No. 5T32DE07133 made this chapter possible. Specifically included herein is the research work of Mark Lumley, PhD, Wayne State University; Linda Abeles, PhD, Gainesville, Florida; Lisa Pistone, PhD, West Virginia University Health Science Center; Elizabeth Onufrak, MS, University of Florida; and Lauren Kaplan-Cohn, PhD, Miami, Florida. The collaborative efforts of the pediatric surgery staff of Shand's Teaching Hospital, including George Singleton, MD, Gerald Merwin, MD, Shirley Graves, MD, Richard Kaplan, MD, and Nicholas Cassissi, MD, and the assistance of Angel Seibring and Paul Greenbaum, Ph.D. are greatly appreciated.

REFERENCES

Billings, A. G. & Moos, R. H. (1981). The role of coping responses and social resources in alternating the stress of life events. *Journal of Behavioral Medicine, 4,* 139-157.

Blount, R. L., Corbin, S. M., Sturges, J. W., Wolfe, V. V., Prater, J. M., & James, L. D. (1989). The relationship between adults' behavior and child coping and distress during BMA/LP procedures: A sequential analysis. *Behavior Therapy, 20,* 585-601.

Bothe, A., & Goldston, R. (1972). The child's loss of consciousness: A psychiatric view of pediatric anesthesia. *Pediatrics, 50,* 252-263.

Burstein, S., & Meichenbaum, D. (1979). The work of worrying in children undergoing surgery. *Journal of Abnormal Child Psychology, 7,* 121-132.

Bush, J. P., Melamed, B. G., Sheras, P. L., & Greenbaum, P. E. (1986). Mother-child patterns of coping with anticipatory medical stress. *Health Psychology, 5,* 137-157.

Dahlquist, L. M., Gil, K. M., Armstrong, F. D., DeLawyer, D. D., Greene, P., & Wuori, D. (1986). Preparing children for medical examinations: The importance of previous medical experience. *Health Psychology, 5,* 249-259.

Escalona, S. (1953). Emotional development in the first year of life. In M. J. Senn (Ed.), *Problems of infancy and childhood.* New York: Foundation Press.

Field, T., Alpert, B., Vega-Lahr, N., Goldstein, S., & Perry, S. (1988) Hospitalization stress in children: Sensitizer and repressor coping styles. *Health Psychology, 7,* 433-445.

Greenbaum, P. E., Melamed, B. G., Cook, E. W. III, Abeles, L. A., & Bush, J. P. (1988). Sequential analysis in predicting parenting patterns which put children at risk during routine medical procedures. *Child and Family Behavior Therapy, 10*, 9–18.

Gross, A. M., Stern, R. M., Levin, R. B., Dale, J., & Wojinilower, D.A. (1983). The effects of mother-child separation on the behavior of children experiencing a diagnostic medical procedure. *Journal of Consulting and Clinical Psychology, 51*, 783–785.

Jacobsen, P. B., Manne, S. L., Gorfinkle, K., Schorr, O., Rapkin, B., & Redd, W. H. (1990). Analysis of child and parent behavior during painful medical procedures. *Health Psychology, 9*, 559–578.

Janis, I. L. (1958). *Psychological stress.* New York: Wiley.

Jay, S. M., Ozolins, M., Elliot, C. H., & Caldwell, S. (1983). Assessment of children's distress during painful medical procedures. *Health Psychology, 2*, 133–147.

Kaplan, D. M., Smith, A., Grobstein, R., & Fischman, S. E. (1973). Family mediation of stress. *Social Work, 18*, 60–69.

Kaplan-Cohn, L. R. (1983). *The influence of a mother's health locus of control and anxiety on information-seeking during her child's medical examination.* Unpublished master's thesis, University of Florida.

Katz, E. R., Kellerman, J., & Siegel, S. E. (1982). *Self-report and observational measurement of acute pain, fear, and behavioral distress in children with leukemia.* Paper presented at the annual meeting of the Society of Behavioral Medicine, Chicago.

Knight, R. B., Atkins, A., Eagle, C. J., Evans, N., Finkelstein, J. W., Fukushima, D., Katz, J., & Werner, H. (1979). Psychological stress, ego defenses, and control production in children hospitalized for elective surgery. *Psychosomatic Medicine, 41*, 40–49.

Lumley, M. (1987). *Age, previous experience, and presurgical behavior as predictors of a child's reaction to anesthesia induction.* Unpublished master's thesis, University of Florida.

Lumley, M., Abeles, L., Melamed, B., Pistone, L., & Johnson, J.H. (1990). Coping outcomes in children undergoing stressful medical procedures: The role of child-environment variables. *Behavioral Assessment, 12*, 223–238.

Manne, S. L., Redd, W. H., Jacobsen, P. B., Garfinkle, K., Schorr, O., & Rapkin, B. (1990). Behavioral intervention to reduce child and parent distress during venipuncture. *Journal of Consulting and Clinical Psychology, 58*, 565–572.

Melamed, B. G. (1990). Stress and coping in pediatric psychology. In J. Johnson & S. Johnson (Eds.), *Advances in child health psychology.* Gainesville: University of Florida Press.

Melamed, B. G., & Bush, J. (1986). Maternal-child influences during medical procedures. In S. Auerbach & S. Stolberg (Eds.), *Crisis intervention with children and families.* Washington, DC: Hemisphere.

Melamed, B. G., Dearborn, M., & Hermecz, D. A. (1983). Necessary considerations for surgery preparation: Age and previous experience. *Psychosomatic Medicine, 45,* 517–525.

Melamed, B. G., Lumley, M. A. (1988). Hospital Fears Rating Scale. In A. Hersen and A. S. Bellack (Eds.), *Dictionary of behavioral assessment techniques.* New York: Plenum.

Melamed, B. G., Myers, R., Gee, C., & Soule, L. (1976). The influence of time and type of preparation on children's adjustment to hospitalization. *Journal of Pediatric Psychology, 1,* 31–37.

Melamed, B. G., & Ridley-Johnson, R. (1988). Psychological preparation of families for hospitalization. *Journal of Developmental and Behavioral Pediatrics, 9,* 96–101.

Melamed, B. G., & Siegel, L. J. (1975). Reduction of anxiety in children facing hospitalization and surgery by use of filmed modeling. *Journal of Consulting and Clinical Psychology, 43,* 511–521.

Melamed, B. G., Siegel, L. J., & Ridley-Johnson, R. (1988). Coping with stress. In T. M. Fields, P. M. McCabe, & N. Schneiderman (Eds.), *Stress and coping* (Vol. 2). Hillsdale, NJ: Erlbaum.

Onufrak, E. J. (1989). *Effect of coping style and quality of previous medical experience on children's response to hospital information.* Unpublished master's thesis, University of Florida

Onufrak, E. J., & Melamed, B. G. (1991, April). *Effects of coping style and quality of previous medical experience on children's response to hospital information.* Paper presented at the Florida Conference on Child Health Psychology, Gainesville.

Peterson, L. (1989). Coping by children undergoing stressful medical procedures: Some conceptual methodological and therapeutic issues. *Journal of Consulting and Clinical Psychology, 57,* 380–387.

Peterson, L., & Toler, S. (1986). An information seeking disposition in child surgery patients. *Health Psychology, 5,* 343–358.

Pinto, R. P., & Hollandworth, J. G. (1989). Using videotape modeling to prepare children psychologically for surgery. Influence of parents and costs versus benefits of providing preparation services. *Health Psychology, 8,* 79–95.

Pistone, L. (1989). *Child response to venipuncture: The influence of mother–child interactions, age, and prior experience on distress.* Unpublished doctoral dissertation, University of Florida.

Routh, D. K., & Sanfilippo, M. D. (1991). Helping children cope with painful medical procedures. In J. P. Bush & S. W. Harkins (Eds.), *Children in pain: Clinical and research issues from a developmental perspective.* New York: Springer-Verlag.

Shaw, E. G., & Routh, D. K. (1982). Effects of mother's presence on children's reactions to aversive procedures. *Journal of Pediatric Psychology, 7,* 33–42.

Spielberger, C. D., Gorusch, R. L., & Lushene, R. (1970). *State-trait anxiety inventory.* Palo Alto, CA: Consulting Psychologists Press.

Venham, L. L., Gaulin-Kremer, E., Munster, E., Bengston, D., & Cohan, J. (1980).

Interval rating scales for children's dental anxiety and uncooperative behavior. *Pediatric Dentistry*, 2, 195-202.

Vernon, D. T., Foley, J., & Schulman, J. L. (1967). Effects of mother-child separation and birth order on young children's responses to two potentially stressful experiences. *Journal of Personality and Social Psychology*, 5, 162-174.

Visintainer, M., & Wolfer, J. (1975). Psychological preparation for surgical pediatric patients: The effect on children's and parents' stress responses and adjustment. *Pediatrics*, 56, 187-202.

Wallston, B. S., Wallston, K. A., Kaplan, G. D., & Maider, S. A. (1976). Development and validation of the Health Locus of Control Scale. *Journal of Consulting & Clinical Psychology*, 44, 580-585.

Zastowny, T., Kirschenbaum D., & Meng, A. (1986). Coping skills training for children. Effects on distress before, during and after hospitalization. *Health Psychology*, 5, 231-247.

CHAPTER 8

Patterns of Children's Coping with Short-Term Medical and Dental Stressors: Nature, Implications, and Future Directions

SUZANNE M. MILLER, HOWARD D. SHERMAN, CHRISTOPHER COMBS, and LINDA KRUUS
Temple University

The romantic view of childhood as a time of carefree larking contrasts with the growing recognition that children's lives are far from stress-free idylls. Although parents can sometimes buffer their offspring, particularly in middle-class settings, some stressors are an inevitable part of the growth process. As the course of development unfolds, youngsters must somehow learn to deal with stressors as diverse as protecting themselves from older siblings or neighborhood bullies, adjusting to the birth of younger siblings, and facing up to their physical and intellectual limitations relative to other children. In some unfortunate cases, more aversive stressors are superimposed against this backdrop, including serious or prolonged illness or injury, parental abuse or neglect, loss of loved ones, and other forms of unexpected trauma.

Traditionally, the phenomenon of children's coping with threat has been relatively ignored. Recently, this situation has begun to change, consistent with a greater attention to issues in developmental psychopathology generally (Lewis & Miller, 1990). In particular, researchers have become interested in exploring and delineating children's natural coping efforts in the face of medical and dental stressors. Medical and dental stressors—especially those of an acute nature—not only require a good deal of adjustment on the part of children, but offer an ideal research arena to study the development of coping. The stressor is relatively objective and standardized, and provides an opportunity to study self-regulatory processes at all key phases: anticipatory, impact, and postimpact.

In this chapter, we explore what is known about the process of coping in children undergoing short-term, aversive medical or dental procedures. The studies reviewed here are not an exhaustive sampling, but they do represent the major published findings in this area. They have been selected on the basis of two criteria. First, they bear on the nature and implications of children's spontaneous patterns when coping with medical and dental stress situations. Second, they focus on children primarily in the 7- to 12-year age range—referred to as "middle childhood"—which is considered to be a relatively distinct period in cognitive development (Flavell, 1977). In comparison with younger children, those in middle childhood demonstrate thinking that is more highly organized, less stimulus-bound, and less stereotypic. On the other hand, in comparison with older children, they show less cognitive flexibility and less ability to think abstractly, beyond their immediate situation and experience.

The chapter is organized as follows: We first examine how coping has been operationalized in the literature, focusing on both more "micro" and more "macro" approaches to children's self-regulatory patterns under threat. We then go on to review issues in the assessment of children's coping, in terms of the methods used (self-report vs. observational) and times of assessment (before, during, and after the stressor). Following this, we explore the impact of coping processes for adaptation and adjustment in the face of identified threat. We then highlight data from a recent study on children's coping with the stress of dental treatment, which help to further delineate the interrelations among dispositional coping style, ongoing coping strategy, and subsequent adaptation. Finally, we present some suggestions and guidelines for future research.

CATEGORIZATION OF COPING CONSTRUCTS

Like adults' coping, children's self-regulatory patterns can be categorized in a number of ways. To date, the literature on children's coping reflects two main divergencies in approach. Some researchers have attempted to categorize subjects' coping efforts in terms of relatively specific, more "micro"-level coping methods, such as distraction, information seeking, and relaxation. Here, coping is thought to involve multiple, discrete techniques. Other researchers have used a more "macro"-level approach, in which coping is conceptualized according to a single, global dimension. Examples include degree of defensiveness, approach–avoidance, or willingness to cognitively process threat-relevant stimuli. Although the assessment of global coping dimensions often draws on the observations or reports of specific coping activities, the data are only used to create the larger categories. Thus, no separate, fine-grained assessment of specific coping methods is undertaken. We review each of these approaches in turn.

Specific Coping Modes

Table 8.1 provides an overview of the studies focusing on specific coping modes. It describes the samples under study, the methods used to assess coping, the times of assessment, and the coping categories used. As can be seen, three of the studies assessed healthy children and obtained hypothetical or recalled accounts of their strategies for coping with medical/dental threats (Band & Weisz, 1988; Brown, O'Keeffe, Sanders, & Baker, 1986; Peterson, Harbeck, Chaney, Farmer, & Thomas, 1990). Another four studies assessed the process of coping in the face of an actual medical or dental stressor (Curry & Russ, 1985; Prins, 1985; Robins, 1987; Savedra & Tesler, 1981). The most striking features of this research are the diversity of strategies investigated and the relatively modest degree of consistency from study to study. No single coping method was targeted in all of the available studies.

The most widely assessed methods were distraction, mentioned in some form in five studies (Band & Weisz, 1988; Brown et al., 1986; Curry & Russ, 1985; Peterson et al., 1990; Prins, 1985); reinterpretation, mentioned in five studies (Band & Weisz, 1988; Brown et al., 1986; Curry & Russ, 1985; Peterson et al., 1990; Prins, 1985); seeking support for emotional or instrumental reasons, mentioned in four studies (Band & Weisz, 1988; Curry & Russ, 1985; Robins, 1987; Savedra & Tesler, 1981); and seeking information, mentioned in four studies (Curry & Russ, 1985; Peterson et al., 1990; Prins, 1985; Savedra & Tesler, 1981). One (potentially) "inappropriate" behavior, escape or avoidance, was also listed in four studies (Band & Weisz, 1988; Brown et al., 1986; Peterson et al., 1990, Savedra & Tesler, 1981). In one case, however, the reference was to having thoughts or wishes to avoid the situation (Brown et al., 1986), whereas in the others the reference was to actual avoidance or escape behaviors.

The remaining coping modes were each explored in only a limited number of studies. These included relaxation, mentioned in three studies (Brown et al., 1986; Peterson et al., 1990; Prins, 1985), and aggression, mentioned in three studies (Band & Weisz, 1988; Peterson et al., 1990; Savedra & Tesler, 1981). A coping method examined in only two of the studies was thought stopping (Brown et al., 1986; Prins, 1985). Sensory focus (i.e., thinking about or focusing upon the sensations one is expe-

Table 8.1. Studies Exploring Specific Coping Modes

Study	Sample	Assessment times and methods	Assessment categories
		Hypothetical/recalled medical or dental stressors	
Band & Weisz (1988)	n = 73 6 yrs.: n = 24 (12 F, 12 M) 9 yrs.: n = 25 (16 F, 9 M) 12 yrs.: n = 24 (15 F, 9 M) Race, Socioeconomic status (SES) not reported	Anticipatory/Impact: Children were interviewed about their coping responses, coping goals, and self-rated efficacy for six situations, including going to the doctor to get a shot.	Children's specific responses were content-analyzed and then placed into one of three categories: 1. Primary control—influencing the environment by bringing objective conditions into line with one's wishes. Comprises the specific categories of direct problem solving (e.g., acting to improve the situation); problem-focused crying (e.g., crying to get help); problem-focused aggression (e.g., attacking those causing the problem); and problem-focused avoidance (e.g., avoiding the situation). 2. Secondary control—accommodating to external conditions by modifying one's own subjective psychological state. Comprises the specific responses of social/spiritual support (e.g., seeking social support); emotion-focused crying (e.g., crying to release emotion); emotion-focused aggression (e.g., kicking a door); cognitive avoidance (e.g., distraction); and pure cognition (e.g., reframing, daydreaming). 3. Relinquished control—no apparent goal-directed behavior, and no apparent effort to augment rewards or decrease punishments (i.e., a failure to cope). Specific response: doing nothing (making no effort to deal with the stressful situation).

Brown, O'Keeffe, Sanders, & Baker (1986)	$n = 487$ Age levels: 8–9; 10–11; 12–13; 14–15; 16–18 M = 43%; F = 52% gender unreported = 5% Race, SES not reported	*Anticipatory/Impact:* Children gave written answers to open-ended questions about thoughts just before and during an imagined dental injection and two nonmedical stressors. Thoughts about anticipatory and impact phases were merged in data analysis.	Children's specific responses were content-analyzed and then categorized into one primary category, based on the proportion of coping to catastrophizing responses: 1. *Coping*—positive self-talk; attention diversion; relaxation/deep breathing; thought stopping. 2. *Catastrophizing*—focusing on negative affect/pain, escape/avoidance, fear of unlikely consequences, fear of inappropriate behavior by self or dentist.
Peterson, Harbeck, Chaney, Farmer, & Thomas (1990)	$n = 60$ Ages 4.17–9.58 ($\bar{X} = 5.89$) M = 32; F= 28 Race, SES not reported	*Anticipatory:* Children were interviewed about whether (1) they would ask questions or remain quiet before an injection; and (2) whether they would advise a friend to ask questions, etc., before a blood test. *Impact:* Children participated in two medical role-play situations (involving getting an injection and having blood drawn) and were *interviewed* on what they (1) were doing or thinking when they received an injection; (2) would advise a friend to do when receiving a blood test.	Children were dichotomized into *information-seeking* versus *information-avoiding*, based on their answers to each separate anticipatory assessment question. Children's specific responses were content-analyzed and then categorized as follows: 1. *Reactive coping (catastrophizing)/Stimulus blocking (avoidance)*—examples: complaining, whining, worrying. 2. *Reactive coping (catastrophizing)/Stimulus approach (approach)*—examples: aggression, active non-cooperation. 3. *Proactive coping (planning)/Stimulus blocking (avoidance)*—examples: distraction, relaxation. 4. *Proactive coping (planning)/Stimulus approach (approach)*—examples: information seeking, thinking about sensations. 5. *Midpoints of both dimensions*—example: passive or neutral behavior. (cont.)

Table 8.1. (*cont.*)

Study	Sample	Assessment times and methods	Assessment categories
		In vivo dental stressor	
Curry & Russ (1985)	$n = 30$ Ages 8–10 ($\bar{X} = 9.5$) M = 18; F = 12 White = 16; Non-white = 14 SES: lower class, lower middle class	*Impact*: Children were observed during dental restoration by independent observer.	Children's behaviors were rated in terms of three specific modes and then summed to yield a *behavioral coping* category. This included the following: 1. *Information seeking*—question asking; vigilant behavior (e.g, looking, feeling, etc.). 2. *Support seeking*—verbal requests; physical contact with dentist or assistant. 3. *Direct efforts to maintain control*—active participation in treatment process; trying to set limits.
		Postimpact: Children were interviewed immediately after treatment and asked about (1) thoughts, (2) self-statements, (3) wishes, during (1) exploratory exam; (2) injection; (3) placement of rubber dam; (4) cavity preparation.	Children's specific responses were content-analyzed and summed to yield a *cognitive coping* category. This included the following: 1. *Reality-oriented working through*—accurate thoughts about procedure; planning for coping. 2. *Positive cognitive restructuring*—thinking about positive outcomes of dental experience. 3. *Defensive reappraisal*—superstitious thoughts; attempts to deny, directly or through fantasy transformation, the aversive aspects of situation. 4. *Emotion-regulating cognitions*—self-statements or thoughts in effort to alleviate fear, discomfort (e.g, "Don't worry"). 5. *Behavior-regulating cognitions*—self-statements or thoughts in effort to regulate behavior (e.g, "Be still"). 6. *Diversionary thinking*—distraction.

Prins (1985)

n = 40
Ages: 8–12 ($\bar{x}$ = 10.2)
M = 16; F = 24
Race, SES nc reported

Anticipatory: Children were interviewed prior to dental restoration about how they cope with dental treatment.

Children's specific responses were content-analyzed and grouped into these categories:

1. *Self-speech* (What do you think/say to self?): positive, neutral, and negative.
2. *Self-regulation* (Do you have a trick/strategy to be less fearful?; If no, can you think of a trick/strategy you could use?):
   a. *Behavioral self-regulation*:
      (1) Regulating breathing, muscle tension, other motoric responses.
      (2) Directing attention away from threatening stimuli—focusing on neutral stimuli, or closing eyes.
      (3) Seeking information (asking questions).
      (4) Influencing dentist's behavior (trying to get dentist to stop).
   b. *Cognitive self-regulation*:
      (1) Thinking about something funny or pleasant.
      (2) Cognitively manipulating the aversive stimuli (e.g., denial of pain/discomfort, or relativizing—thinking of children who have much worse dental/medical treatments).
      (3) Thought stopping.
      (4) Emphasizing/affirming one's own competence.
      (5) Stressing long-term consequences of getting versus not getting treatment.
3. *Use of a coping plan* (Do you make a plan to cope with fear?)—yes versus no.
4. *Use of self-reinforcement* (Do you compliment yourself for success in coping?)—yes versus no.
5. *Attributions of self-regulation failure* (Why don't self-control methods work sometimes?)—external versus internal attributions.

(*cont.*)

Table 8.1. (cont.)

Study	Sample	Assessment times and methods	Assessment categories
		In vivo medical stressor (hospitalization/surgery)	
Robins (1987)	n = 27 Ages 6-17 ($\bar{X}$= 12.6) M = 18 (67%); F = 9 (39%) White = 21 (78%); Black = 6 (22%) SES not reported	*Anticipatory:* Children were administered 16 Thematic Apperception Test (TAT)-like cards depicting general (nonmedical) themes and instructed to produce stories prior to orthopedic surgery. *Postimpact:* TAT-like cards were readministered before discharge.	Children's specific responses were content-analyzed into *adaptive scales* and compared to norms for the following: 1. Reliance on Others. 2. Support from Others. 3. Support by Child (Self-Sufficiency). 4. Problem Identification. 5. Limit Setting. 6. Resolution 1 (Unrealistic Solution). 7. Resolution 2 (Constructive Solution). 8. Resolution 3 (Insightful Solution).
Savedra & Tesler (1981)	n = 33 Ages 6-12 M = 18; F = 15 Race, SES not reported	*Anticipatory/Postimpact:* Children were observed using a 10-second time-sampling procedure, summed across 5-minute intervals, at six different points during experience: admission to ward; first blood test; immediate presurgery period; first 4 hours on ward (after return from recovery room); day after surgery (morning and evening); and daily, second day after surgery until discharge (rotating between morning, afternoon, and evening of each day).	For each time period, observed behaviors were totaled and grouped into three categories to reflect three different levels of involvement: 1. *Inactive*—child is silent and nonparticipating; sits or lies motionless or nearly so; may exhibit vacant staring, blank facial expression, and apathy. 2. *Precoping or orienting*—the process of familiarizing self with the environment. Behaviors include looking and listening for information, actively manipulating and exploring, or verbal interaction (e.g., asking questions). 3. *Active coping:* (a) *Attempts to control*—offers, expresses, suggests, gives (verbally or nonverbally), acts autonomously (actions not suggested or directed by others).

(b) *Cooperates*—complies, allows, accepts, offers no resistance, agrees with, compliments, rewards, thanks, congratulates others for initiating action.

(c) *Resists*—withdraws, leaves, leans, steps, or turns away. Implies that action is taken because situation is undesirable.

(d) *Suspends*—avoids situation, by sensory withdrawal or by accepting or rejecting offered resource conditionally or tentatively.

(e) *Ignores*—does not respond to requests, offers, or resources. Continues current activity, ignoring person attempting interaction. Action seems deliberate, rather than failure to perceive stimulus.

(f) *Negates*—rejects, denies, disagrees, says no, pushes hand or object away.

(g) *Attacks*—attempted or actual physical or verbal attack.

riencing) was listed only once (Peterson et al., 1990). This is surprising, given that this strategy has been found to be effective for adults (see Ahles, Blanchard, & Leventhal, 1983) and has emerged as a prominent form of informational preparation in medical and dental stress situations (Miller, Combs, & Stoddard, 1989; Siegel & Peterson, 1980). Other methods examined in only one study were acting brave (Peterson et al., 1990), cognitively emphasizing or affirming one's own competence (Prins, 1985), complaining (Peterson et al., 1990), crying in order to accomplish some objective (Band & Weisz, 1988), and ignoring offers or requests (Savedra & Tesler, 1981). Some methods discussed in the adult literature were omitted altogether. For example, "white-knuckling," or deliberately stiffening or tensing muscles when experiencing pain or discomfort, was not assessed (see Chaves & Brown, 1987). It may have been tapped by "influencing one's motor behavior," described as "regulating one's breathing pattern and muscle tension" (Prins, 1985, p. 646). However, it was not specified whether this would include muscle tensing, as well as relaxing.

Cross-study comparison is often difficult because of terminological differences from study to study, along with insufficient detail about the coping methods assessed. For example, Peterson et al. (1990) included a category of "self-instruction," but the criteria for this category were not delineated. Therefore, we cannot ascertain whether it would map onto any of the categories used in other studies, such as "positive self-talk" (Brown et al., 1986) or "emotion-regulating cognitions" (Curry & Russ, 1985). As another example, Prins (1985) identified a strategy termed "relativizing," described as comparing oneself to children who had worse medical problems. Relativizing did not appear in pure form in any other study, but it may have been included in various other categories: "pure cognition" (Band & Weisz, 1988), "positive self-talk" (Brown et al., 1986), and either "positive cognitive restructuring" or "defensive reappraisal" (Curry & Russ, 1985). In addition, the studies differ with respect to how fine-grained or specific the coping methods were. For example, distraction was sometimes described in rather global terms (e.g., techniques to distract oneself; Band & Weisz, 1988) and sometimes in more specific terms (e.g., imagery, thinking about some non-stress-related subject in a self-distractive way, relaxation, self-instruction, thinking of later rewards, and pretending the stressor doesn't hurt; Peterson et al., 1990).

Some investigators made a distinction between coping "cognitions" and coping "behaviors" (Curry & Russ, 1985; Prins, 1985). Although no precise definitions were offered, the former would appear to reflect modes of thinking that affect how an event is processed (e.g., fantasizing), while the latter would appear to reflect more overt, observable behaviors (e.g., asking questions). However, there is clearly overlap among these categories. Furthermore, the grouping of strategies was not consistent from study to study. For example, viewing a pleasant picture in the dentist's office was sometimes considered to be a cognitive strategy ("diversionary thinking") and sometimes a behavioral strategy ("influencing attention").

An important—yet relatively neglected—question is whether any of the different methods of coping tend to cohere. Among the seven studies that assessed children's use of specific coping methods, only Curry and Russ (1985) directly investigated this issue. Unfortunately, they divided the coping methods into "cognitive" and "behavioral" categories (not further defined) and only assessed coherences within each category. For those coping methods clustered into the "behavioral" category (seeking information, seeking support, and attempting to maintain control), they found that children who tended to seek information during a dental session also tended to seek support. Children who tended to try to maintain control over the situation, on the other hand, were not necessarily likely to seek either information or support. This finding parallels results in the adult literature (Miller, Brody, & Summerton, 1988). Each of the three methods in the "behavioral" category was positively associated with the total number of responses for this category.

For those methods placed in the "cognitive" category (reality-oriented working through, positive cognitive restructuring, defensive reappraisal, emotion-regulating cognitions, behavior-regulating cognitions, and diversionary thinking), children who tended to use diversionary thinking (distraction) were significantly less likely to use defensive reappraisal (denial, superstitious thinking, cognitive reframing). No other specific coping methods in the cognitive category were associated. Three of the six specific methods in this category (behavior-regulating cognitions, emotion-regulating cognitions, and positive cognitive restructuring) were positively associated with total number of cognitive responses.

Although the majority of studies did not assess the empirical coherences among specific coping modes, most of them collapsed the fine-grained categories into more overarching categories, based on theoretical assumptions. These included stimulus approach versus stimulus avoidance (Peterson et al., 1990); coping versus catastrophizing (Brown et al., 1986; Peterson et al., 1990); inactive coping versus precoping (information seeking) versus active coping (Savedra & Tesler, 1981); and primary control versus secondary control versus relinquished control (Band & Weisz, 1988). Like the specific categories themselves, the overarching categories were in some cases not fully defined or explained. Furthermore, there appears to be a good deal of inconsistency in how the specific techniques were grouped. Fantasizing, for example, was placed in the category of "distraction" methods by Peterson et al. (1990). In the Band and Weisz (1988) study, fantasizing was considered an example of a type of coping termed "pure cognition," which is conceptually distinct from their distraction category. "Pure cognition" in turn was collapsed by

Band and Weisz into an overarching category entitled "secondary control," which refers to attempts to change one's accommodation to a situation.

Information seeking—a major focus in much of the research—was classified as a "behavioral coping" method (Curry & Russ, 1985) and a "behavioral self-regulation" method (Prins, 1985). Both of these categories included efforts to maintain or exert control. However, Prins also included distraction and regulating one's breathing in the behavioral category, whereas Curry and Russ included support seeking. Hence, the overall categories are very different. Peterson et al. (1990) treated information seeking as a unitary, global dimension in the appraisal (anticipatory) stage of coping. In contrast, in the encounter (impact) stage, they posited an alternate, more complex model, consisting of two orthogonal dimensions: proactive coping (i.e., the adaptive use of a plan to reduce stress) versus reactive coping (i.e., catastrophizing) and stimulus approach (i.e., attempts to alter threat-relevant stimuli) versus stimulus blocking (i.e., attempts to shield oneself from threat-relevant stimuli).

In this model, a child high on proactive coping and stimulus blocking would be described as engaging in distraction or relaxation, whereas a child high on proactive coping and stimulus approach would be described as focusing attention on the event or its sensations. In contrast, a child high on reactive coping and stimulus blocking would be described as complaining, worrying, or whining; a child high on reactive coping and stimulus approach would be described as attempting to alter the threatening situation to reduce his or her vulnerability through active noncooperation or aggression. A child near the midpoints on both the proactive–reactive and stimulus blocking–stimulus approach dimensions would be believed to display neutral coping, marked by passive behaviors. So, in the encounter phase, information seeking would be placed primarily—but not entirely—in the category entailing plan-oriented approaches to threat-relevant stimuli. In contrast, the asking of questions in a fearful manner would be classified as "worry/whining."

The model proposed by Peterson et al. (1990) has a number of advantages. It focuses attention on the possible differences between coping modes during the anticipatory and impact stages, and thus highlights temporal and situational influences in the coping process. It also provides a unified theoretical–empirical approach by linking specific types of coping to overarching dimensions. However, a number of questions remain unanswered at this point. In particular, it is unclear whether the dimension of information seeking versus information avoiding fully characterizes the anticipatory stage of coping. In addition, it is unclear whether the specific coping methods cluster well into the overarching coping dimensions that have been posited.

Overall, it is apparent that there is little similarity in the overarching coping categories posited in these studies. Furthermore, the categories were largely derived on theoretical grounds, rather than through systematic data-analytic methods. Hence, instead of allowing the data to drive the grouping of strategies, the investigators imposed categories "from the top down." The use of multidimensional scaling and other statistical methods would have helped to determine whether the coping categories that were created actually reflected naturally occurring coherences in children's self-regulatory patterns.

Global Coping Modes

Table 8.2 summarizes the samples, assessment times and methods, and coping categories of the studies tapping more global coping modes. In this approach, coping is viewed in terms of a single, continuous dimension, although the dimension under study has varied somewhat from study to study. Burstein and Meichenbaum (1979) focused on high versus low "defensiveness," operationalized in terms of children's readiness to play with medical versus nonmedical toys and by scores on a defensiveness questionnaire. Less defensive children were considered to be more open to processing threat-relevant information, and thereby to perform the "work of worrying" more efficiently. Similarly, Tarnow and Gutstein (1983) assessed the concept of "self-preparation," described as an active rehearsal process involving both information seeking and efforts to gain mastery over the situation. Self-preparation was operationalized in terms of the child's willingness to become involved in play with medical objects, role play, and informational preparation.

Hubert, Jay, Saltoun, and Hayes (1988) identified a dimension of behavioral involvement with threatening medical stimuli, operationalized by approach (willingness to look, touch, ask questions, and initiate involvement) versus avoidance (turning away, trying to escape or change the situation) of threat-relevant stimuli during informational preparation. LaMontagne (1984, 1987) used a related concept, "active" coping versus "avoidant" coping, operationalized in terms of the child's knowledge about his or her medical condition, willingness to seek additional information, and willingness to discuss the surgery. Peterson and Toler (1986) assessed the disposition to seek versus avoid threat-relevant information in a medical setting. Operationalization was in terms of component information-seeking behaviors, such as asking questions, taking part in discussion, thinking about the medical procedure, planning for coping, and willingness to advise a friend to seek information in that setting.

Finally, Knight et al. (1979) targeted high versus low "effectiveness" of ego defenses. This was operationalized as a composite of affective

Table 8.2. Studies Exploring Global Coping Modes

Study	Sample	Assessment times and methods	Assessment categories
		In vivo medical stressor (bone marrow aspiration) [BMA])	
Hubert, Jay, Saltoun, & Hayes (1988)	n = 43 Ages 3–11 ($\bar{X}$= 6.24) M = 26; F = 17 White = 46%; Hispanic = 33%; black = 7%; Asian = 14% SES not reported	*Impact:* Children were observed during informational preparation for first BMA. Ratings taken at five times: preparation materials in room; rationale for BMA given; positioning, washing, and touching of demo doll; demonstration of local numbing by injection; and demonstration of BMA.	*Approach-avoidance* (summed across five time points), was rated on a 1–5 Likert scale: 1 = *Avoidance*—turns away, tries to escape or change situation. 5 = *Approach*—looks, touches, questions, initiates involvement.
		In vivo medical stressor (hospitalization/surgery)	
Burstein & Meichenbaum (1979)	n = 20 Ages 4.8–8.6 ($\bar{X}$= 7.1) M = 10; F = 10 Race, SES not reported	*Anticipatory:* Children were observed during play with a medical toy and a nonmedical toy (matched for attractiveness) during 6-minute play periods. Play was assessed at home 1 week before surgery and in hospital evening before surgery. Children were interviewed about the tendency to deny common weaknesses. *Postimpact:* Play was assessed at home 1 week after surgery.	*Play preference*—total amount of time spent with medical versus nonmedical toys. *Defensiveness*—scored from 0 to 27 (on 27-item questionnaire), with higher score indicating greater defensiveness (denial of common weaknesses). *Play preference*—total amount of time spent with medical versus nonmedical toys in each play period.

| Knight, et al. (1979) | $n = 25$
Ages 7–11
$M = 19$; $F = 6$
Race, SES not reported | *Anticipatory:* Children were interviewed (immediately after being informed of surgery in 2 weeks) and the day before surgery to assess "defense effectiveness." The interviewer rated child's self-report and observed behavior during the interview.
The Rorschach Test, administered by a clinical psychologist, was used as a separate measure of defense effectiveness.

Postimpact (just before discharge): Clinical interview only. | 1. *Defense effectiveness*—assessed by the following methods:
  a. The interview was rated 1–5 on a Likert-type scale (1 = Good defense effectiveness, 5 = Poor defense effectiveness), based on the interviewer's observations of the child's affective distress, functional intactness, and defense reserve.
  b. The Rorschach Test was interpreted by two clinical psychologists (blind to nature of study) to arrive at a separate measure of defense effectiveness.
2. *Child's interview responses* were categorized by the interviewer into intellectualization; intellectualization with isolation; mixed pattern; denial; denial with isolation; displacement; projection. |
| LaMontagne (1984) | $n = 51$
Ages = 8–12 ($\bar{X} = 10.7$)
$M = 25$; $F = 26$
Race, SES not reported | *Anticipatory:* Children were interviewed prior to minor elective surgery. | *Avoidant–active coping* was rated on a 1–10 Likert scale:
1–3 = *Avoidant coping group*—child has limited knowledge of medical problem and procedure, is hesitant to discuss these topics.
4–7 = *Middle coping group*—child gives evidence of both coping modes.
8–10 = *Active coping group*—child shows detailed knowledge about medical problem, surgery, and post-op course; shows readiness to discuss these topics and/or seeks additional information. |

(cont.)

Table 8.2. (cont.)

Study	Sample	Assessment times and methods	Assessment categories
LaMontagne (1987)	$n = 42$ Ages 8-18 ($\bar{X} = 13.39$) M = 23; F = 19 Race, SES not reported.	*Anticipatory:* Children were interviewed prior to minor elective surgery.	*Avoidant-active coping* (see LaMontagne, 1984, above)

Peterson & Toler (1986)	$n = 59$
	Ages 5-11 ($\bar{X} = 7.27$)
	M = 33; F = 26
	Race: all white
	SES: mainly middle class
		Anticipatory: Children and parents were interviewed at admission about children's typical coping (parents) and procedural knowledge (children). Children were interviewed before surgery about their information-seeking versus information-avoiding tendencies.	1. *Information seeking—child self-report;* 9 items (summed) inquired about information seeking (e.g., does child ask questions if worried; does child recommend question asking to a friend in similar situation; what has child asked about while in hospital; what did child think about before, during, and after blood test; what thoughts made child feel better).
			2. *Procedural knowledge—child self-report;* 15-items (summed) assessed the amount of information child had concerning hospital and surgical procedures upon admission.
			3. *History of coping—parent report;* four separate scores:
			  (a) Parent method for preparation of child. Likert scale: 1 (tell child all details beforehand) to 5 (tell child only at time of procedure).
			  (b) Child's usual method of coping. Likert scale: (concentrates, wants procedural and sensory details) to 5 (prefers distraction).

172

(c) Child's typical behaviors regarding medical situations (several subparts—e.g., is upset if you talk about the procedure), scored yes–no.

(d) Degree of distress registered by child in four common medical situations (e.g., going to the dentist, getting a shot).

4. *Information seeking—parent observation*; a visual analogue scale, yielding two scores:

(a) Child's verbal discussion of medical procedures

(b) Question asking.

1. *Information seeking—rater observation*:

(a) Child's discussion of blood test, during blood test (rating scale unspecified).

(b) Child's question asking during blood test (rating scale unspecified).

(c) Information-seeking checklist; ten items (summed) assessed information approaching (e.g., child is curious about what is happening) versus information avoiding (e.g., child blocks out what is happening).

Impact (blood test): Children were observed by rater.

(cont.)

Table 8.2. (cont.)

Study	Sample	Assessment times and methods	Assessment categories

Tarnow & Gustein (1983)	$n = 34$
	Ages 4–5 ($n = 16$); and 6–9 ($n = 18$)
	M = 19; F = 15
	White = 29; black = 5
	SES: mean parent educational level = 13.2 yrs.
		Postimpact (postsurgery): Children were observed by parents during removal of the IV tube and assessment of temperature and blood pressure.
		
		Anticipatory: Children were observed prior to tonsillectomy, using two boxes, one filled with actual hospital equipment (e.g., surgical masks, syringes) and one with nonmedical toys. Three different conditions were assessed: (1) Child was given both boxes, and invited to play with any or all contents of boxes; (2) child pretended experimenter was a child having an operation and "taught" him or her what would happen; and (3) parents prepared child informationally for surgery using the medical objects in room.
			1. *Information seeking—parent observation;* a visual analogue scale yielding two scores:
			  (a) Child's verbal discussion of medical procedures.
			  (b) Child's question asking.
			
			*Involvement–noninvolvement—*each 5-minute observation interval was separately rated for level of active involvement with medical equipment on a 0–3 Likert scale:
			0 = complete lack of involvement.
			3 = active involvement in an integrated fashion.

distress, intactness of normal psychological functioning (in such areas as intellectual capabilities, social behavior, appetite, and sleep), and defense reserve (the ability to remain calm and respond appropriately when confronted with increasingly threatening descriptions of the medical procedure).

In these studies, then, individuals who approached threatening stimuli and remained more active were distinguished from those who avoided such stimuli and remained more uninvolved. Such an approach may thus collapse coping modes together that may actually be conceptually and empirically distinct (e.g., efforts to predict vs. efforts to control). In research with adults, individuals who monitor for medical threats have been shown to be less—not more—likely to prefer to play an active role in their medical care (e.g., Miller et al., 1988). The use of such global categories may blur these distinctions. Furthermore, important subtleties of the coping process may be lost, such as the way in which different strategies are combined together and the situational and individual factors that influence the use and effectiveness of these strategies. Finally, concepts such as "defensiveness" and "defense effectiveness" appear to incorporate adaptational outcomes into the coping construct. That is, the nature and efficacy of coping strategies are not kept separate. This makes a "clean" exploration of the impact of diverse self-regulatory processes on adaptational outcomes difficult.

METHODS AND PERIODS OF ASSESSMENT

Two major methods have been used to assess coping: self-report and observation. Seven of the studies described above used self-reports alone to assess coping (Band & Weisz, 1988; Brown et al., 1986; LaMontagne, 1984, 1987; Peterson et al., 1990; Prins, 1985; Robins, 1987); three used direct observation alone (Hubert et al., 1988; Savedra & Tesler, 1981; Tarnow & Gutstein, 1983), and four combined self-report and observational techniques (Burstein & Meichenbaum, 1979; Curry & Russ, 1985; Knight et al., 1979; Peterson & Toler, 1986). The self-report format has a number of advantages, including an emphasis on identifying subtle attentional strategies. Furthermore, it allows for an evaluation of the child's metacognitive appraisals of his or her coping efforts, such as self-speech, planning, self-reinforcement, and attributions for failure (Prins, 1985). To be maximally informative, information should be obtained about the use of a comprehensive range of coping strategies (e.g., "What tricks or strategies do you use to be less fearful?"; cf. Prins, 1985, p. 642), how helpful they are, how difficult they are to enact, and whether the child is aware of other strategies he or she would not use (Peterson et al., 1990; Prins, 1985). Moreover, children who have limited verbal skills or who are not inclined to respond to the questions need to be probed sufficiently. Therefore, the interview guidelines should not allow "Do not know" to be accepted at face value as a response. Having the child talk out loud during the experience, respond to imagined or role-play vignettes, and report at multiple assessment points can help to pin down the nature and function of strategies utilized.

The observational format also has a number of advantages. It bypasses children's self-report and focuses on what they actually do under stress. Furthermore, it allows for ratings by more than one observer, thus increasing the reliability of the behavioral data under consideration. For example, in one study, two observers independently rated the children's approach–avoidance behaviors during informational preparation for a bone marrow aspiration procedure. There was a high degree of agreement between them (Hubert et al., 1988). Coping strategies that can be anchored more behaviorally also present fewer problems for validation than those that are more cognitive or abstract in character. For instance, observers' ongoing reports of a child's question asking can be compared to videotapes of the child's actual question asking in the relevant situation. Although certain variables (such as timidity) may inhibit a child who wants to ask questions from doing so, this problem can be partially circumvented by separating out predictions of what the child wants to do, expects to do, and has actually done.

Using interview and observational methods together is optimal, since the combination draws on the strengths of both and cancels out their weaknesses. Unfortunately, only a handful of the studies discussed above explored the interrelations between self-report and observational methods. In one study, children were asked how they had coped with their (just completed) blood test, whether they asked questions about aspects of the experience that worried them, and what coping advice they would give to a friend in a similar circumstance (Peterson & Toler, 1986; see also Toler, 1985). Self-reported information-seeking scores were significantly associated with several other measures of information seeking, including parental reports of the child's typical tendency to ask questions and participate in medical-related discussion during common medical procedures; observational ratings by parents of the child's question asking and discussion during hospitalization; observational ratings by the researcher of the child's question asking and discussion during blood drawing; and the child's medical knowledge at admission.

In contrast, parental observations of other coping behaviors—such as assertiveness with medical staff, level of activity during medical procedures, and visual observation of ongoing medical procedures—were not associated with children's reports of information seeking. Thus, although the identification of an information-seeking approach appears to be valid, attention to threat may not be a unitary construct. At least in children, visual and verbal modes of information seeking may not necessarily cohere or tap into the same process (Miller, Combs, & Kruus, in press).

A second major aspect of assessment is that of the time(s) at which coping is assessed. Children's encounters with medical and dental stressors are typically differentiated into anticipatory, impact, and post-impact (recovery) stages of coping. As Peterson et al. (1990) point out, there are no clear demarcations among these three stages of coping in response to a given stressor. Moreover, as a child enters the post-impact stage of one stressor, he or she may simultaneously enter the anticipatory stage of another stressor. For example, in one study, children were assessed during informational preparation for a bone marrow aspiration (Hubert et al., 1988). The period immediately after the preparation was, in some sense, the post-impact period. However, this was also the anticipatory period before the actual aspiration procedure. Despite the difficulties, it is useful to try to draw boundaries among the different stages and to explore differences and convergences across the measurement points.

Several of the studies used multiple assessment points, at times both before and after surgery (Burstein & Meichenbaum, 1979; Knight et al., 1979; Peterson & Toler, 1986; Robins, 1987; Savedra & Tesler, 1981). However, only three explored the nature of coping coherences across different times of assessment. Burstein and Meichenbaum (1979) used a questionnaire measure of psychological defensiveness, which assessed the tendency of children to deny common weaknesses and failings. Children with high defensiveness scores were less likely to play with medical-related toys at an initial play session (at home, 1 week before hospitalization), but there was no relationship between defensiveness and play preference on two subsequent occasions (in hospital the evening before surgery and at home 1 week after surgery). Play in the hospital was severely diminished, with neither relevant nor irrelevant toys eliciting interest, in comparison to play at both home sessions. This coincided with higher levels of self-reported anxiety at the in-hospital session. Hence, anxiety may have depressed the appearance of certain types of coping. During higher-stress periods, then, it may be more beneficial to assess children's coping via more structured methods.

Savedra and Tesler (1981) assessed the presence or absence of a number of specific coping behaviors at six different points during hospitalization and surgery: first hour of arrival on the hospital ward, first blood drawing, presurgery, first 4 hours after return to the ward from the recovery room, the day following surgery, and daily for the duration of the hospital stay (all daily assessments were averaged for this last time category). Results showed that only 21% of the 5-minute assessment intervals were characterized by a single observed coping behavior, 32% were characterized by two different coping behaviors, another 32% by three different coping behaviors, and the remaining 15% by four or five types of coping behaviors. Moreover, the preponderance of different types of coping varied from assessment period to assessment period. Admission was characterized by information seeking and attempts to control; blood drawing was typified by cooperation; and preoperative coping was dominated by information seeking. This is consistent with research in the adult literature, showing that individuals demonstrate considerable variability in the types of coping strategy at their disposal (Folkman & Lazarus, 1980) and that different aspects of the stressor may activate distinct coping profiles (Suls & Fletcher, 1985).

Peterson et al. (1990) provided the most comprehensive assessment of coping during the anticipatory and impact stages. Children who sought information during the anticipatory stage of coping were more likely to use a "proactive" (planful) coping technique during the impact stage, either of an avoidant nature (e.g., distraction, relaxation) or of an approach-oriented nature (e.g., information seeking, sensory focus), than were children who had avoided information during the anticipatory stage. Hence, attention to information prior to the stressor tended to cohere with more deliberate, organized modes of coping during the impact stage. Perhaps children who initially seek information give themselves the opportunity to appraise the situation and to prepare a mode of response that they feel comfortable with.

Although the available research is limited, the findings to date suggest that it may be possible to reliably identify dimensions such as information seeking and level of defensiveness. Moreover, there may be some coherences across different modes of measurement (self-report vs. observational) and some stability in coping over time. However, the coping measures also appear to show a certain degree of situational and temporal specificity. Agreement across different modes of assessment appears to be highest when the measures are obtained close together in time, under a similar set of stimulus conditions. In the adult literature, the benefits of avoidant versus confrontive coping appear to vary as a function of time and severity of the stressor (Miller, in press). It is not yet possible, however, to draw firm conclusions about children's coping, since the studies have not really been designed to tease apart more subtle temporal and situational influences on self-regulation.

COPING AND ADAPTATION

In addition to whether coping modes can be identified in young children undergoing medical and dental stressors, a critical question is whether coping patterns have implications for the course of adjustment in these contexts. Yet only one of the studies focusing on specific coping methods explored the impact of these micro-level patterns for adaptation. Robins (1987) found that total number of coping responses obtained on a projective test, assessed prior to surgery, was associated with less parent-rated anxiety and withdrawal in the immediate postsurgery period. In addition, one of the presurgery subscale scores, constructive limit setting, was found to be positively associated with long-term (1-month) overall psychological adjustment.

The remaining studies all looked at adaptational outcomes as a function of more global coping dimensions. Burstein and Meichenbaum (1979) found that lower prehospital defensiveness and greater preference for medical-related toys 1 week before surgery were predictive of lower anxiety 1 week after surgery. However, play behavior assessed at the hospital the evening before surgery did not predict postsurgery adjustment. Similarly, Tarnow and Gutstein (1983) found that children who showed a greater preference for medical equipment (both when alone and in surgery-related role play on admission to the hospital) were rated by their parents as showing a greater decrease in symptoms of distress after surgery, but not in symptoms of fear. On the other hand, children who were initially more involved in their parents' efforts to prepare them for surgery subsequently showed a greater reduction in parent-rated fear, but not in parent-rated distress.

Hubert et al. (1988), studying hospitalized children during informational preparation for their first bone marrow aspiration, found that children tending to approach threat-relevant stimuli (as rated by an observer using a global approach–avoidance scale) were also rated by the observer as less distressed during the informational preparation and during the actual aspiration shortly afterward. In addition, they were rated by their primary nurse as being less distressed on the ward during the first 2 days of hospitalization. No association was found between approach or avoidant coping style and either heart rate change or the child's own ratings of fear or pain.

Peterson and Toler (1986) assessed information seeking (described in terms of making plans, expressing appropriate concern, asking questions, and observing the medical procedure) and found it to be associated with only 3 of 11 stress variables (asking of questions during anesthesia induction, observed distress in anticipation of the blood test, and parent-rated fearfulness after surgery). Question asking, however, should be considered more of a validation variable than a stress variable in the context of this study. The remaining two stress variables were predicted marginally, suggesting that information seeking had very little predictive power in terms of adaptation.

Finally, Knight et al. (1979) found no correlation between either an interview measure of defense effectiveness (defined as a composite of affective distress; intactness of such psychological functions as intellectual functioning, social behavior, eating, and sleeping; and ability to remain calm and respond appropriately when challenged by increasingly threatening descriptions of medical stimuli) or a Rorschach Test index of defense effectiveness and urinary cortisol levels, when assessed 1–2 weeks before surgery. At the second assessment (in hospital the day before surgery), greater defense effectiveness (as assessed on both interview and Rorschach measures) was correlated with lower cortisol levels. Greater defense effectiveness prior to surgery also predicted better post-surgery adaptation, as rated by hospital ward personnel at discharge. A third administration of the clinical interview at discharge similarly found defense effectiveness to be associated with better ward adjustment ratings. In terms of observer ratings, children who had been judged to cope primarily by intellectualization, intellectualization with isolation, or a "mixed" pattern (not further explained) tended to show lower cortisol levels. By contrast, a pattern of denial, denial with isolation, displacement, or projection was associated with higher levels of cortisol.

Overall, findings on the relationship of coping to adaptation must be viewed as preliminary. The results suggest that children may adapt better when they prepare themselves for and master the experience (Tarnow & Gutstein, 1983); when they use psychological defenses of intellectualization, intellectualization with isolation, or a mixed pattern (Knight et al., 1979); and when they are less defended (Burstein & Meichenbaum, 1979) and seek out threat-relevant information (Peterson & Toler, 1986; Hubert et al., 1988). Peterson (1989) has suggested that successful coping methods are all characterized by a tendency to cope actively with the stressor. Although this provides a parsimonious approach to the research on coping, helping to tie together a diverse set of studies, the notion of active versus avoidant coping is not yet well delineated. Indeed, each of these types of coping appears to be complex and may entail a number of different components, which cut across the two self-regulatory modes. For example, as Peterson et al. (1990) point out, planfulness may be a component of either approach or avoidant coping. A child can act intentionally to seek information or intellectualize the situation (reflecting a planful, "active" coping approach), or, on the other hand, to avoid information or distract from the situation (reflecting a planful, "avoidant" coping approach). A child who intentionally (planfully) distracts himself or herself may actually fare better than one who obsessively and involuntarily enmeshes himself or herself in threat-relevant information.

Unfortunately, little is known about whether and how children consciously appraise a stressful situation and their potential responses to the situation, or how they make decisions about the best course of action to follow. Prins (1985) found that 40% of children interviewed prior to a dental restoration had some type of plan (e.g., "Be brave," "Don't cry," "I am going to squeeze the chair if it becomes difficult"). However, when they were asked in a separate question what specific coping methods they would use with the dentist, only 12.5% of those children who reported a plan also reported specific coping methods that were consistent with their plan. Clearly, much remains to be learned about the ways in which children formulate coping plans, the nature of these plans, their execution, and their perceived and actual efficacy.

In a related vein, the effectiveness of a given strategy may depend on the extent to which it enables the child to fully process and come to terms with the threat. Research in a variety of contexts suggests that efficient emotional processing of threat is critical for the successful regulation of stress (Foa & Kozak, 1986; Miller, in press). Confrontive coping may sometimes facilitate and sometimes impede this process. Individuals who seek information to the degree that they become sensitized to threat may be unable to habituate, because they continually redose themselves with threat-relevant thoughts and images. Conversely, those who block out information to the degree that they completely fail to confront threat-relevant stimuli may be engaged in pathological avoidance.

EXTENSION OF THE CONSTRUCT NETWORK

Our research with adults has suggested that there are two main attentional modes for dealing with health-related and non-health-related stressors. The first mode, "monitoring," entails information seeking and scanning for threat-relevant cues. The second mode, "blunting," involves attempts to cognitively avoid cues about threat. Furthermore, individuals differ in their dispositional tendencies to seek or avoid threatening information. Monitors typically prefer to scan for threat-relevant information, even in uncontrollable situations. In contrast, blunters generally prefer to distract themselves, particularly when the threat is uncontrollable. We have devised and validated a self-report instrument to identify monitors and blunters (Miller, 1987).

In a series of field and laboratory-based studies, we have found that monitors tend to show more sustained arousal, anxiety, concerns, and discomfort than blunters, particularly in the face of short-term stressors. They also tend to cope by engaging in greater vigilance and in less distraction and relaxation. In addition, monitors are typically more dissatisfied with the amount of information usually provided and fare better when voluminous information is made available than when it is withheld (Miller, 1990, in press). In ongoing work, we have been attempting to explore—in a more fine-grained manner—the nature of these processes in young children. Specifically, we have focused on youngsters in the age range of 7–12 years who must undergo an aversive dental treatment. Coping efforts have been assessed in several different ways, at various points in the situation (Miller, Sherman, Combs, Kruus, & Caputo, 1991).

To begin with, we have devised and are piloting a self-report instrument for use with children that closely parallels the adult version. The Child Behavioral Style Scale (CBSS) consists of four hypothetical stress-inducing situations of an uncontrollable nature. Two of these situations (a doctor and a dentist scenario) are highly similar to the dental situation actually under study. For example, the children are asked to imagine that their mothers have taken them to the doctor's office because they are sick. Each scenario is followed by eight options, half of which reflect a monitoring or information-oriented approach (e.g., "Would you think about what the doctor is going to do to you?") and half of which reflect a blunting or information-avoidant approach (e.g., "Would you think about something else to get your mind off being sick?").

The scale is administered in an interview format, to control for any differences in reading comprehension. Children are asked to indicate, for each option, whether or not they would engage in it. The scale yields two scores: a Monitoring score, based on the total of all the information-seeking items endorsed, and a Blunting score, based on the total of all the blunting items endorsed. Initial findings show that the internal reliability of the Monitoring subscale is adequate, but the internal reliability of the Blunting subscale is low. This parallels research with adults, showing that the Monitoring score is often a more cohesive and potent predictor of behavior than the Blunting score (Miller et al., 1988). Hence, the preliminary analyses reported here were conducted on the basis of scores on the Monitoring subscale. We are currently revising the instrument in an attempt to improve the internal reliability.

Among the existing studies, only Peterson and Toler (1986) obtained ratings (from the parent) of the children's typical information-seeking style. These ratings cohered with children's actual attentional strategies, as assessed by their self-reports of information seeking in response to a medical stressor. To explore these patterns further, we obtained measures of self-reported coping strategy in response to the dental situation itself and compared them with our coping style measure. On arrival at the dentist's office, children were asked two global questions to predict their own attentional strategies (i.e., "When you are with the dentist, how much do you think you will pay attention to what is happening?" and "When you are with the dentist, how much do you think you will daydream, try to sleep, or think about other things?")

Preliminary analyses have been conducted on a subset of the data, controlling for age, sex, race, and number of previous visits. The results showed that measures of dispositional style were related to children's predictions of coping strategy under actual threat. Children disposed to monitor were significantly more likely to say that they intended to pay attention when they were with the dentist. Thus, reports of typical coping dispositions were found to cohere with children's coping intentions when directly threatened with an aversive event.

Following the dental treatment, children rated the extent to which they had used each of 15 specific coping modes. A factor analysis was then performed, yielding five independent factors. These included two vigilance-type factors: (1) Sensory Vigilance (paying attention to what the dentist was doing, paying attention to how everything looked and sounded, paying attention to how much it hurt, and paying attention to the feel of the dentist's hands and instruments) and (2) Question Asking (asking the dentist questions). There were also two avoidance-type factors: (1) Internal Distraction (daydreaming/trying to sleep, closing one's eyes, making a tight fist, and thinking about other things) and (2) External Distraction (keeping one's eyes on something else in the room and keeping one's mind off what the dentist was doing by paying attention to other things). Finally, there was a factor of Emotion Regulating, involving relaxation (relaxing oneself), focusing on the positive (telling oneself how nice one's teeth will look), self-instruction (telling oneself not to think about what the dentist is doing), and fantasizing (pretending one is somewhere else or doing something different from what is happening).

As discussed above, most of the existing studies have identified specific categories largely on conceptually derived grounds. Strikingly, many of the theoretically generated categories turn out empirically to contain different components of the factor-analysis-derived categories in our study. Furthermore, in some instances more than one theoretically generated category maps onto a given empirically generated category. Thus, at least in the dental context, the conceptually derived categories prove to be empirically impure and to cut across several of the identified factors. This suggests that they may be overly broad and thereby may be obscuring important patterns in the data.

Children who were more likely to display a monitoring dispositional style reported after the procedure that they had engaged in more sensory vigilance (e.g., watching the dentist, focusing on what they were feeling and how much it hurt). Similarly, comparisons across situational coping measures revealed that children who predicted (on arrival at the dentist's office) that they would pay attention later reported having engaged in greater amounts of sensory vigilance. Conversely, children who predicted that they would distract themselves subsequently reported that they had engaged in less sensory vigilance. Children's predictions of their intentions to distract themselves during the procedure were related to their subsequent internal, although not external, distraction efforts.

Overall, there appears to be a degree of correspondence between children's hypothetical reports of how they generally tend to cope (i.e., their degree of monitoring) and their on-site predictions of how they intend to cope in a given stressful situation. This parallels our research with adults and suggests that it may also be possible to begin to identify individual differences in coping styles at a fairly formative stage of development. When linkages between either coping style or specific predictions of coping strategy and actual coping behaviors used are considered, a mixed information-seeking cluster appears to emerge. Children who are dispositionally inclined to monitor and who specifically predict that they will monitor actually engage in more sensory vigilance, although they do not report engaging in greater question asking.

We were also interested in examining the relationships among observer ratings of the child's coping strategies in the situation and the child's own self-reports. Toward these ends, parents were asked before the treatment to predict the extent to which their child would pay attention to (monitor) the situation and the extent to which the child would try to distract from (blunt) what was happening. Following the treatment, the dentist was asked to indicate the extent to which the child had asked questions, paid attention, and engaged in self-distraction. Initial findings showed that the association between observational and self-report ratings varied, depending on the measure, the observer, and the time of assessment.

Parents' predictions of their children's coping modes were unrelated to the children's corresponding pretreatment predictions or to the children's posttreatment reports of coping strategy. In contrast, the dentists' ratings of what children actually did during the procedure were related to both self-reported and observed coping. Specifically, children who were rated by the dentist as having paid greater attention during the treatment reported subsequently that they had engaged in greater sensory vigilance (paying attention to what the dentist was doing and to how everything looked, sounded, and felt). In addition, children who were rated by their dentists as having engaged in greater internal distraction and less question-asking (verbal information seeking) during treatment were more likely to report later that they had made use of emotion-regulating strategies (e.g., relaxation, calming self-statements, fantasizing).

Finally, an important issue was to determine whether and how dispositional coping style and ongoing coping strategy might moderate indices of adjustment. Measures of anxiety were obtained from a number of sources, including the child, the parent, the dentist, and an independent observer. In addition, each child was videotaped while in the dentist's chair. These recordings were subsequently scored to yield an index of the child's disruptiveness during the treatment, using a modified version of the Behavior Profile Rating Scale (Melamed, Weinstein, Hawes,

& Katin-Borland, 1975). This measure can be considered to assess a child's overt, behavioral signs of fear during impact.

Our preliminary results suggest that the impact of coping modes may well depend on the type of strategy, the informant, and the adaptational outcome under consideration. Using the measure of dispositional coping style, monitoring showed a nonsignificant trend to be associated with self-reports and observer ratings of increased anxiety before, during, and after the procedure. Thus, as in adult populations, monitoring in the face of threat—particularly of an acute nature—appears to be anxiety-inducing (Miller, 1990). This makes sense, since high monitors generally remain more cognitively alert for and focused on threat. Monitors also tend to interpret potential threats more negatively than blunters do (Miller, Combs, & Kruus, in press). Interestingly, children who predicted before the treatment that they would daydream or try to fall asleep also showed greater anxiety, according to both self-report and the ratings of the observer.

In addition, there were some associations between the children's reports of the coping strategies they had used during the procedure and adjustment. Self-reports of greater question asking were related to greater anxiety as measured by the child's own ratings, the dentist's ratings, and the observer's ratings. Videotape recordings also showed that children who reported asking more questions were more disruptive during treatment. The use of internal distraction was similarly associated with high anxiety, according to the child's self-report. In contrast, the use of emotion-regulating strategies led to lower self-reported anxiety.

Children's coping, when assessed from the dentists' perspective, complemented these patterns. Children rated by the dentists as having paid greater attention were judged to be more anxious and disruptive during the treatment, according to the dentists' observations and ratings of videotaped behaviors. Further, children rated by the dentists as having asked more questions showed greater self-reported, dentist-rated, and observer-rated anxiety, as well as greater disruptiveness. On the other hand, children who were sucessfully able to tune out (according to the dentist) tended to show less anxiety.

Overall, these results suggest a complex relationship between coping and adjustment. One type of intrusive monitoring (question asking) and one type of extreme blunting (daydreaming/trying to sleep) were both strongly related to poorer outcomes. Overreliance on such strategies may be particularly insidious in the face of exposure to more severe or prolonged stressors (Miller, in press). Strategies such as reinterpretation (i.e., framing the event in a more positive light)—which allows for processing of the stressor but does so in a more diluted, less threatening fashion—may be optimal.

FUTURE DIRECTIONS

Taken together, some tantalizing leads have begun to emerge that help to determine what the real issues are, at both the micro and macro levels. It is clear that it is possible to identify distinctive coping patterns in young children. However, some primary questions still need to be addressed. One major challenge is to delineate what patterns are basic to the coping process, to outline their nature and structure, and to determine when these patterns are stable over time and consistent across situations. Although there is some evidence that coping may be an important aspect of the adaptational process, its exact role in the path to adjustment still needs to be clarified. Future research should continue to explore coping patterns, looking in a comprehensive manner at specific coping modes assessed by both self-report and observational methods, at various points in time during the stressful encounter.

Attention should also be given to issues of differential adaptiveness, planfulness, and emotional processing, particularly with respect to different points in the developmental course. As children mature, they undergo changes in their cognitive capacity that may affect the types of strategies that do and do not work for them, as well as changes in their ability to understand and evaluate their own coping efforts. In addition to age, a number of other factors may plausibly influence the coping process. These include sociodemographic factors, prior experience, gender, and interpersonal processes. These factors may also have an impact on adaptation. For example, a number of studies have shown that older children appear to adjust better to medical and dental stressors than do younger children, at least in the short term (Hubert et al., 1988; Peterson & Toler, 1986; Robins, 1987). Since factors such as age may affect adaptation via their influence on the coping process, it is important to explore the nature of these interactions.

A key dimension that is emerging in the adult literature, and that may have some relevance here, has to do with the notion of flexibility in coping. Some individuals appear to have a wide repertoire of strategic responses, which they are able to execute at will and target to the demands of the situation at hand. Others rigidly persist at strategies that are ineffective, either because of the effort involved in enacting them or because of the toll they take on adjustment. At present, virtually nothing is known about children's flexibility in coping, the ways in which notions of flexibility arise, or the types of children who are able to adapt themselves easily to the demands of a given situation.

In addition, it is unclear how flexibility may interact with potential mechanisms such as approach–avoidance orientation, passivity–activity, intentionality, and emotional processing. To help untangle these issues, the assessment of coping strategies must become increasingly fine-grained and situation-specific. What children actually do (or report doing) in a given stressful encounter must be differentiated from what they plan to do, how hard it is for them to do it, and how helpful they perceive their strategy to be. Moreover, studies with adult populations suggest that individuals may have dispositional tendencies to cope with stress in a given way. Our initial data suggest that, as is the case with adults, certain types of coping choices may reflect more stable tendencies, which may interact with situational factors (e.g., amount of information available) to determine adaptiveness (Miller et al., 1989). The key for the future will be to determine how best to describe and measure potential dispositional and situational moderators of ongoing experience, as well as their interaction (Miller, 1990).

Little is also known about so-called "failures" in coping. Although this is a potentially important dimension, it may be difficult to get a handle on what precisely is occurring when children seem to fold passively in response to threat. In studies that include only behavioral observation, it is difficult to know whether a child who does not appear to be coping behaviorally may in fact be coping cognitively. For example, a child who looks passive may in fact be exerting considerable effort to remain silent and motionless, because he or she thinks the stressor will hurt less that way. In studies that include only self-report, behavioral actions may be overlooked.

Apart from these larger conceptual and methodological issues, some technical issues merit attention. A methodological limitation of a number of the studies is the use of very small sample sizes. Indeed, in 6 out of the 14 studies examined in this chapter, the sample size was quite limited (Burstein & Meichenbaum, 1979, $n = 20$; Curry & Russ, 1985, $n = 30$; Knight et al., 1979, $n = 25$; Robins, 1987, $n = 27$; Savedra & Tesler, 1981, $n = 33$; Tarnow & Gutstein, 1983, $n = 34$). This may have resulted in insufficient power to find effects, particularly since relatively few subjects were distributed across both genders and a wide age range.

One route to enhancing our knowledge base about the nature and generality of basic coping strategies in children—and their role in the evolution and adaptiveness of the coping process in medical and dental contexts—is to draw on the contributions of related literatures. For example, researchers in other areas have explored basic issues in attention, information encoding, and memory that may have implications for coping under stress. We know a good deal about the way in which children process information and develop strategic behaviors for mastering such tasks as reading (Brown, Bransford, Ferrara, & Campione, 1983), delaying gratification for the sake of larger rewards (Mischel, Shoda, & Rodriguez, 1989), and dealing with failure experiences (Dweck & Leggett, 1988). We need to get a better handle on how such person learning variables facilitate or impede the process of children's coping with medical and dental stressors, and how they affect children's ability to successfully negotiate one of life's more troublesome—but universal— challenges.

Acknowledgments

This research was supported in part by grant CA46591 from the National Cancer Institute to the first author. Its contents are solely the responsibility of the authors and do not necessarily represent the official views of the National Cancer Institute. We thank Anand Athavale, Gregg Hurst, Rosemary Murphy, Richard Sommers, and Kimberly Sproat for their help.

REFERENCES

Ahles, T. A., Blanchard, E. B., & Leventhal, H. (1983). Cognitive control of pain: Attention to the sensory aspects of the cold pressor stimulus. *Cognitive Therapy and Research, 7*, 159–178.

Band, E. B., & Weisz, J. R. (1988). How to feel better when it feels bad: Children's perspectives on coping with everyday stress. *Developmental Psychology, 24*, 247–253.

Brown, A. L., Bransford, J. D., Ferrara, R. A., & Campione, J. C. (1983). Learning, remembering, and understanding. In J. H. Flavell & E. M. Markman (Vol. Eds.), *Handbook of child psychology*, (4th ed.): *Vol. 3. Cognitive development* (pp. 77–166). New York: Wiley.

Brown, J. M., O'Keeffe, J., Sanders, S. H., & Baker, B. (1986). Developmental changes in children's cognition to stressful and painful situations. *Journal of Pediatric Psychology, 11*, 343–357.

Burstein, S., & Meichenbaum, D. (1979). The work of worrying in children undergoing surgery. *Journal of Abnormal Child Psychology, 7*, 121–132.

Chaves, J. F., & Brown, J. M. (1987). Spontaneous cognitive strategies for the control of clinical pain and stress. *Journal of Behavioral Medicine, 10*, 263–276.

Curry, S. L., & Russ, S. W. (1985). Identifying coping strategies in children. *Journal of Clinical Child Psychology, 14*, 61–69.

Dweck, C. S., & Leggett, E. L. (1988). A social-cognitive approach to motivation and personality. *Psychological Review, 95*, 256–273.

Foa, E. B., & Kozak, M. J. (1986). Emotional processing of threat: Exposure to corrective information. *Psychological Bulletin, 99*, 20–35.

Folkman, S., & Lazarus, R. S. (1980). An analysis of coping in a middle-aged community sample. *Journal of Health and Social Behavior, 21*, 219–239.

Flavell, J. H. (1977). *Cognitive development*. Englewood Cliffs, NJ: Prentice-Hall.

Hubert, N. C., Jay, S. M., Saltoun, M., & Hayes, M. (1988). Approach-avoidance and distress in children undergoing preparation for painful medical procedures. *Journal of Clinical Child Psychology, 17*, 194–202.

Knight, R. B., Atkins, A., Eagle, C. J., Evans, N., Finkelstein, J. W., Fukushima, D., Katz, J., & Weiner, H. (1979). Psychological stress, ego defenses, and cortisol production in children hospitalized for elective surgery. *Psychosomatic Medicine, 41*, 40–49.

LaMontagne, L. L. (1984). Children's locus of control beliefs as predictors of preoperative coping behavior. *Nursing Research, 33*, 76–79, 85.

LaMontagne, L. L. (1987). Children's preoperative coping: Replication and extension. *Nursing Research, 36*, 163–167.

Lewis, M., & Miller, S. M. (Eds.). (1990). *Handbook of developmental psychopathology*. New York: Plenum.

Melamed, B. G., Weinstein, D., Hawes, R., & Katin-Borland, M. (1975). Reduction of fear-related dental management problems with use of filmed modeling. *Journal of the American Dental Association, 90*, 822–826.

Miller, S. M. (1987). Monitoring and blunting: Validation of a questionnaire to assess styles of information-seeking under threat. *Journal of Personality and Social Psychology, 52*, 345–353.

Miller, S. M. (1990). To see or not to see: Cognitive informational styles in the coping process. In M. Rosenbaum (Ed.), *Learned resourcefulness: On coping skills, self-regulation and adaptive behavior* (pp. 95–126). New York: Springer.

Miller, S. M. (in press). Monitoring and blunting in the face of threat: Implications for adaptation and health. In L. Montada, S. H. Filipp, & M. Lerner (Eds.), *Life crises and losses in the adult years*. Hillsdale, NJ: Lawrence Erlbaum.

Miller, S. M., Brody, D. S., & Summerton, J. (1988). Styles of coping with threat: Implications for health. *Journal of Personality and Social Psychology, 54*, 142–148.

Miller, S. M. Combs, C., & Kruus, L. (in press). Tuning in and tuning out: Confronting the effects of confrontation. In H. W. Krohne (Ed.), *Attention and avoidance: Strategies in coping with aversiveness*. New York: Springer-Verlag.

Miller, S. M., Combs, C., & Stoddard, E. (1989). Information, coping, and control in patients undergoing surgery and stressful medical procedures. In A. Steptoe & A. Appels (Eds.), *Stress, personal control and health* (pp. 107–129). Chichester, England: Wiley.

Miller, S. M., Sherman, H. D., Combs, C., Kruus, L., & Caputo, G. C. (1991). *Emotional correlates of cognitive coping patterns*. Unpublished manuscript, Temple University.

Mischel, W., Shoda, Y., & Rodriguez, M. L. (1989). Delay of gratification in children. *Science, 244*, 933–938.

Peterson, L. (1989). Coping by children undergoing stressful medical procedures: Some conceptual, methodological, and therapeutic issues. *Journal of Consulting and Clinical Psychology, 57*, 380–387.

Peterson, L., Harbeck, C., Chaney, J., Farmer, J., & Thomas, A. M. (1990). Children's coping with medical procedures: A conceptual overview and integration. *Behavioral Assessment, 12*, 197–212.

Peterson, L., & Toler, S. M. (1986). An information seeking disposition in child surgery patients. *Health Psychology, 5*, 343–358.

Prins, P. J. M. (1985). Self-speech and self-regulation of high- and low-anxious children in the dental situation: An interview study. *Behaviour Research and Therapy, 23,* 641–650.

Robins, P. M. (1987). Coping responses and adaptational outcomes of children undergoing orthopedic surgery. *Journal of Clinical Child Psychology, 16,* 251–259.

Savedra, M., & Tesler, M. (1981). Coping strategies of hospitalized school-age children. *Western Journal of Nursing Research, 3,* 371–384.

Siegel, L. J., & Peterson, L. (1980). Stress reduction in young dental patients through coping skills and sensory information. *Journal of Consulting and Clinical Psychology, 48,* 785–787.

Suls, J., & Fletcher, B. (1985). The relative efficacy of avoidant and nonavoidant coping strategies: A meta-analysis. *Health Psychology, 4,* 249–288.

Tarnow, J. D., & Gutstein, S. E. (1983). Children's preparatory behavior for elective surgery. *Journal of the American Academy of Child Psychiatry, 22,* 365–369.

Toler, S. M. (1985). The relationship between preoperative information and coping styles in children undergoing surgery. (Doctoral dissertation, University of Illinois, Urbana). *Dissertation Abstracts International, 45,* 3634B.

CHAPTER 9

Stress, Coping, and Metabolic Control Among Youngsters with Diabetes

ALAN M. DELAMATER
University of Miami School of Medicine

It is well known that potent stress has major effects on metabolism in normal, nondiabetic individuals by increasing production of hormones that result in elevated levels of blood glucose. It is not surprising, therefore, that stress can have deleterious effects on diabetic individuals, who are unable to metabolize glucose because of a relative or absolute insulin deficiency. Conventional wisdom among patients with diabetes, their family members, and health care professionals is that stress is indeed a significant contributing factor in disruption of metabolic control. Presumably, stress affects metabolic control directly via physiological mechanisms (i.e, counterregulatory hormones), indirectly by interfering with regimen compliance, or through both pathways. Of course, whether or not a stressor has adverse effects for individuals depends on how the event is perceived and how effectively they cope with the stressor (Lazarus & Folkman, 1984).

The purpose of this chapter is to review the empirical literature regarding the effects of psychological stress and coping styles among children and adolescents with Type I diabetes mellitus. Because the literature focusing on these issues in diabetic youths is relatively small, relevant findings from the adult literature are also considered. First, the effects of stress are discussed; this discussion covers studies employing experimentally induced stressors in the laboratory, studies using questionnaire methodologies, and studies conducted in patients' natural environments with self-monitoring of stress and blood glucose. The effects of coping on health outcomes are then reviewed, including studies concerned with identifying predictors of coping styles, as well as research examining the effects of interventions (e.g., stress management training) to improve coping. Methodological issues and directions for future research are discussed at the conclusion of each of the major sections of the chapter.

EFFECTS OF PSYCHOLOGICAL STRESS

Laboratory-Based Studies

A number of early studies investigated the effects of acute experimentally induced stress on a variety of physiological variables in adult diabetic patients. Reviews of this literature have noted the inconsistency of findings and have identified several methodological problems, including heterogeneous or biased samples, lack of experimental control over stressors, failure to control for effects of insulin and carbohydrate ingestion, and need for reliable measures and appropriate statistical tests (Barglow, Hatcher, Edidin, & Sloan-Rossiter, 1984; Lustman, Carney, & Amado, 1981).

Recent controlled laboratory studies have clearly shown that adult patients with Type I diabetes do have an enhanced glycemic response to physiological levels of epinephrine (Berk et al., 1985; Shamoon, Hendler, & Sherwin, 1980). Therefore, if psychological stress is severe enough, it can be expected to result in metabolic decompensation. Two recent studies with improved methodologies have been conducted with adult patients with Type I diabetes. Kemmer et al. (1986) found that whereas acute psychological stress caused significant increases in cardiovascular responses and catecholamines, the experimental stressors (mental arithmetic and public speaking) did not have an adverse impact on metabolic control. Studies by Carter, Gonder-Frederick, and colleagues (Carter, Gonder-Frederick, Cox, Clarke, & Scott, 1985; Gonder-Frederick, Carter, Cox, & Clarke, 1990) have shown the importance of individual differences in the stress–blood glucose relationship: Blood glucose changes were found to be idiosyncratic but reliable, with some patients demonstrating increases while others had decreases in blood glucose.

Few controlled investigations have been conducted on the physiological effects of psychological stress in youngsters with diabetes. Results of clinical studies by Baker and colleagues (Baker, Barcai, Kaye, & Haque, 1969; Baker, Minuchin, Milman, Liebman, & Todd, 1975) suggest that diabetic youths have a more rapid increase of blood ketones following epinephrine infusion than do normal children, and that beta-adrenergic blockade may prevent hyperglycemia due to stress. These investigators also have proposed that family stress may precipitate ketoacidosis in "psychosomatic" children directly via physiological mechanisms (Minuchin, Rosman, & Baker, 1978); however, these studies used small, select samples of children and families, thereby limiting the generalizability of the findings.

My colleagues and I (Delamater, Bubb, et al., 1988) evaluated the physiological effects of acute psychological stress in a sample of 31 adolescents. Patients were studied in the morning after an overnight fast and prior to insulin injection. A number of cardiovascular, hormonal, and metabolic variables were measured before and after three 10-minute stressors (a cognitive quiz and two family interaction tasks) administered over 80 minutes. Significant increases in subjective stress ratings and cardiovascular responses were observed, but significant hormonal and metabolic changes as a result of the stressors were not observed. Mean stress reactivity was similar in subgroups of patients defined by levels of metabolic control. However, post hoc analyses of subgroups based on individual differences in stress reactivity suggested that those who showed increases in blood glucose to the family interaction tasks were in chronically poor metabolic control.

Another laboratory study of the physiological effects of psychological stress in adolescents was conducted recently by Gilbert, Johnson, Silverstein, and Malone (1989). Thirty 11- to 18-year-old patients (15 in good and 15 in poor metabolic control) and 15 nondiabetic controls participated in a 32-minute session during which three stressors (a venipuncture and two 3-minute public speaking tasks) were administered. Diabetic patients were tested after taking their usual insulin doses the night before and morning of the experiment. Heart rate and skin conductance were measured throughout the experimental session, and metabolic measures were obtained at the beginning and end; self-report stress ratings were obtained after each stressor. Results showed similar stress reactions in all three groups and no evidence of metabolic decompensation as a result of the stressors.

Stabler et al. (1987) conducted a study in order to determine whether individual differences in Type A behavior could account for differential glycemic response to stress. Twenty-one 8- to 16-year-old diabetic patients participated in the study; 10 were rated as Type A and 11 as Type B on the Matthews Youth Test for Health. On the morning of the experiment, children had their usual breakfast and insulin at home. Blood glucose was measured at the clinic at 11 A.M., followed by a standard meal. Two hours later, another blood glucose test was conducted and patients played a stressful video game for 10 minutes, after which blood glucose was again measured.

Although there were no differences in blood glucose prior to the stress condition, Type A children had significantly higher blood glucose after the stress. The 10-minute stressor increased Type A children's mean blood glucose by approximately 14 mg/dl, whereas Type B children's blood glucose decreased by about 50 mg/dl—an unexpected finding. The differences observed in glycemic stress responses of Type A and Type B children were apparently not due to differences in postprandial metabolism. However, given that insulin administration was not controlled for the morning of the experiment, this could potentially be accounted for by differences in long-lasting (i.e., NPH) insulin, particularly if Type A patients had less. Conclusions about hyperglycemic responses to stress in Type A diabetic children must be reserved until further studies with larger samples are conducted.

Questionnaire Studies

Studies investigating the relationship of stressful experiences of daily life to metabolic control among adults have shown associations between increased stress and glycosuria (Bradley, 1979) and elevated glycosylated hemoglobin (GHb, a measure of average blood glucose in the preceding 2-3 months) levels (Cox, Taylor, Nowacek, Holley-Wilcox, & Pohl, 1984; Frenzel, McCaul, Glasgow, & Schafer, 1988). Anxiety and depression have also been associated with GHb levels in adults (Mazze, Lucido, & Shamoon, 1984).

Several studies have been reported concerning life stress and metabolic control among diabetic youths. Chase and Jackson (1981) studied 84 children and adolescents ages 6-18 years, and found frequency of stressful life events in the preceding 3 months (as measured by the Coddington [1972] Life Events Record) to be associated with elevated GHb ($r = .41$), triglyceride ($r = .45$), and cholesterol ($r = .30$) levels. Analyses by age group (6-11, 12-14, and 15-18 years) indicated significant correlations only for older adolescents. The mean stress scores for a subgroup of 12 children with one or more hospitalizations for diabetic ketoacidosis (DKA) during the preceding 3 months were significantly higher than those for youths without DKA.

In a study of 141 youths from 10 to 17 years of age attending a summer camp, Brand, Johnson, and Johnson (1986) found negative life stress during the past year (as measured by the Johnson & McCutcheon [1980] Life Events Checklist) to be associated with worse metabolic control, reflected by higher urine ketones ($r = .18$). Further analyses indicated that this relationship varied as a function of age, sex, and locus of control. Partial correlational analyses revealed that negative life events were associated with urine ketones in young (10-12 years of age) male patients ($r = .41$) with internal locus of control ($r = .57$). It should be noted these subgroups were composed of fairly small samples ($n = 26$ and $n = 28$, respectively). Stress was not related to measures of GHb in this study, however.

My colleagues and I (Delamater, Smith, Lankester, & Santiago, 1988b) investigated the relationship between stressful life events, as well as general and diabetes-specific everyday stress or hassles, and metabolic control as determined by GHb in a sample of 47 adolescents. Patients were administered the Life Events Checklist and newly developed questionnaires measuring general hassles in the past month (General Stress Questionnaire, or GSQ) and diabetes-related hassles (Diabetes Stress Questionnaire, or DSQ). The GSQ and DSQ each contain 65 items, which are rated on a 4-point scale indicating the degree of stress ("not at all" to "very much"). Internal consistency and test–retest reliability were satisfactory for both the GSQ and DSQ total scores and rationally derived subscales.

Results showed significant relationships between GHb and both frequency ($r = .42$) and intensity ($r = .31$) of negative life events during the past year, as well as frequency ($r = .34$) and intensity ($r = .31$) of positive life events. Significant correlations were also obtained between GHb and the total DSQ score ($r = .31$), as well as its subscales for stress related to glucose testing, dietary compliance, insulin use, and relationships with parents (all p's $< .04$). Significant relationships were not observed between GHb and GSQ scores, age, sex, diabetes duration, socioeconomic status, or self-reported and parent-rated measures of regimen compliance. Analyses of sex differences revealed greater frequency and intensity of positive life events and more diabetes-related stress among girls. Whereas positive life events were associated with GHb among only girls, frequency of negative life events was related to GHb for both boys and girls. However, diabetes-related stress was associated with GHb only for boys. These results suggest that stress is a significant correlate of metabolic control among diabetic adolescents and that sex differences and type of stress are significant determinants of this relationship.

It is apparent that the family environment and relationships can be significant sources of stress for children and adolescents (La Greca, 1988). Thus another line of research in the pediatric diabetes literature has focused on family factors in relation to regimen compliance and metabolic control. A number of studies have shown that family functioning is correlated with youths' regimen compliance and metabolic control (e.g., Anderson, Miller, Auslander, & Santiago, 1981; Hanson, Henggeler, & Burghen, 1987a). Because the role of the family is covered in detail in another chapter in the current volume (see Hanson, Chapter 10), it is not covered further in this chapter.

Naturalistic Studies

Besides attempts to induce stress in the laboratory or reliance on patients' retrospective ratings of stress, another methodology to study the stress-blood glucose relationship uses self-monitoring of stress and blood glucose levels by patients on a daily basis in their natural environments. This methodology has the advantages of greater external validity; decreased time intervals between stressors and ratings of their effects; and mulitple measurements over time, permitting evaluation of individual differences. A recent study conducted with adults showed significant stress effects for 7 of 15 patients; the mean (across all patients) percentage of variance in blood glucose accounted for by stress, independent of diet and exercise effects, was 10% (Halford, Cuddihy, & Mortimer, 1990). Only a few studies using this type of methodology have been conducted so far with diabetic youths.

Hanson and Pichert (1986) observed a significant association between negative daily stress and mean blood glucose over a 3-day period among 39 youngsters (mean age = 13.8 years) at a summer diabetes camp. The correlation between negative cumulative stress (i.e., frequency and intensity of stressors) and blood glucose was .38 with the effects of diet and exercise partialed out, and .27 with those effects not considered. This study was noteworthy from a methodological perspective because subjects completed a daily measure of stress (a 36-item questionnaire), blood glucose was measured four times for each of the 3 days, and the analyses statistically controlled for the effects of carbohydrate ingestion and exercise.

We (Tomakowsky, Delamater, Boardway, & Gutai, 1991) examined the relationship of daily stress and emotions to blood glucose in an intensive study of eight adolescents (mean age = 15 years) conducted over a 2-month period. Patients were instructed to self-monitor daily stress (on a scale of 1–7) and emotions (coded positive or negative) prior to blood glucose measurement. Memory reflectance meters were used to measure blood glucose; meters were equipped with electronic logbooks that recorded time of day and blood glucose, as well as stress and emotion ratings. The mean number of observations recorded per subject was 71 (range = 22–122).

Analysis of variance (subject × emotion × time of day) showed significant effects of subject, time of day (A.M. vs. P.M.), a subject × time interaction, and a subject × emotion interaction, indicating individual differences in the relationship between emotions and blood glucose. Individual analyses revealed a significant main effect of negative emotion (higher blood glucose) for one subject and a significant time × emotion interaction for another subject (with higher blood glucose associated with negative emotions after noon). Multiple-regression analyses, controlling for time of day, showed significant effects of stress on blood glucose for one of eight subjects (higher blood glucose with increased stress), with 11% of the variance in blood glucose accounted for by stress after time of day was controlled for. These findings indicate that individual differences are important in understanding the relation of stress and negative emotions with blood glucose levels among diabetic adolescents, and they provide support for the hypothesis that some patients exhibit increased blood glucose to stress and negative emotions.

Methodological Issues and Future Research

The effects of stress in diabetic individuals have been investigated in laboratory studies with experimentally induced stressors; by means of questionnaire ratings of retrospective stress levels in correlational studies; or through self-monitoring of stress and blood glucose in the natural environment in prospective studies. Each of these methodologies has certain advantages and disadvantages. Although laboratory methods allow better experimental control, the external validity of stressors may be limited. Questionnaire ratings may be subject to bias and imprecision related to the retrospective nature of the measures, but have the advantage of covering a relatively large span of time, which is a benefit in correlational studies with measures of long-term metabolic control. Studies in the patients' natural environments have more ecological validity, but ultimately rely upon the accuracy of self-monitoring in fairly motivated and compliant individuals. Patients who participate in extensive self-monitoring protocols may therefore not be representative of diabetic patients in general.

Most of the research on stress effects in diabetic youths has relied on questionnaire methods. Despite the fact that different measures have been used, most of these studies have shown a significant relationship between life stress or diabetes-specific stress and metabolic control. In general, correlations in the .20–.40 range have been reported. Thus, the magnitude of the relationship is not statistically impressive, accounting for about 10% of the variance in GHb. Results from naturalistic self-monitoring studies also indicate that about 10% of the variance in blood glucose can be accounted for by stress. However, it is important to note that this effect is averaged across many subjects; in some there are no effects of stress, whereas others may show a more substantial and clinically significant effect.

The notion that individual differences are important in understanding the relationship between stress and blood glucose has received strong support in both experimental and naturalistic studies with adults. Yet only three experimental studies and two naturalistic studies with diabetic youths have been reported. Results have been consistent with the adult studies, but more research in this area is needed, especially with these methodologies. Both laboratory-based experimental and naturalistic studies must control for the effects of carbohydrate intake, insulin use, exercise levels, and time of day (i.e., diurnal effects) in sorting out the effects of stress on blood glucose. This research should be directed toward identification of subgroups of patients who appear to be stress-responsive—both those whose blood glucose increases and those who show decreases with stress. For example, there is some evidence that Type A behavior may be associated with increased blood glucose response to stress. This notion has theoretical support as well, in that Type A behavior in nondiabetics is associated with increased sympathetic arousal under certain conditions; activation of the sympathetic nervous system would have counterregulatory effects on blood glucose via stress hormones. More research into this possibility is needed in studies of diabetic youths.

Little is known about the types of stressors that may have an impact on metabolic control. A developmental perspective would be helpful in developing a taxonomy of stressors that have potential significance among diabetic youths of various ages, disease duration, gender, and socioeconomic status. This really is a measurement issue as well as a conceptual issue. Besides the life events approach, for which standardized instruments are available, disease-specific measures of stress offer investigative advantages. Work in this area is just beginning. It would be informative and clinically valuable to know the expected effects of various stressors for subgroups of children defined by age and relevant demographic factors.

The nature of the stress–blood glucose relationship has not been entirely worked out in terms of the mechanisms involved. At this point, there appears to be more support for the idea that stress has a direct effect on metabolic control via physiological mechanisms, rather than exerting its impact via disrupted regimen compliance. Of course, either or both may operate in individual cases. Controlled laboratory investigations using epinephrine infusions to physiological levels would be helpful in documenting the impacts of stress on blood glucose with both diabetic and nondiabetic youths, as in previous studies with adults. In addition, more studies are needed to explore the possibility that stress has adverse effects on metabolic control via regimen noncompliance.

EFFECTS OF COPING

It is clear that the effects of stress in patients with chronic illness depend upon how events are appraised and how effectively individuals respond to the stressor (Felton & Revenson, 1984; Lazarus & Folkman, 1984). For example, in a study of diabetic adults, avoidant coping was associated with poorer metabolic control (Frenzel et al., 1988). In this section, empirical research focusing on coping processes—that is, appraisal, attributions, perceived control, and specific ways of coping or coping styles—is reviewed according to the type of methodology employed. In addition, studies concerned with predictors of coping, cognitive factors related to health outcomes, and interventions to improve coping in diabetic youths are discussed.

Questionnaire Studies

My colleagues and I (Delamater, Kurtz, Bubb, White, & Santiago, 1987) investigated the relationship of stress and coping to metabolic control in a study of 27 youths (mean age = 15 years). Patients completed the Ways of Coping Checklist (Folkman & Lazarus, 1980) in relation to a recent personal stressor, and also completed measures of anxiety and hassles. Although the stress measures were unrelated to the measure of metabolic control (GHb), the Ways of Coping Checklist differentiated patients in good versus poor metabolic control: Those in poor control scored significantly higher on the Wishful Thinking ($r = .49$) and Avoidance/Help Seeking ($r = .46$) subscales, as well as on total coping ($r = .43$). Cognitive appraisal was also related to metabolic control status, with patients in poor control reporting an inhibited pattern. These findings are suggestive of a pattern of avoidance and inhibition among youths in poor metabolic control; however, this study was limited by a relatively small sample and a possible confound of the coping measure with type of stress referred to in completing the checklist (more patients in poor control reported a diabetes-related stressor).

In a subsequent study (Delamater, Smith, Lankester, & Santiago, 1988a), 47 adolescents completed the Ways of Coping Checklist once with reference to a recent stressful diabetes-related event and then again with reference to a non-diabetes-related stressor. Although general and disease-specific coping measures were significantly correlated (all r's > .51), the diabetes-specific coping measures were more strongly related to GHb. Worse metabolic control was associated with higher scores on Self-Blame ($r = .49$), Keeps to Self ($r = .32$), and Wishful Thinking ($r = .29$) in coping with diabetes-related stress; a higher score on Seeking Social Support in coping with general stress was also associated with worse metabolic control ($r = .38$). These findings are consistent with our previous results (Delamater et al., 1987), lending support to the concept that the ways in which young patients cope with stress are important factors in their metabolic control. Further support for the importance of this avoidant pattern of coping with diabetes-related stress was provided in a recent study of 60 adolescents (Delamater et al., 1990). A composite coping variable was created—"maladaptive coping"—by summing the scores on the Detachment, Keeps to Self, Self-Blame, and Wishful Thinking subscales from the Ways of Coping Checklist; maladaptive coping correlated significantly with GHb ($r = .41$).

Hanson et al., (1989) investigated coping styles in relation to health outcomes and predictors of coping styles in a sample of 135 diabetic youths (mean age = 14.5 years). Besides completing measures of life stress and family environment, patients completed the Adolescent— Coping Orientation for Problem Experiences (A-COPE; Patterson & McCubbin, 1987), a 54-item questionnaire in which frequencies of specific coping behaviors are rated. Second-order factor analysis revealed two coping styles: (1) utilizing personal and interpersonal resources, and (2) ventilation and avoidance. Although coping was unrelated to the measure of metabolic control (GHb), the ventilation and avoidance style was significantly associated with regimen compliance, with more frequent use of this coping style related to worse compliance. Mulitiple-regression analysis revealed that this coping style was predicted by older age, lower family cohesion, and higher levels of stress; lower family adaptibility was also related to this coping style among youths with longer diabetes duration.

Another study by these investigators (Hanson, Henggeler, & Burghen, 1987b), including 104 adolescents, showed that social competence of the adolescent buffers the relationship between stress and metabolic control, such that youths with higher levels of social competence are protected from the adverse effects of stress on metabolic control. Stress was not associated with regimen compliance, but parental support of the regimen was related to improved compliance. Thus, these findings support the view that stress exerts its adverse effects directly on metabolic control (presumably through physiological mechanisms) rather than indirectly through regimen compliance. Furthermore, these data indicate the important role of individual differences in psychosocial functioning in mediating the relationship between stress and metabolic control.

In the Hanson and Pichert (1986) study of daily stress and metabolic control of adolescents at camp (see "Effects of Psychological Stress," above), additional data were provided concerning the role of perceptions of adjustment to stressors. On each of the 3 days of data collection, participants rated their adjustment to each stressor on a scale from 0 to 5 ("very poorly" to "very well"), reflecting perceptions of the adequacy of their coping efforts. After the effects of diet and exercise were controlled for, adjustment to stress was marginally associated with average blood glucose levels ($r = -.37$); this relationship was significant in the analyses of the 17 boys in the sample ($r = -.52$), suggesting that perception of control over stress is associated with improved glucose levels.

Although not focusing on specific types of coping responses to stress, several other studies using questionnaire or rating methods have concerned cognitive factors relevant to the coping process among diabetic youths, particularly beliefs about the controllability of events and the ability to have an impact on them. Self-efficacy (Bandura, 1977) and learned helplessness (Seligman, 1975) are two cognitive constructs pertinent to coping reserach. Self-efficacy among diabetic adolescents was studied by Grossman, Brink, and Hauser (1987). These investigators developed a diabetes-specific self-efficacy scale and showed in a study of 68 patients that self-efficacy was significantly associated with average blood glucose levels ($r = .31$), as well as a total medical index score ($r = .25$) comprised of blood glucose, urine glucose, urine acetones, and 24-hour glycosuria measures. We (Kuttner, Delamater, & Santiago, 1990) investigated the relationships among the learned helplessness attributional style, depression, regimen compliance, and metabolic control in a study of 50 adolescents. Learned helplessness was significantly associated with depression and metabolic control ($r = .31$ with GHb), but was not related to measures of regimen compliance.

Interview Studies

Semistructured interviews were used by Tennen, Affleck, Allen, McGrade, and Ratzan (1984) to examine relationships among causal attributions, perceived control over health outcomes, coping, and metabolic control in a study of 32 children (mean age $= 11$ years). Ratings on all variables were made by physicians and nurses. Results showed that perceived control was not related to overall coping. However, children who made behavioral (i.e., internal or self-blame) attributions concerning the cause of their diabetes were rated as coping better with their illness and as being in better metabolic control. In addition, children in better metabolic control were rated as coping more successfully. The significance of these findings is limited by several methodological problems, however. For example, the coping measure had low reliabilities and was potentially biased by rater knowledge of metabolic control. The importance of causal attributions about the origin of diabetes is theoretically not as significant as the role of attributions about current levels of functioning.

Two longitudinal studies have investigated coping strategies of children during their adjustment to newly diagnosed diabetes. Kovacs, Brent, Steinberg, Paulauskas, and Reid (1986) interviewed 74 preadolescents and their parents soon after diagnosis and two additional times during the first year of diabetes. Cognitive and behavioral coping strategies were identified and then related to measures of psychological adjustment. Common behavioral strategies included involving friends in various aspects of diabetes management and seeking information about diabetes; common cognitive strategies included wishful thinking ("I wish I did not have it"), shock and bewilderment ("Why me?"), and thoughts of forbidden foods. A global index of coping was unrelated to age, sex, or various measures of psychological adjustment throughout the first year.

Jacobson et al. (1990) studied the effects of coping and psychosocial adjustment on regimen compliance in a prospective study of 61 newly diagnosed patients (9–16 years old) over the first 4 years of diabetes. Measures of coping and adjustment were obtained shortly after diagnosis. Coping measures included locus of control, defense mechanisms, and adaptive strengths; the latter two were rated by examiners from a semi-structured interview. Psychosocial adjustment was assessed by ratings provided by parents and patients, using standardized measures of self-esteem, behavior problems, social competence, and diabetes-specific adjustment. Regimen compliance ratings were made by health care team members after outpatient visits; the 4-year mean of compliance ratings was used in the analysis. Regression analysis indicated that, after patient age was controlled for, higher levels of compliance were predicted by better psychosocial adjustment and more mature defense mechanisms. Although these results suggest the importance of initial coping styles and psychosocial adjustment as predictors of regimen compliance among newly diagnosed children, several methodological problems qualify the findings, including low interrater reliabilities for the coping and compliance measures, and possible confounding of these measures with knowledge of metabolic control.

Band (1990) explored the role of cognitive development in children's coping with diabetes. Thirty-two pre-formal-operational (mean age = 8.8 years) and 32 formal-operational (mean age = 14.6 years) youths participated in structured interviews addressing how they coped in relation to three broad issues (staying well, being happy, and having diabetes in general) and five specific stressors of diabetes (diet, insulin injections, insulin reactions, glucose testing, and hemoglobin A1 tests). Children described their coping strategies and rated the controllability of stressors and the effectiveness of their coping efforts. Coping responses were coded as primary (concerned with influencing the objective events or conditions) or secondary (concerned with influencing subjective state), and also as instrumental, cognitive, or social–emotional. Adequate reliabilities were obtained for the coping ratings. Medical adjustment was measured by physician or nurse ratings (on a scale of 1–5) of five indices: GHb, glucose test records, compliance with diet, cooperation with the regimen, and overall ease of managing the diabetes.

Coping responses were analyzed first for developmental effects and then in relation to the measure of medical adjustment. Results showed greater secondary coping among formal-operational children, with more cognitive strategies than pre-formal-operational children, who exhibited greater use of instrumental strategies. Cognitive-developmental differences were not observed in perceived control or coping efficacy. Both cognitive development and coping style (primary–secondary) main effects on medical adjustment were observed: Better adjustment was associated with primary coping and pre-formal-operational children. Although subjects with diabetes of less than 1 year's duration were excluded from the study, this finding may be confounded by diabetes duration, because younger children generally have better regimen compliance and metabolic control. Confidence in the role of primary coping in overall medical adjustment would be greater with an analysis controlling for the effects of both age and duration. It should be noted that although the medical adjustment measure had high internal consistency, interrater reliabilities were not reported. Furthermore, this measure confounded regimen compliance and metabolic control with raters who may be biased by knowledge of either.

In another report based on these same subjects, Band and Weisz (1990) explored the relationship among cognitive development, coping styles, diabetes knowledge, and psychosocial adjustment. Two measures of child adjustment were provided by parent ratings: a general measure (the Conners Parent Rating Scale), and a diabetes-specific measure created for the study (the Socio-behavioral Adjustment Scale, consisting of seven items addressing specific self-care behaviors and social behavior). Results of multiple-regression analyses showed that perceived control over stress predicted somatic problems in pre-formal-operational children; perceived coping efficacy predicted conduct problems in formal-operational children; and perceived coping efficacy and primary–secondary coping predicted diabetes-specific adjustment in social behavior. Relatively little variance was accounted for in these analyses, however. In general, these findings are qualified by the low internal consistency of the diabetes-specific adjustment measure and the rather high probability of statistically significant findings' being due to chance. However, these reports underscore the importance of developmental factors in understanding the relationships among coping and disease-related variables.

Studies of Coping Interventions

If we assume that stress is a significant factor in control of diabetes and that coping styles influence the impact of stress on compliance and metabolic control, interventions to improve coping with stress would be expected to have beneficial effects for diabetic individuals. Stress management training has been explored with diabetic patients, although most studies have been conducted with adults and have employed few patients in either case studies or small-group designs. Coping interventions with adults have primarily used relaxation procedures; the few studies available with youths have used anxiety management training, including the use of relaxation, or social coping skills training.

Interventions to reduce stress through electromyographic biofeedback and home relaxation practice resulted in decreased insulin requirements in two case studies with adults (Fowler, Budzynski, & Vandenbergh, 1976; Seeburg & DeBoer, 1980). Fifteen weekly sessions of biofeedback-assisted relaxation reduced the daily range of blood glucose in a study of five adults, but did not improve GHb average glucose levels, or insulin requirements (Landis et al., 1985). In a study of 10 adults in poor metabolic control who practiced biofeedback-assisted progressive muscular relaxation, compared with 10 matched patients who were treated conventionally, relaxation therapy did not improve glucose tolerance after 1 week of frequent practice, nor did it improve GHb levels or insulin dose requirements after 6 weeks of home practice (Feinglos, Hastedt, & Surwit, 1987). More positive effects of relaxation on metabolic control have been shown for adult patients with Type II diabetes (Lammers, Naliboff, & Straatmeyer, 1984; Surwit & Feinglos, 1983).

Relatively few investigations of stress management training have been reported with diabetic youths. In a study of five poorly controlled adolescent girls, anxiety management training (including relaxation) was associated with improved metabolic control as measured by urine glucose tests (Rose, Firestone, Heick, & Faught, 1983). Subjective reports of anxiety and tension, however, showed no changes. These findings are limited by possible sampling bias and imprecise measure of metabolic control, however. In addition, it is not clear that the anxiety management training was related to improved glycemic control, because regimen compliance apparently improved as well.

An alternative approach to coping with diabetes stress is social coping skills training. Five diabetic children were successfully trained in the use of effective social skills to cope with difficult diabetes-related interpersonal stressors, as demonstrated by in vivo assessment of behavior at a fast-food restaurant (Gross, Johnson, Wildman, & Mullett, 1981). In a subsequent study, six children receiving social coping skills training were compared with five who received only conventional treatment; although treated children showed significant improvements in diabetes-related social skills, they did not evidence improved metabolic control (Gross, Heimann, Shapiro, & Schultz, 1983). A similar type of peer group program targeting social situations related to regimen noncompliance was investigated by Kaplan, Chadwick, and Schimmel (1985) in a randomized study of 21 adolescents. Results showed that patients who participated in the program had significant improvements in both compliance and metabolic control.

Methodological Issues and Future Research

Whether or not stress has an adverse impact on metabolic control depends on both the nature of the stressor and the ways in which individuals cope. Research must therefore address both of these factors in explicating the stress–blood glucose relationship. However, research on the effects of coping often fails to discriminate stressful environmental events, appraisal, coping responses, and psychological outcomes, thus creating a confusing state of affairs in our understanding of the process of stress and coping among diabetic youths. For example, psychological adaptation and regimen compliance have both been considered as indices of "coping" in some studies.

In research on coping among diabetic youths, it is important to be clear about the construct itself. The problem of confounding measures of stress, coping, and psychological outcomes has been articulated previously (Lazarus, DeLongis, Folkman, & Gruen, 1985). Not only must coping measures be distinct from measures of stress and outcomes and be sensitive to the interactive environmental–individual process, but understanding of children's coping also requires measurement of social context and developmental variables (Compas, 1987). Study of children's coping behaviors is a particularly complex methodological issue; this situation is certainly made more challenging when considering coping issues in diabetic youths.

Coping can be understood in terms of its functions—either problem-focused or emotion-focused. There is good evidence that emotion-focused coping is associated with poor psychosocial adjustment in studies of adults (Folkman & Lazarus, 1980; Rohde, Lewinsohn, Tilson, & Seeley, 1990) and children (Compas, Malcarne, & Fondacaro, 1988) without chronic illness. Studies of adults with chronic illness have also provided data associating emotion-focused coping with poor health outcomes (Felton & Revenson, 1984; Frenzel et al., 1988). From the types of coping strategies employed, a pattern of avoidance, escapism, and wishful fantasy emerges. Consistent with these findings, several questionnaire studies with diabetic youths have shown a significant relationship between these avoidant coping styles (including self-blame) and poor metabolic control. Ineffective or maladaptive coping itself has been associated with increased stress levels, so it is at this point difficult to determine the process by which stress and coping affect regimen compliance and metabolic control. Future research addressing these issues could profit by prospective designs utilizing structural equation modeling.

Developmental studies have shown that emotion-focused coping strategies increase with age in nondiabetic children and adolescents (Compas et al., 1988; Curry & Russ, 1985), and, not surprisingly, among diabetic children as well (Band, 1990; Band & Weisz, 1990). Because regimen compliance and metabolic control generally worsen as children become older, it is important to control for the effects of age and duration in studies relating coping styles to health outcomes.

Emotion-based coping and avoidance in particular may not always be associated with adverse effects. Under some conditions (e.g., when stressors are uncontrollable), such coping may serve an adaptive function. Research directed toward controllability of various stressors would also be informative, as preliminary work suggests that perceptions of increased control over stressors are associated with improved blood glucose levels (Hanson & Pichert, 1986).

Given that a number of individual factors may act to increase the probability that a child feels stressed and is predisposed to react in certain ways (Compas, 1987), future research should focus on identifying moderators and mediators of the stress–blood glucose relationship. Such studies to predict coping behavior and outcomes must consider relevant aspects of both the environment (e.g., family support) and the individual (e.g., temperament, self-efficacy). In the pediatric diabetes literature, very little progress has been made in this area. It is known, however, that variables such as social competence appear to buffer the effects of stress on metabolic control (Hanson et al., 1987b). More studies identifying factors that may protect youths from the adverse effects of stress, as well as factors that may potentiate the stress effects, are needed.

One line of research from the general literature on children's coping that may be particularly pertinent to diabetes is coping in achievement contexts (e.g., Dweck & Wortman, 1982). This research has shown different coping strategies and attributions in "helpless" and "mastery-oriented" children. Diabetes management is essentially an achievement context, so similar coping patterns should hold in youths who have achieved success with the regimen and the challenge of attaining good metabolic control. Those who fail in this task should be more likely to feel helpless and to make attributions accordingly. Initial work with learned helplessness in diabetic youths has supported this idea (Kuttner et al., 1990).

Another perspective on children's coping focuses on interpersonal cognitive problem solving (Spivack & Shure, 1982). Although this research considers a limited mode of coping behavior, it has clear relevance to diabetes, in that so many of the stressors of diabetes and barriers to compliance are social in nature. Preliminary work in this area shows that interventions to improve social coping skills may benefit diabetic youths (Gross et al., 1983; Kaplan et al., 1985). In general, the literature on coping skills training in diabetic youths is very sparse, with no controlled studies of the effects of stress management procedures such as relaxation therapy and cognitive restructuring, and only a few reports of social coping skills training.

CONCLUSIONS

Psychological stress does appear to be related to metabolic control problems among diabetic youths. Only a subgroup of patients may actually be "stress responders," however. The available findings indicate that stress is associated with increases in blood glucose, but that some patients may show decreases in blood glucose with stress. The mechanism of this effect is not clear, but is most likely related to the effects of counterregulatory stress hormones. Effects of stress on blood glucose may be influenced by environmental (e.g., family supportiveness) and individual physiological (e.g., prestress blood glucose and insulin levels) and psychosocial (e.g., social competence) variables, as well as by attributions (e.g., learned helplessness) and specific coping responses (e.g., avoidant, escapist coping). The interaction of these factors over time is important to understanding the process of stress and coping in relation to regimen compliance and metabolic control. Further research of this process and controlled studies of interventions to improve coping are needed.

REFERENCES

Anderson, B. J., Miller, J. P., Auslander, W. F., & Santiago, J. V. (1981). Family characteristics of diabetic adolescents: Relationship to metabolic control. *Diabetes Care, 4*, 586–594.

Baker, L., Barcai, A., Kaye, R., & Haque, N. (1969). Beta adrenergic blockade and juvenile diabetes: Acute studies and long-term therapeutic trial. *Journal of Pediatrics, 75*, 19–29.

Baker, L., Minuchin, S., Milman, L., Liebman, R., & Todd, T. (1975). Psychosomatic aspects of juvenile diabetes mellitus: A progress report. *Modern Problems in Pediatrics, 12*, 332–343.

Band, E. B. (1990). Children's coping with diabetes: Understanding the role of cognitive development. *Journal of Pediatric Psychology, 15*, 27–41.

Band, E. B., & Weisz, J. R. (1990). Developmental differences in primary and secondary control coping and adjustment in juvenile diabetes. *Journal of Clinical Child Psychology, 19*, 150–158.

Bandura, A. (1977). Self-efficacy: Towards a unifying theory of behavior change. *Psychological Review, 84*, 191–215.

Barglow, P., Hatcher, R., Edidin, D. V., & Sloan-Rossiter, D. (1984). Stress and metabolic control in diabetes: Psychosomatic evidence and evaluation of methods. *Psychosomatic Medicine, 46*, 127–144.

Berk, M. A., Clutter, W. E., Skor, D., Shah, S. D., Gingerich, R. R., Parvin, C. A., & Cryer, P. E. (1985). Enhanced glycemic responsiveness to epinephrine in insulin-dependent diabetes mellitus is the result of the inability to secrete insulin. *Journal of Clinical Investigation, 75*, 1842–1851.

Bradley, C. (1979). Life events and the control of diabetes mellitus. *Journal of Psychosomatic Research, 23*, 159–162.

Brand, A. H., Johnson, J. H., & Johnson, S. B. (1986). Life stress and diabetic control in children and adolescents with insulin-dependent diabetes. *Journal of Pediatric Psychology, 11*, 481–495.

Carter, W. R., Gonder-Frederick, L., Cox, D. J., Clarke, W. L., & Scott, D. (1985). Effect of stress on blood glucose in IDDM. *Diabetes Care, 8*, 411–412.

Chase, H. P., & Jackson, G. G. (1981). Stress and sugar control in children with insulin-dependent diabetes mellitus. *Journal of Pediatrics, 98,* 1011–1013.

Coddington, R D. (1972). The significance of life events as etiologic factors in the diseases of children. II: A study of a normal population. *Journal of Psychosomatic Research, 16,* 205–213.

Compas, B. E. (1987). Coping with stress during childhood and adolescence. *Psychological Bulletin, 101,* 393–403.

Compas, B. E., Malcarne, V. L., & Fondacaro, K. M. (1988). Coping with stressful events in older children and young adolescents. *Journal of Consulting and Clinical Psychology, 56,* 405–411.

Cox, D. J., Taylor, A. G., Nowacek, G., Holley-Wilcox, P., & Pohl, S. L. (1984). The relationship between psychological stress and insulin-dependent diabetic blood glucose control: Preliminary investigations. *Health Psychology, 3,* 63–75.

Curry, S. L., & Russ, S. W. (1985). Identifying coping strategies in children. *Journal of Clinical Child Psychology, 14,* 61–69.

Delamater, A. M., Albrecht, D. R., Opipari, L., Quick, J., Hale, P., Postellon, D., & Gutai, J. (1990). Racial differences in psychosocial functioning of adolescents with Type I diabetes mellitus. *Diabetes, 39*(Suppl. 1), 9A.

Delamater, A. M., Bubb, J., Kurtz, S., Kuntze, J., Smith, J., White, N., & Santiago, J. V. (1988). Physiologic effects of acute psychological stress in adolescents with Type I diabetes mellitus. *Journal of Pediatric Psychology, 13,* 69–86.

Delamater, A. M., Kurtz, S. M., Bubb, J., White, N., & Santiago, J. V. (1987). Stress and coping in relation to metabolic control of adolescents with Type I diabetes. *Journal of Developmental and Behavioral Pediatrics, 8,* 136–140.

Delamater, A. M., Smith, J. A., Lankester, L., & Santiago, J. V. (1988a, April). *Relationship of coping responses to metabolic control of adolescents with diabetes.* Paper presented at the First Florida Conference on Child Health Psychology, Gainesville.

Delamater, A. M., Smith, J. A., Lankester, L., & Santiago, J. V. (1988b, April). *Stress and metabolic control in diabetic adolescents.* Paper presented at the annual meeting of the Society of Behavioral Medicine, Boston.

Dweck, C. S., & Wortman, C. B. (1982). Learned helplessness, anxiety, and achievement motivation: Neglected parallels in cognitive, affective, and coping responses. In H. W. Krohne & L. Laux (Eds.), *Achievement, stress, and anxiety.* Washington, DC: Hemisphere.

Feinglos, M., Hastedt, P., & Surwit, R. S. (1987). Effects of relaxation therapy on patients with Type I diabetes mellitus. *Diabetes Care, 10,* 72–75.

Felton, B., & Revenson, T. (1984). Coping with chronic illness: A study of illness controllability and the influence of coping strategies on psychological adjustment. *Journal of Consulting and Clinical Psychology, 52,* 343–353.

Folkman, S., & Lazarus, R. S. (1980). An analysis of coping in a middle-aged community sample. *Journal of Health and Social Behavior, 21,* 219–239.

Fowler, J. E., Budzynski, T. H., & Vandenbergh, R. L. (1976). Effects of an EMG biofeedback relaxation program on the control of diabetes. *Biofeedback and Self-Regulation, 1,* 105–112.

Frenzel, M. P., McCaul, K. D., Glasgow, R. E., & Schafer, L. C. (1988). The relationship of stress and coping to regimen adherence and glycemic control of diabetes. *Journal of Social and Clinical Psychology, 6*, 77-87.

Gilbert, B. O., Johnson, S. B., Silverstein, J., & Malone, J. (1989). Psychological and physiological responses to acute laboratory stressors in insulin-dependent diabetes mellitus adolescents and nondiabetic controls. *Journal of Pediatric Psychology, 14*, 577-592.

Gonder-Frederick, L. A., Carter, W. R., Cox, D. J., & Clarke, W. L. (1990). Environmental stress and blood glucose change in insulin-dependent diabetes mellitus. *Health Psychology, 9*, 503-515.

Gross, A. M., Heimann, L., Shapiro, R., & Schultz, R. (1983). Social skills training and hemoglobin A1c levels in children with diabetes. *Behavior Modification, 7*, 151-184.

Gross, A. M., Johnson, W. G., Wildman, H., & Mullet, N. (1981). Coping skills training with insulin dependent pre-adolescent diabetics. *Child Behavior Therapy, 3*, 141-153.

Grossman, H. Y., Brink, S., & Hauser, S. T. (1987). Self-efficacy in adolescent girls and boys with insulin-dependent diabetes mellitus. *Diabetes Care, 10*, 324-329.

Halford, W. K., Cuddihy, S., & Mortimer, R. H. (1990). Psychological stress and blood glucose regulation in Type I diabetic patients. *Health Psychology, 9*, 516-528.

Hanson, C. L., Cigrang, J. A., Harris, M. A., Carle, D. L., Relyea, G., & Burghen, G. A. (1989). Coping styles in youths with insulin-dependent diabetes mellitus. *Journal of Consulting and Clinical Psychology, 57*, 644-651.

Hanson, C. L., Henggeler, S. W., & Burghen, G. A. (1987a). Model of associations between psychological variables and health-outcome measures of adolescents with IDDM. *Diabetes Care, 10*, 752-758.

Hanson, C. L., Henggeler, S. W., & Burghen, G. A. (1987b). Social competence and parental support as mediators of the link between stress and metabolic control in adolescents with insulin dependent diabetes mellitus. *Journal of Consulting and Clinical Psychology, 55*, 529-533.

Hanson, S. L., & Pichert, J. W. (1986). Perceived stress and diabetes control in adolescents. *Health Psychology, 5*, 439-452.

Jacobson, A. M., Hauser, S. T., Lavori, P., Wolfsdorf, J., Herskowitz, R., Milley, J., Bliss, R., Gelfand, E., Wertlieb, D., & Stein, J. (1990). Adherence among children and adolescents with insulin-dependent diabetes mellitus over a four-year longitudinal follow-up: I. The influence of patient coping and adjustment. *Journal of Pediatric Psychology, 15*, 511-526.

Johnson, J. H., & McCutcheon, S. (1980). Assessing life stress in older children and adolescents: Development of the Life Events Checklist. In I. G. Sarason & C. D. Spielberger (Eds.), *Stress and anxiety* (Vol. 7, pp. 111-125). Washington, DC: Hemisphere.

Kaplan, R. M., Chadwick, M. W., & Schimmel, L. E. (1985). Social learning intervention to promote metabolic control in Type I diabetes mellitus: Pilot experimental results. *Diabetes Care, 8*, 152-155.

Kemmer, R., Bisping, R., Steingruber, H., Baar, H., Hardtmann, R., Schlaghecken, R., & Berger, M. (1986). Psychological stress and metabolic control in patients with Type I diabetes mellitus. *New England Journal of Medicine*, *314*, 1078-1084.

Kovacs, M., Brent, D., Steinberg, T., Paulauskas, S., & Reid, J. (1986). Children's self-reports of psychological adjustment and coping strategies during first year of insulin-dependent diabetes mellitus. *Diabetes Care*, *9*, 472-479.

Kuttner, M., Delamater, A. M., & Santiago, J.V. (1990). Learned helplessness in diabetic youths. *Journal of Pediatric Psychology*, *15*, 581-594.

La Greca, A. M. (1988). Children with diabetes and their families: Coping and disease management. In T. M. Field, P. M. McCabe, & N. Schneiderman (Eds.), *Stress and coping across development* (pp. 139-159). Hillsdale, NJ: Erlbaum.

Lammers, C., Naliboff, B., & Straatmeyer, A. (1984). The effects of progressive relaxation on stress and diabetic control. *Behaviour Research and Therapy*, *22*, 641-650.

Landis, B., Jovanovic, L., Landis, E., Peterson, C., Groshen, S., Johnson, D., & Miller, N. (1985). Effect of stress reduction on daily glucose range in previously stabilized insulin-dependent diabetic patients. *Diabetes Care*, *8*, 624-626.

Lazarus, R. S., DeLongis, A., Folkman, S., & Gruen, R. (1985). Stress and adaptational outcomes: The problem of confounded measures. *American Psychologist*, *40*, 770-779.

Lazarus, R. S., & Folkman, S. (1984). Coping and adaptation. In W. D. Gentry (Ed.), *Handbook of behavioral medicine* (pp. 282-325). New York: Guilford Press.

Lustman, P., Carney, R., & Amado, H. (1981). Acute stress and metabolism in diabetes. *Diabetes Care*, *4*, 658-659.

Mazze, R. S., Lucido, D., & Shamoon, H. (1984). Psychological and social correlates of glycemic control. *Diabetes Care*, *7*, 360-366.

Minuchin, S., Rosman, B., & Baker, L. (1978). *Psychosomatic families: Anorexia nervosa in context*. Cambridge, MA: Harvard University Press.

Patterson, J. M., & McCubbin, H. I. (1987). Adolescent coping style and behaviors: Conceptualization and measurement. *Journal of Adolescence*, *10*, 163-186.

Rohde, P., Lewinsohn, P. M., Tilson, M., & Seeley, J. R. (1990). Dimensionality of coping and its relation to depression. *Journal of Personality and Social Psychology*, *58*, 499-511.

Rose, M. I., Firestone, P., Heick, H.M.C., & Faught, A. K. (1983). The effects of anxiety management training on the control of juvenile diabetes mellitus. *Journal of Behavioral Medicine*, *6*, 381-395.

Seeberg, K. N., & DeBoer, K. F. (1980). Effects of EMG biofeedback on diabetes. *Biofeedback and Self-Regulation*, *5*, 289-293.

Seligman, M. E. (1975). *Helplessness: On depression, development, and death*. San Francisco: W. H. Freeman.

Shamoon, H., Hendler, R., & Sherwin, R. S. (1980). Altered responsiveness to cortisol, epinephrine, and glucagon in insulin-infused juvenile-onset diabetics: A mechanism for diabetic instability. *Diabetes, 29,* 284–291.

Spivack, G., & Shure, M. B. (1982). The cognition of social adjustment: Interpersonal cognitive problem-solving thinking. In B. B. Lahey & A. E. Kazdin (Eds.), *Advances in clinical child psychology* (Vol. 5, pp. 323–372). New York: Plenum Press.

Stabler, B., Surwit, R. S., Lane, J., Morris, M. A., Litton, J., & Feinglos, M. N. (1987). Type A behavior pattern and blood glucose control in diabetic children. *Psychosomatic Medicine, 49,* 313–316.

Surwit, R. S., & Feinglos, M. N. (1983). The effects of relaxation on glucose tolerance in non-insulin-dependent diabetes mellitus. *Diabetes Care, 6,* 176–179.

Tennen, H., Affleck, G., Allen, D. A., McGrade, B. J., & Ratzan, S. (1984). Causal attributions and coping with insulin-dependent diabetes. *Basic and Applied Social Psychology, 5,* 131–142.

Tomakowsky, J., Delamater, A. M., Boardway, R., & Gutai, J. (1991, March). *Daily stress, emotions, and blood glucose levels in diabetic adolescents.* Paper presented at the 12th Annual Meeting of the Society of Behavioral Medicine, Washington, DC.

Developing Systemic Models of the Adaptation of Youths with Diabetes

CINDY L. HANSON
Diabetes Research Group
California School of Professional Psychology, San Diego

Several current theories in child clinical psychology and developmental psychology propose that child adaptation is best understood when it is viewed within its systemic context (Henggeler & Borduin, 1990; Lerner, 1989; Mash, 1989). That is, child adaptation is associated closely with transactions occurring within and between the multiple systems (e.g., family, peer, school, health care) in which children are embedded. Moreover, the reciprocal nature of these transactions is emphasized. Although there are important differences between the various system models (e.g., the broad-based social learning approach, the behavioral–systems perspective, the multisystemic model, the ecological–systems approach), most systems theorists agree that poor psychosocial and health outcomes in the child reflect dysfunctional relationships, an inadequate fit, and/or adaptational breakdowns within or between the interrelated systems.

Within the field of pediatric psychology, researchers are beginning to develop more broad-based models of health and adaptation in children and adolescents (e.g., Hanson, 1990; Kazak, 1989; Wallander, Varni, Babani, Banis, & Wilcox, 1989). Although a historical overview of systemic approaches to health and illness is beyond the scope of this chapter (see, e.g., Engel, 1977; Schwartz, 1982), a systems approach is consistent with current developmental and family emphases in pediatric psychology and with its broadening consideration of systemic variables, such as sibling relationships, peer relations, and social support (La Greca, 1990b; Wallander, 1991). From a systems perspective, stress and coping are best understood by examining the interrelations among the developmental and individual characteristics of the child and the various organizational contexts within which the child is embedded. From this perspective, treatment efforts often involve changes within and between ecological systems.

A primary contention of this chapter is that building models that integrate biological, psychosocial, health care, and social systems is essential for understanding the interactive and contextual nature of health and adaptation. The type of model building involved in a systems approach, however, is time-consuming and costly. Nevertheless, the long-term benefits include a more complete understanding of the critical components necessary for developing efficacious preventive and therapeutic interventions in pediatric psychology. Our research group is in the process of developing multidimensional and longitudinal models of the psychosocial health and physical well-being of youths with insulin-dependent diabetes mellitus (IDDM). Figure 10.1 is a pictorial representation of a systems model that integrates our empirical findings across studies and samples. The vast majority of the associations illustrated are based on regression/beta coefficients that were derived with the consideration of important covariates. The dotted arrows represent five indirect associations between psychosocial constructs and health outcomes. Note that not all of the associations in the model have been tested within the same study. The model represents findings from multiple studies, many of which are described subsequently.

IDDM is one of the most prevalent and serious chronic illnesses in youths (LaPorte & Tajima, 1985). Kaplan (1990) suggests that only two behavioral outcomes are ultimately important in health care: longevity and quality of life. IDDM can significantly impair both outcomes because it often leads to serious major organ system complications (e.g., retinopathy and blindness, nephropathy, neuropathy, myocardial infarction, stroke). Because research seems to suggest that poor glycemic control is associated with severe short-term and long-term complications (Danowski, Ohlsen, & Fisher, 1980; Orchard et al., 1990; Pirart, 1978), the primary goal of health care interventions has been the attainment of good metabolic control. To achieve this goal, treatment has focused on promoting adherence to a complex and difficult treatment regimen. The role of contextual factors in promoting positive health outcomes is an empirical priority.

The purpose of this chapter is to describe our programmatic research efforts in developing multidimensional models of the health outcomes and psychosocial adaptation of youths with IDDM. A brief overview of the stages involved in developing models is described first, followed by a more in-depth discussion of our findings in the areas of family relations, coping processes, and life stress. Last, our current project and plans for the future are briefly highlighted.

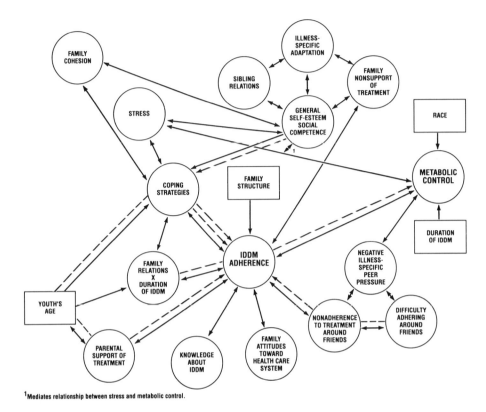

¹Mediates relationship between stress and metabolic control.

Figure 10.1. Cross-sectional associations between psychosocial factors and health outcomes (adherence and metabolic control) in youths with insulin-dependent diabetes mellitus (IDDM).

DEVELOPING AND VALIDATING MODELS OF HEALTH AND ADAPTATION

As a framework for conceptualizing programmatic research, Patterson (1986) has delineated 10 stages in building causal models:

1. Field observation and clinical experience to generate an *a priori* model.
2. Tailoring of measures for constructs (multiple modes and agents).
3. Assessment of a sample of families.
4. Structural equation modeling.
5. Revision of measures.
6. Assessment of a new sample.

7. Structural equation modeling.
8. Replication.
9. Longitudinal investigation of developmental sequences.
10. Experimental manipulation to determine causal status.

As the list indicates, the first stage entails the generation of preliminary hypotheses based on current literature and clinical experience. The second stage involves the development of instruments to measure the constructs identified in the first stage. The use of multiple respondents and multiple indices of a particular construct is essential in such development. During stage 1 of our own model-building process, we reviewed the literature on youths with IDDM (Hanson & Henggeler, 1984) and determined that there was empirical support for a multisystemic theoretical model of the psychosocial and physical adaptation of youths with IDDM. Therefore, we proceeded to stage 2 and developed an assessment battery to measure the pertinent constructs identified during stage 1.

During stage 3, the researcher uses the assessment instruments to examine relationships among key constructs in an appropriate sample. Stage 4 involves the use of statistical analyses to perform modeling techniques based on the results of the assessment in stage 3. During stage 3 of our process, the assessment battery was used to evaluate approximately 130 adolescents with IDDM and their families. We developed a path-analytic cross-sectional model in stage 4 (described later) that delineated the associations between health outcomes (i.e., adherence and metabolic control) and five key constructs: life stress, adolescent social competence, family relations, family knowledge about IDDM, and adolescent age (Hanson, Henggeler, & Burghen, 1987a). As noted previously, it is important at this stage to use multiple respondents and/or multiple indices of a particular construct whenever possible. For example, the parents' knowledge about IDDM may be as important to the health of a youth as the youth's knowledge of appropriate care (La Greca, 1988). Most of the constructs in our model were assessed with multiple measures and included information from multiple perspectives. For example, the construct of "family relations" was derived through factor analysis and included measures of four variables: marital adjustment, family cohesion, family adaptability, and parental support. Respondents included both parents for marital adjustment, and both parents and adolescents for the other three measures.

In the model we developed during stage 4 (Hanson et al., 1987a), we tested whether the five key psychosocial constructs (family relations, family knowledge about IDDM, adolescent social competence, life stress, adolescent age) were linked directly with metabolic control or linked indirectly through their associations with adherence behaviors. Newbrough, Simpkins, and Maurer (1985) had hypothesized that psychosocial constructs have indirect effects on metabolic control via their direct effects on adherence behaviors. For example, positive family relations are hypothesized to improve adherence, which then promotes good metabolic control. An additional issue that had not been addressed in previous research was the associations among the psychosocial constructs themselves in predicting health outcomes. For example, perhaps family functioning has a positive effect on health outcomes because it is associated with low stress and/or positive social competence in the child. When the influences of stress and social competence are controlled, perhaps the linkage between family functioning and health status is minimal.

The findings from this preliminary model developed during stage 4 showed that family relations were related indirectly to metabolic control through adherence behaviors, as hypothesized by Newbrough et al. (1985). The association found between family relations and adherence behaviors supports the assumptions of several investigators that positive family functioning covaries with favorable outcomes related to treatment adherence, which then relates to good metabolic control. Our findings for life stress and social competence, however, did not support the indirect model of associations. As discussed later in this chapter, the data revealed that life stress was directly associated with metabolic control; it was not indirectly associated with metabolic control via adherence behaviors, as proposed by Newbrough et al. (1985). In addition, social competence buffered the relationship between high life stress and poor metabolic control. Although family relations and stress covaried, each contributed unique variance in predicting metabolic control in our model.

The direct link between knowledge about IDDM and adherence behaviors in the model justifies the view that families of children with IDDM should be well informed regarding the most appropriate management of the disease; however, knowledge about IDDM was not linked directly or indirectly to metabolic control. Perhaps a certain level of knowledge is important, but beyond this base level, knowledge of diabetes management does not itself facilitate improved metabolic control. The knowledge measure used in the study (Johnson et al., 1982) assessed basic knowledge about the disease and problem-solving skills in daily management decisions. It is likely that both components are necessary to promote adherence to treatment. In addition, the effective *use* of the knowledge base is necessary (La Greca, 1988). Readers are referred to Hanson and Onikul-Ross (1990) for a discussion of developmentally appropriate expectations and behaviors regarding the youths' knowledge and parent–child sharing of adherence responsibilities and tasks.

Other findings in the model developed during stage 4 are consistent with developmental transitions occurring during adolescence. In our model, adolescent age had both direct and indirect effects on adherence.

In support of the direct link between adolescent age and adherence, several investigators have reported that older adolescents are less adherent to treatment (e.g., Johnson, Silverstein, Rosenbloom, Carter, & Cunningham, 1986). The mechanisms to explain this relationship had not been empirically demonstrated (La Greca, 1990a). Our data enabled us to offer some additional hypothetical as well as empirically based explanations to help clarify the association between the youths' age and adherence. In a separate study (Hanson, Cigrang, et al., 1989), we found that the relationship between older adolescent age and poor adherence was more strongly associated with the negative *coping behaviors* of older adolescents than with older adolescent *age* per se. In addition, we found that adolescent age is directly linked with parental support of treatment, which in turn is associated with treatment adherence (Hanson, Henggeler, & Burghen, 1987c). Thus, the mechanisms by which older adolescent age is associated with poor treatment adherence can be empirically explained by the indirect relationships of age to (1) coping strategies and (2) parental support of treatment. Other variables probably mediate the relationship between older age and poor adherence as well. For example, as adolescents become older and more independent, the decisions that they make regarding their behaviors are less likely to be based on health reasons and more likely to be based on social and self-esteem reasons (Chassin, Presson, & Sherman, 1987). Unfortunately, some of the non-healthy behaviors that develop during adolescence can affect health outcomes in the future, and the behavioral patterns themselves can extend into adulthood as well.

The other link between adolescent age and adherence behaviors in our model was an indirect one via family relations. Older adolescents had less positive family relations, which in turn were linked with lower adherence. These findings are consistent with some of the changes in family relations during adolescence, including more distancing of family relations, increased conflict over daily issues (e.g., schoolwork, chores, general irritations) (Montemayor, 1982; Montemayor & Hanson, 1985), and less perceived cohesiveness among older adolescents and their parents (see review by Collins, 1990). The decreased parental support (Hanson et al., 1987c) and parental responsibility for adherence tasks during adolescence (Anderson, Auslander, Jung, Miller, & Santiago, 1990; La Greca, 1988) are necessary for the youths' emancipation and successful independent functioning; however, they also relate to lowered adherence. Although some of these changes in family relations (e.g., less cohesiveness, less support) may precipitate lower adherence, poor adherence can also cause strain and less cohesiveness in the parent–teenager relationship.

It is noteworthy that a direct association between adherence and metabolic control has not been consistently demonstrated in youths (Johnson,

Freund, Silverstein, Hansen, & Malone, 1990) or adults (Glasgow, McCaul, & Schafer, 1987). In part, this is because adherence is a multifaceted construct, and some aspects of adherence are not expected to relate to levels of metabolic control (e.g., the *frequency* of testing blood glucose [unless one adjusts the dosages according to the blood glucose values], having a source of sugar readily available for hypoglycemia). Even good adherence to the treatment regimen will not relate to metabolic control if a youth is underinsulinized or if hormonal changes during puberty cause a significant deterioration in glucose control. Glycosylated hemoglobin levels also reflect mean levels of blood glucose, so youths who have blood sugar values that fluctuate above and below the ideal zone can have glycosylated hemoglobin levels similar to those of youths who have relatively stable blood glucose levels falling in the target zone. Moreover, the association between adherence and blood glucose levels is complicated by individual variability in response to behaviors related to the treatment regimen (e.g., diet, exercise). Researchers are only beginning to unveil the complexities of the relationship between adherence and metabolic control (e.g., Glasgow, 1991; Glasgow et al., 1987; Johnson et al., 1990).

Although our preliminary model developed in stage 4 was the first *empirically* derived model of the linkages between psychosocial variables and the health outcomes of adolescents with IDDM, the model has several limitations. First, the model is limited to the conceptual domains that were assessed in the study. Some potentially important variables were not considered (e.g., coping behaviors of the youths). Second, the model was based on adolescents and may not be applicable to younger children. Third, the model was based on cross-sectional rather than longitudinal data, so the temporal effects of the findings cannot be explored. Fourth, although the observed correlations between the psychosocial measures and the health outcome measures were generally equal to or greater than those observed by other investigators, a large part of the variance remains unexplained. Fifth, it seems likely that additional refinements in the measurement of constructs such as adherence may further increase the explanatory power of the model.

In Patterson's (1986) outline of the model-building process, constructs that have not contributed a significant amount of variance to the model are deleted in stage 5, and new constructs are added to the revised assessment battery. During stage 6, the assessment battery is administered to a new sample. With our second large-scale assessment of a different sample of families, our initial research studies through stage 6 included over 250 youths with IDDM assessed at different times. Results from some of these studies are described subsequently. With funding from the National Institutes of Health (Hanson, 1989), we are conducting a longitudinal assessment of approximately 250 youths and their families to further develop and empirically test our cross-sectional findings of the linkages between psychosocial variables and health outcomes. Efforts to improve our preliminary model have entailed three new components: (1) the inclusion of elementary-school-age children, (2) the inclusion of new measures to assess constructs that were not evaluated in the initial studies, and (3) the use of a longitudinal design. With the longitudinal design, we will be able to generate models to evaluate developmental trends and the differential effects of psychosocial variables, such as family and peer relations, on young children compared to adolescents.

Stage 8 entails the third cross-sectional replication of the model, if improvement of the model is needed. Such replication can be conducted on the cross-sectional data obtained during the early years of the longitudinal project. The longitudinal findings at stage 9 provide the evaluation of developmental changes over time and facilitate decisions regarding the need for further alterations in the model. The final stage involves experimental manipulation that is based on the causal model. Specifically, we will develop intervention strategies based on the findings from the longitudinal causal analyses and design a comparative treatment outcome study in which one of the treatments is based on the causal model. Prior to controlled treatment studies, however, a determination of the variables that covary with changes in psychosocial and health outcomes is essential.

THE FAMILY ENVIRONMENT

In this section, the interrelations between normal developmental processes of the youth and family, family relations, and the psychosocial and health outcomes in youths with IDDM are discussed. These studies were conducted in stages 3 through 6 of our model-building process and were based on samples of youths and families that were heterogeneous in their demographic, psychosocial, and health status characteristics. The high participation rates also enhanced the external validity of the findings. Our findings suggest that the developmental changes that occur among families of youths with IDDM are associated with important psychosocial and health outcomes in the youths. Moreover, variations in family functioning at different times during the course of the illness are associated with the youths' overall physical and psychosocial well-being.

Family Structure and Demographics

Although children with IDDM and their families are not generally at risk for psychosocial dysfunction, we hypothesized that the additional stress of living with a chronic illness might place children from single-parent households at increased risk for poor health outcomes, because of the substantial time, energy, and financial resources that may be less available in single-parent families (Hanson, Henggeler, Rodrigue, Burghen, & Murphy, 1988). Contrary to our hypotheses, children from single-parent families actually adhered better to treatment than, and did not differ in metabolic control from, their father-present counterparts. These strengths and positive outcomes exhibited by children from single-parent families are consistent with the developmental research indicating that the loss of a father can promote the development of responsible behavior in adolescents (Kurdek, 1981; Rohrlich, Ranier, Berg-Cross, & Berg-Cross, 1977; Weiss, 1979).

Because of the higher prevalence and severity of complications from diabetes, as well as higher mortality rates of African-Americans, we examined race and gender differences in metabolic control among youths with IDDM (Hanson, Henggeler, & Burghen, 1987b). We found that African-American female adolescents had worse metabolic control than either white males and females or African-American males. In addition, we examined psychosocial constructs (e.g., knowledge about IDDM, adherence to treatment, family relations, stress, social support) that might explain the poor health status of African-American females. No between-group differences were found to account for the poor health status of African-American females. Further research is needed to determine the factors that contribute to the poor health status of African-Americans with IDDM (see also Gavin & Goodwin, 1990).

Family Attitudes toward the Health Care System and Diabetes

Another relatively unexplored area of research is that of the relationships between the family and the health care system and the ways in which these interrelations are associated with health outcomes. In one of our initial studies (Hanson, Henggeler, Harris, et al., 1988), we explored whether health outcomes were associated with parents' and youths' satisfaction with physicians' personal qualities, physicians' professional competence, and the cost and convenience of medical care. In general, family members had favorable views of physicians' personal qualities and professional competence, and held relatively neutral attitudes regarding the cost and convenience of care. The youths' adherence to treatment was positively related to the youths' satisfaction with the personal qualities of physicians and to parental satisfaction with the professional competence of physicians. Thus, when youths perceived physicians as caring or parents viewed physicians as skillful, the youths tended to be more adherent to treatment.

Future research might evaluate specific variables that are linked with family members' satisfaction with the caring behaviors and professional competence of physicians and other health care professionals. Consistent with a "goodness-of-fit" model of adaptation, health outcomes should be superior when the youths' and parents' interpersonal styles complement the physicians' style. For example, families that are more authoritarian and rigid in style may respond more favorably to physicians who are more autocratic with regard to medical recommendations; likewise, flexible families may respond more favorably to health care professionals who are more democratic and authoritative in their style. The evaluation of other systemic characteristics that mediate the relationship between the family and the health care system would also be useful.

Family and Marital Relations

Several empirical investigations have examined the associations between global family relations and the health of youths with IDDM (e.g., Anderson, Miller, Auslander, & Santiago, 1981; Cederblad, Helgesson, Larsson, & Ludvigsson, 1982; Hauser et al., 1990; Klemp & La Greca, 1987). In our evaluation of family and marital factors (Hanson, Henggeler, Harris, Burghen, & Moore, 1989), we addressed some of the methodological issues (e.g., multiple perspectives, validity of the instruments) and potential confounds (e.g., spurious correlations because of highly interrelated factors, controlling for the effects of demographic characteristics) that had not been considered previously. Although our correlational results were generally consistent with earlier findings, the results changed when we evaluated how disease duration interacted with family relations in predicting metabolic control. Under conditions of short disease duration, family relations (i.e., flexible family relations, high family cohesion, and high marital satisfaction) were strongly linked to good metabolic control, but these associations were attenuated with increased duration of IDDM. Because duration of the disease and age are highly correlated, we speculated that our findings might reflect the ongoing normative developmental processes of emancipation. The competing influences of peer relations and the increased time spent away from home by older youths might lessen the effects of family relations on the youths' metabolic control. When empirically testing this hypothesis, we discovered that the duration of IDDM, not the youths' age, mediated the effects of family relations on metabolic control.

Because of the correlational nature of the study, it is not known whether these family factors contributed to a deterioration in the health of the youths early in the course of the disease, or whether the youths' poor health contributed to low cohesiveness and rigidity in family relations, as well as to parental marital dissatisfaction. From a multisystemic perspective, a recursive bidirectional model of effects is hypothesized. For example, the relationship between poor metabolic control and family rigidity may reflect attempts by parents to provide increased structure to stabilize the youths' poor control. On the other hand, family rigidity may create stress within the family or inhibit adaptive problem-solving, and thus may exacerbate metabolic control.

Importantly, the results suggest that future investigations need to consider (1) the associations between pertinent developmental variables, such as duration of IDDM, and health outcomes; (2) the *unique* effects of family relations on health outcomes; and (3) the interactions between developmental and family variables in mediating psychosocial and health outcomes.

General versus Illness-Specific Family Relations

Different models of association are hypothesized regarding the relationships between health outcomes and illness-specific versus general family relations (e.g., family cohesion). Some models posit that illness-specific interactions are stronger predictors of health outcomes than general family relations, though the findings are inconsistent (Schafer, Glasgow, McCaul, & Dreher, 1983; Schafer, McCaul, & Glasgow, 1986). For adolescents, research demonstrates that general family relations are associated with health outcomes and quality of life (Anderson et al., 1981; Hanson, Henggeler, et al., 1989; Hauser et al., 1990). From a systems perspective, general family relations are hypothesized to have direct or indirect associations with health and psychosocial outcomes. For example, as mentioned earlier, we (Hanson et al., 1987a) found a direct relationship between general family functioning and adherence, and an indirect relationship between general family functioning and metabolic control. In a subsequent study, we examined the issue of whether negative diabetes-specific parent–child interactions represented isolated problems specific to the management of the disease, or whether they were indicative of more pervasive problems for the youths and families (Hanson, Harris, Rodrigue, Cigrang, & McKee, 1989). Our results indicated that high levels of negative diabetes-specific interactions were related to worse adjustment to the illness by the youths, lower perceived competence, and more behavioral problems. In addition, families with high levels of negative diabetes-specific interactions were characterized by higher levels of general family conflict and marital strife. These findings suggest that illness-specific negative interactions need to be evaluated within the larger context of general family functioning, because interventions that focus solely on reducing parent–child tension surrounding disease management issues may not be meeting the more extensive needs of the families.

Sibling Relations

Positive affective ties between siblings can provide significant sources of emotional support throughout siblings' lives (Dunn & Kendrick, 1982), whereas excessive sibling conflict and rivalry may interfere with psychosocial adaptation (Bryant, 1982). We examined the associations between sibling relations and various aspects of the youths' general psychosocial adaptation (e.g., behavioral, emotional, and social competencies) and illness-specific adaptation (e.g., metabolic control, adherence to treatment, acceptance of the illness) (Hanson et al., in press).

Three aspects of the study addressed relative voids in the literature. First, the linkages between sibling relations and the functioning of chronically ill youths have rarely been addressed. Second, studies on the sibling relations of adolescents have focused on the correlates of sibling structural and constellation variables (e.g., birth order, sibling age), rather than on describing the types of sibling relations that are linked with youths' adaptation. Third, it is possible that associations between sibling relations and child adaptation may be attenuated when the influences of family functioning are controlled. Alternatively, parent-child dyads and sibling dyads may represent interrelated and *independent* systems within the family, and each may contribute unique variance to the youths' psychosocial and health outcomes.

Our findings showed that sibling relations, especially sibling conflict, were associated with several important dimensions of the youths' adaptation. These findings are particularly noteworthy because sibling relations added variance above and beyond that contributed by demographic characteristics, sibling constellation variables, and important dimensions of family relations. Thus, our findings suggest that in conjunction with the larger family system, the sibling dyad contributes an independent source of variance in predicting the youths' illness-specific and general psychosocial adaptation. For example, low marital satisfaction predicted sibling conflict (perhaps via marital conflict), but it was sibling conflict rather than marital satisfaction that predicted the youths' adjustment (acceptance of illness, externalizing behaviors). Likewise, sibling conflict added unique variance in predicting the youths' general self-esteem, above and beyond the effects of family cohesion. It is also likely that the associations between family relations (e.g., marital dyad, family cohesion) and sibling conflict are reciprocal. Although low levels of sibling conflict do not necessarily promote positive marital and family relations, high levels of sibling conflict undoubtedly take a toll on marital and familial relations. Although there are many systems-oriented treatment approaches, and sibling behavior may be targeted in some of these, most intervention models place little emphasis on sibling relations. In general, adolescents engage in conflict as frequently with siblings as with parents, and the issues over which they disagree and the coping strategies to resolve the issues appear similar (Csikszentmihalyi & Larson, 1984; Montemayor & Hanson, 1985). The importance of youths' coping strategies in dealing with conflict and other daily stressors within the context of the family environment is discussed next.

THE CONTEXTUAL NATURE OF COPING

Coping has been viewed as an end product of adaptation to an illness (e.g., positive adjustment or self-esteem) or as a set of behavioral, emotional, or cognitive strategies engaged in as a response to stress. Youths with chronic illnesses have often been assumed to be at risk for psychosocial difficulties because of the daily disruptions and demands of the disease. From this perspective, researchers have evaluated differences between healthy and chronically ill youths. Instead of assuming that differences imply deficits, researchers from an adaptational model of stress and coping interpret differences as adaptations to particular person-environment contexts; thus, the aspects of child competence and the family strengths that promote adaptation are emphasized (Hanson et al., 1990). Understanding the adaptational processes involved in stress and coping among children and adolescents necessitates an examination of contextual factors (Compas, 1987a; Montemayor & Flannery, 1990).

An evaluation of developmental differences in coping behaviors among children and adolescents with varying durations of the disease and across different contexts is also needed (see, e.g., Compas, 1987a; Hanson, Cigrang, et al., 1989). As IDDM progresses, the stressors of the illness vary as a function of the disease duration and the youths' developmental level (e.g., Hamburg & Inoff, 1983). Coping strategies that promote health and well-being early in the course of the disease may differ from those employed as the duration lengthens. Likewise, the effectiveness and the types of strategies chosen are mediated by the youths' developmental age. In general, developmental issues related to the health of youths with IDDM (Anderson, 1987; Johnson, 1987; La Greca, 1987) have received scant attention, in part because longitudinal studies are necessary to study developmental changes. A more thorough discussion of developmental issues related to adaptation and coping in youths with IDDM is presented in Hanson and Onikul-Ross (1990).

Coping during Early Childhood

Positive coping and happiness in young children (approximately 2 to 6 years of age) is highly dependent on their perceived sense of social acceptance, self-worth, and energy level (Harter, 1987). Harter concluded that parental support is a much stronger predictor of self-worth in these young children than are the competencies of the children. Consistent with their developmental level, young children experience parental support via the activities they share with their parents (e.g., playing with the children, reading bedtime stories) (Harter, 1989). For the young child, feelings of negative affect and poor adaptation are more likely to result from a lack of support from parents or significant others in the child's life than from having IDDM (Hanson & Onikul-Ross, 1990).

At this young age, social comparisons are used to make sure "one is getting one's fair share and is being treated like the other children" (Harter, 1983, p. 358), rather than for self-evaluative purposes. As such, the child with IDDM may feel unhappy that he or she is not allowed to eat candy like other children, but not being able to eat candy like other children is not shaping the child's perceptions of himself or herself. This is true in part because the young child is unable to reflect on the peers' view of his or her inability to eat candy. For the young child with IDDM, parental expressions of emotional and instrumental support seem most effective in building the child's emerging sense of self, and, concomitantly, successful coping with the disease.

Coping during Middle Childhood

The ability to take others' perspectives and make meaningful social comparisons emerges during middle childhood (approximately 8 to 11 years of age). The child can compare his or her abilities with those of other children and, importantly, is concerned about what peers think of him or her. The child with IDDM may become more concerned about the treatment aspects of the disease, particularly as they relate to public behavior (e.g., experiencing hypoglycemia at school, injecting insulin in front of peers). Because hypoglycemia can cause negative changes in the child's emotions (e.g., crying, anger), the child may be particularly sensitive about his or her blood glucose becoming "too low" in front of peers, especially because the ability to control one's negative emotions is an important determinant of self-worth at this age (Harter, 1983, 1988). In addition, the child may feel ashamed of the hypoglycemic reaction because of his or her new third-person awareness of the self. The child with IDDM may also be ridiculed for the hypoglycemic reaction or for other behaviors surrounding IDDM care, but he or she is certainly not alone in receiving negative feedback from peers, because verbal assaults (e.g., insults) tend to increase during middle childhood (Hartup, 1983).

A child may have negative feelings about having IDDM or the tasks related to care of the disease, but these feelings do not necessarily generalize to other aspects of his or her life, because children at this age do not integrate their competencies across the specific domains (e.g., scholastic competence, athletic competence, physical appearance) to form perceptions of themselves. If a child is feeling poorly about several areas of his or her life, *including* IDDM, the child may be expected to have low self-worth and depressed affect. From this developmental framework, a model of associations that includes an evaluation of both illness-specific and general psychosocial adaptation is critical.

Coping during Adolescence

The increasing importance of others' opinions to the child's self-worth becomes reflected by the fact that physical appearance is the most powerful predictor of self-worth for children 8 to 15 years of age and social acceptance is second, especially for young adolescents (Harter, 1990). Harter has found that self-perceptions in the domain of physical appearance correlate most highly with global self-esteem throughout the life span. The effects of IDDM on adolescents' well-being are probably mediated by issues related to the youths' physical appearance and social acceptance. Youths with IDDM are not typically disfigured unless there are concomitant complications, such as dermatological problems (e.g., Feingold & Elias, 1990). Arranging the youths' insulin injections and glucose-testing tasks so that they do not interrupt daily activities with peers may be less than ideal physiologically; however, the positive effects on perceptions of self-worth and social acceptance are important for both behavioral and physiological outcomes. For example, perceptions of positive self-regard and competence appear to buffer the negative effects of life stress on physiological outcomes (i.e., metabolic control) (Hanson et al., 1987c). In addition, if quality of life is impaired, changes are often necessary in the treatment regimen in order to enhance long-term maintenance of adherence behaviors (Glasgow, in 1991).

The opinions of significant others substantially affect adolescents' global sense of self-worth (Harter, 1990; Maccoby & Martin, 1983). As Harter (1987) has demonstrated, parental attitudes are critical in the development of positive self-worth in children, with classmate support and parental judgments becoming more nearly parallel in their significance during older childhood and early adolescence. Among older adolescents, classmate support becomes more important than parental support in perceptions of global self-worth (Harter, 1990). Interestingly, classmate support is even more salient in perceptions of self-worth than is close friendship support, and this is true across the life span. Harter proposes that close friendships provide needed support, but that the larger social mirror is more important in enhancing self-image. A youth with IDDM may feel comfortable with conducting the daily tasks related to diabetes care and adhering to the meal plan while in the presence of close friends, but may have considerable difficulty in the presence of classmates, with whom fears of negative attitudes are more prominent.

During early adolescence the youth begins to internalize standards and values, and can incorporate the opinions of others into his or her self-concept (Harter, 1990). Incorporating the often conflicting opinions of significant others (e.g., parents, peers, teachers, siblings, close friends, romantic partners) into the youths' self-perceptions can be stressful, especially during middle adolescence (approximately 14 to 15 years of age), when youths are often preoccupied with the opinions of others in these multiple networks. Although youths in middle adolescence can detect inconsistencies in self-attributes, they are not able to integrate these opposing self-attributes into a unified sense of self until late adolescence. The youth in middle adolescence may feel independent, carefree, and competent with peers, yet may feel insecure and dependent on parents in regard to the tasks and responsibilities associated with diabetes care. These two disparate images of the self can cause considerable distress for the youth during middle adolescence (Harter, 1990). Harter has also demonstrated that a powerful determinant of self-worth is the extent to which a youth's areas of greater competence match those that he or she values as important, and the areas of lesser competence are viewed with less salience. Valuing areas of greater competence and de-emphasizing areas of lesser competence is especially important for the adolescent who is coping with stressful life changes (e.g., the transitions from elementary school and junior high) (Harter, 1990).

We evaluated the contextual nature of coping, using family relations and life stress as important environmental mediators of coping responses in adolescents with IDDM (Hanson, Cigrang, et al., 1989). From a developmental perspective, we examined disease duration and adolescent age as predictors of the coping styles. Two styles of coping were factor-analytically derived: "utilizing personal and interpersonal resources" (e.g., emotional support from family members; participating in social activities and relationships; relying on personal skills to manage problems) and "ventilation and avoidance" (e.g., getting angry and blaming others for problems; avoiding the problem by minimization; and engaging in negative activities such as drinking, smoking, and using drugs).

Compas, Malcarne, and Fondacaro (1988) found that an "emotion-focused" coping style, similar to our "ventilation and avoidance," was related to emotional and behavioral problems and that its use increased with age in a sample of 10- to 14-year-old youths. Our findings suggest that this type of coping behavior is also used by older adolescents and that its use is associated with nonadherence to the IDDM treatment regimen. Because the ventilation and avoidance coping style was linked with a negative health outcome, we specifically examined the contextual nature of this coping style.

Four important contextual correlates of ventilation and avoidance were identified: older adolescent age, high life stress, low family cohesiveness, and family rigidity. We hypothesized that perhaps ventilation and avoidance coping behaviors were used more frequently among youths with high life stress because the difficulties that they were experiencing were largely uncontrollable (e.g., parents divorced or separated). Initial support for this hypothesis was confirmed with exploratory correlational analyses (Hanson, Cigrang, et al., 1989). Frequent use of ventilation and avoidance coping was associated with stressors related to family strains and responsibilities (e.g., several items related to increased arguments between parents and teenagers; a family member with emotional problems) and school strains and substance use (e.g., a family member's excessive drinking; a child/teenager suspended from school; increased parent–teenager arguments over cigarettes, alcohol, or drugs). Youths may have used ventilation and avoidance in response to the increased parent–child conflict in these families. Research indicates that adolescents use avoidance coping strategies frequently in response to parent-teenager conflict (Montemayor & Hanson, 1985). In addition, the frequent use of ventilation and avoidance by a youth may strain the family environment and increase the occurrence of stressful life events (see e.g., Compas, 1987a, 1987b).

Independent of other individual and environmental conditions, ventilation and avoidance coping strategies were also predicted by low family cohesiveness across the developmental period (i.e., the association between family cohesion and negative coping was not mediated by the youths' age). The relatively strong contribution of family cohesion is consistent with other recent research indicating that the importance of the family does not decrease in magnitude throughout adolescence; rather, the nature of the interactions changes (e.g., see Collins, 1990).

Although family cohesion was an important predictor of ventilation and avoidance coping throughout adolescence, family adaptability (i.e., rigidity) was linked to this coping style only in youths with a long duration of illness. Flexible family relations buffered the expression of maladaptive coping behaviors under conditions of long disease duration. Perhaps family relations become more rigid as the duration of the disease increases, which then results in the more frequent use of this negative coping style. Parents may also increase the structure and rules of the family in an attempt to change the youths' negative coping styles (e.g., yelling or blaming others, avoiding others). In any case, family flexibility is important in mediating the frequent use of ventilation and avoidance coping as disease duration lengthens. As mentioned previously, flexible and cohesive family relations also covaried with positive health outcomes early in the course of the disease (Hanson, Henggeler, et al., 1989). Thus, in two different temporal contexts, flexibility in family relations was associated with positive psychosocial and health outcomes. Cohesion among family members was associated with important in health outcomes during the early stages of the illness (Hanson, Henggeler, et al., 1989) and with reduced levels of negative coping behaviors during adolescence (Hanson, Cigrang, et al., 1989).

Disease duration has been a critical mediator of the links between psychosocial factors (e.g., family relations, coping styles) and health outcomes in our research. In addition to physiological changes that are occurring overtly and covertly with increased disease duration, there are additional stressors because of the *sustained* coping efforts that are necessary to manage the disease effectively (Hanson, 1990). Diabetes involves a double demand: long duration and frequent daily hassles (Wrubel, Benner, & Lazarus, 1981). Perhaps the daily hassles contribute most to the constant demands of living with IDDM (e.g., monitoring glucose levels; experiencing undesirable glycemic levels; monitoring food intake; the regularity needed in the timing of meals and other adherence tasks; monitoring glucose and food intake prior to, during, and after exercise). Band (1990) and others (Cerreto & Travis, 1984) have commented that previous concepualizations presented to children about their diabetes, such as "[Children with diabetes] can live normal lives comparable to those of their peers if they are consistently responsible in the performance of their health care behaviors" (Band, 1990, p. 29), can cause resentment and unhappiness because "there is nothing normal about multiple shots a day and constant monitoring of body systems, diet, and exercise" (Band, 1990, p. 29). The chronic nature of IDDM treatment necessitates that adaptation is viewed as a process over time; in this respect, it is not unlike other stressors, such as parental divorce and remarriage (Emery, 1988).

For youths with IDDM, daily strains are a normal part of their lives. Yet, as Kovacs and her colleagues (Kovacs, Brent, Steinberg, Paulauskas, & Reid, 1986; Kovacs, Feinberg, et al., 1985; Kovacs, Finkelstein, et al., 1985) report, children with IDDM are quite resilient. After approximately 6 months following the diagnosis of the disease, most of the initial emotional distress of the parents and youths in the study was resolved. In fact, youths with IDDM evaluated themselves positively on psychological indices (e.g., self-esteem, depression, anxiety) both at IDDM onset and 1 year later, as compared to the normative data on healthy youths. Thus, it appears that most children adapt quite well following the onset of IDDM and are not necessarily at psychological risk. Studies we have conducted (Hanson et al., 1990) indicate, first, that there are no differences in self-esteem based on age at disease onset and gender, and second, that most youths with IDDM are functioning within the normal range in important areas of self-esteem. It is important to note that prior levels of psychosocial functioning are important determinants of later psychosocial and health-related functioning (Jacobson et al., 1990), and that a period of acute distress and adjustment to the disease is to be expected.

STRESS

Several studies suggest that early adolescence is one of the most stressful times during the life span (Simmons, 1987). From a developmental framework, early adolescence (i.e., between 9–10 years and 14–15 years of age) is a time of tremendous psychosocial change and rapid physical growth, surpassed only by the period of infancy (Lerner & Foch, 1987). There are several normative stressors during this period that cause discomfort (e.g., uncomfortableness with the physical changes of puberty, changes with the transition to junior high, emergence of opposite-sex relationships, changes in the nature of peer and family relationships). One of the peak ages at which IDDM becomes overt (and is diagnosed) is during early adolescence. Whether a youth develops IDDM or already has it during this period, the biological, developmental, and psychosocial changes that are occurring also affect management of the disease (e.g., increased responsibility for adherence tasks, changes in the complexities of daily adherence behaviors associated with changes in peer relationships). During early adolescence, youths also begin to question parental authority and social expectations, and to recognize the arbitrary nature of such rules (Baumrind, 1987). For young adolescents with IDDM, these social-cognitive developmental changes precipitate increased questioning of the necessity and efficacy of adhering to the treatment regimen, especially if nonadherence to the regimen does not create major short-term problems (e.g., hypoglycemia or severe hyperglycemia). In addition, exposure to risk-taking behaviors and new situations (e.g., drugs, sexual behavior, fad diets) characterizes the advent of adolescence (Baumrind, 1987), and also poses additional stressors for youths with IDDM.

Research further suggests that youths who experience multiple stressors concurrently (e.g., a change in schools, a stressful family event, pubertal changes) also experience lowered self-esteem, worse academic performance, less involvement in extracurricular activities, and more problem behaviors (Simmons, 1987). Findings by Compas, Wagner, Slavin, and Vannatta (1986) suggest that major life transitions (e.g., entering new school, new living environment) also represent periods of greatest vulnerability to life stress on psychological symptoms. Compas, Howell, Ledoux, Phares, and Williams (1989) found that major life stressors increased daily hassles, which then predicted psychological symptoms. Based on the work of these investigators, it seems that youths may be at risk for psychological dysfunction when life stress increases the daily strains of the experience, such as during major life transitions or when multiple stressors are being experienced concurrently. Because youths with IDDM experience a greater than normal amount of daily strains in everyday life, it would be particularly interesting to examine whether life stress is most detrimental to their psychological and physical health during critical periods of significant distress (e.g., major life transitions, multiple concurrent stressors).

We examined two issues in regard to the associations between life stress and physical health outcomes (Hanson et al., 1987c). First, we assessed whether the relationships between life stress and health outcomes supported a direct or indirect model of association. That is, we evaluated whether stress and metabolic control were directly linked, or whether stress was indirectly associated with metabolic control via adherence behaviors. To our knowledge, other researchers have not tested the indirect or direct models of association between life stress and metabolic control in youths with IDDM. Chase and Jackson (1981) found an association between life stress and metabolic control in a group of 15- to 18-year-olds, but not in younger age groups. The researchers did not evaluate adherence behaviors, and thus could not evaluate the direct versus indirect models of association. Brand, Johnson, and Johnson (1986) found that urine ketones levels were associated with negative life stress in 10- to 12-year-old children who exhibited an internal locus of control. These authors did not find a relationship between life stress and metabolic control, nor did they evaluate adherence behaviors, so the direct versus indirect models of association with the outcome measure of urine ketones could not be evaluated. S. L. Hanson and Pichert (1986) evaluated 39 youths over 3 days and found a relationship between cumulative negative daily stressors and blood glucose levels, independent of the effects of diet and exercise. Because diet and exercise were not related significantly to blood glucose levels, the findings could not support the direct or indirect models of association. Other investigators have examined the life stress–health outcome relationship in adults with IDDM, but the direct versus indirect models of association were not explored (Barglow, Hatcher, Edidin, & Sloan-Rossiter, 1984; Cox et al, 1984).

In our research (Hanson et al., 1987c), a direct model of associations was supported: High life stress was associated with poor metabolic control independent of adherence behaviors. Tarnow and Silverman (1981–1982) present hypothetical models of how stress can have a negative physiological effect on metabolic control, and O'Leary (1990) discusses other deleterious effects of chronic stress on the immune system. Compas et al. (1989) suggest that the link between life stress and *psychological* adjustment is mediated by daily hassles, and that parental perceptions of stress do not relate to the youths' adjustment; rather, youths' perceptions of stress relate to parental adjustment. In our study, the life stress measure included daily strains (e.g., increased arguments between parent and teenager) as well as major life events, was composed of primarily negative events, and was based on the adolescents' perceptions. These factors may account for the significant association found between life stress and metabolic control in our study. (The effects of acute and of chronic stress on immune and endocrine functioning differ, and studies that have evaluated the effects of acute stress on glycemic control are inconsistent and are not reviewed here. See Delamater, chapter 9, for detailed discussion.)

Note that our findings do not preclude findings of an association between life stress and adherence behaviors in other samples, or perhaps a relationship between life stress and specific adherence behaviors. Nevertheless, the results are significant in empirically supporting the hypothesized direct relationship between life stress and metabolic control in youths. Because the association between adherence and metabolic control was only slightly greater than the association between stress and metabolic control, health care professionals should consider the possibility that problems in achieving good metabolic control are exacerbated by environmental stressors. Further evaluation of this direct association between life stress and metabolic control will be tested with the longitudinal data that we are presently collecting. In addition, individual variability in responsiveness to stress, diet, and exercise as they relate to health outcomes is an area that is largely unexplored and of critical importance (e.g., Halford, Cuddihy, & Mortimer, 1990).

The second purpose of our study (Hanson et al., 1987c) was to evaluate whether parental support or social competence, which reflect important dimensions in the adaptation of chronically ill children, mediated the relationship between high life stress and poor metabolic control, via either a "main effects" or a "buffering effects" model (Cohen & Wills, 1985). In the main effects model, social competence and parental support should have a beneficial effect on the youth's health, regardless of the level of stress in the youth's life. The buffering effects model asserts that the beneficial effects of social competence and parental support emerge under conditions of high stress. Our results supported a buffering effects model for social competence: Social competence buffered the negative link between high stress and poor metabolic control. For adolescents with high social competence, high stress was not associated with poor metabolic control, whereas for adolescents with low social competence, such an association did exist. Although it is possible to view social competence as a mediator of the negative effects of stress on metabolic control, it is also likely that good metabolic control enhanced the adolescents' ability to develop positive social relations and social competence. Parental support was positively associated with adherence, but it was not related to metabolic control. Perhaps parental support did not buffer the effects of stress because the support was specific to adherence behaviors (and the link between stress and metabolic control was not mediated by adherence behaviors). Further evaluation of different types of support (e.g., Cauce, Felner, & Primavera, 1982; Procidano & Heller, 1983) on positive and negative health outcomes is needed.

J. H. Johnson (1986) has suggested that buffers of life stress may have interactive or additive effects when moderating the relationships between life stress and health and adjustment. For example, Johnson cites findings from Lawrence and Russ (1985) suggesting that personal competence and social support together mediate the relationship between life stress and adjustment better than when either variable is considered alone. Although we did not test the buffering effects of social competence and global self-esteem separately, it is noteworthy that the mediator between life stress and poor glycemic control in our study was a composite score of the adolescents' perceptions of both global self-esteem and social competence (Hanson et al., 1987c). We will attempt to replicate these findings from the data that we are collecting for the larger prospective model. The effect of joy and positive events on health is another area in which research is needed (Johnson, 1986; O'Leary, 1990; Siegel & Brown, 1988).

BRIEF OVERVIEW OF CURRENT PROJECT AND FUTURE PLANS

We have received a 5-year longitudinal grant from the National Institute of Diabetes, Digestive, and Kidney Diseases (Hanson, 1989) to conduct a large-scale evaluation of the multisystemic model of health and adaptation in youths with IDDM. The major aim of the longitudinal project is to develop and empirically test our preliminary model, which is based on our initial cross-sectional studies, of the linkages among pertinent psychosocial variables (e.g., family relations, coping, stress, diet, physical activity) and health outcomes in a large sample of youths with IDDM. Approximately 250 families will be assessed three times over the course of 1 year. We will be able to evaluate developmental differences in the variables that relate to health and well-being by examining youths ranging in age from 4 to 20 years. Our long-term goals involve developing intervention strategies based on the longitudinal causal analyses and then testing the model with a controlled treatment outcome study in which one of the treatments is based on the multisystemic empirical model. I look forward to our continued efforts to develop better and more sophisticated models of the adaptation and health of youths with IDDM.

Acknowledgments

I wish to thank the numerous people who have made these studies possible. I thank Scott Henggeler for helping to shape my thinking in this area and for his continued support throughout the entire process. George Burghen's enthusiastic collaboration and expertise have been invaluable. My appreciation is also extended to Russ Glasgow, Suzanne Johnson, and Lizette Peterson for their excellent critiques, guidance, and support. I am grateful for the opportunity to have worked closely with several graduate and undergraduate students, some of whom I now enjoy as colleagues, including Michael Harris, Jeff Cigrang, and Jim Rodrigue. Sincere thanks and gratitude are extended to Angie Schinkel and Michelle De Guire, who have been tremendous in coordinating the current longitudinal project, and to Orville Kolterman, who has been instrumental in providing the additional support necessary to conduct the longitudinal project. Without the help of many youths with IDDM and their families, none of the work would have been possible. I also thank Annette La Greca for inviting me to share our work in this chapter. Preparation of this chapter was supported by the National Institute of Diabetes, Digestive, and Kidney Diseases Grant No. DK 41969 and by the San Diego State University Foundation.

REFERENCES

Anderson, B. J. (1987). Directions for pediatric diabetes research and care. *Newsletter of the Society for Pediatric Psychology, 11,* 3–7.

Anderson, B. J., Auslander, W. F., Jung, K. C., Miller, J. P., & Santiago, J. V. (1990). Assessing family sharing of diabetes responsibilities. *Journal of Pediatric Psychology, 15,* 493–509.

Anderson, B. J., Miller, P., Auslander, W. F., & Santiago, J. V. (1981). Family characteristics of diabetic adolescents: Relationship to metabolic control. *Diabetes Care, 4,* 586–594.

Band, E. B. (1990). Children's coping with diabetes: Understanding the role of cognitive development. *Journal of Pediatric Psychology, 15,* 27–41.

Barglow, P., Hatcher, R., Edidin, D. V., & Sloan-Rossiter, D. (1984). Stress and metabolic control in diabetes: Psychosomatic evidence and evaluation of methods. *Psychosomatic Medicine, 46,* 127–144.

Baumrind, D. (1987). A developmental perspective on adolescent risk taking in contemporary America. In C. E. Irwin, Jr. (Ed.), *New directions for child development: No. 37. Adolescent social behavior and health* (pp. 93–125). San Francisco: Jossey-Bass.

Brand, A. H., Johnson, J. H., & Johnson, S. B. (1986). Life stress and diabetic control in children and adolescents with insulin-dependent diabetes. *Journal of Pediatric Psychology, 11,* 481–495.

Bryant, B. K. (1982). Sibling relationships in middle childhood. In M. E. Lamb & B. Sutton-Smith (Eds.), *Sibling relationships: Their nature and significance across the lifespan* (pp. 87–121). Hillsdale, NJ: Erlbaum.

Cauce, A. M., Felner, R. D., & Primavera, J. (1982). Social support systems in high risk adolescents: Structural components and adaptive impact. *American Journal of Community Psychology, 10,* 417–428.

Cederblad, M., Helgesson, M., Larsson, Y., & Ludvigsson, J. (1982). Family structure and diabetes in children. *Pediatric and Adolescent Endocrinology, 10,* 94–98.

Cerreto, M., & Travis, L. (1984). Implications of psychological and family factors in the treatment of diabetes. *Pediatric Clinics of North America, 31,* 689–710.

Chase, H. P., & Jackson, G. G. (1981). Stress and sugar control in children with insulin-dependent diabetes mellitus. *Journal of Pediatrics, 98,* 1011–1013.

Chassin, L., Presson, C. C., & Sherman, S. J. (1987). Applications of social developmental psychology to adolescent health behaviors. In N. Eisenberg (Ed.), *Contemporary topics in developmental psychology* (pp. 353–374). New York: Wiley.

Cohen, S., & Wills, T. A. (1985). Stress, social support, and the buffering hypothesis. *Psychological Bulletin, 98,* 310–357.

Collins, W. A. (1990). Parent–child relationships in the transition to adolescence: Continuity and change in interaction, affect, and cognition. In R. Montemayor, G. R. Adams, & T. P. Gullotta (Eds.), *From childhood to adolescence: A transitional period?* (pp. 85–106). Newbury Park, CA: Sage.

Compas, B. E. (1987a). Coping with stress during childhood and adolescence. *Psychological Bulletin, 101,* 393–403.

Compas, B. E. (1987b). Stress and life events during childhood and adolescence. *Clinical Psychology Review, 7,* 275–302.

Compas, B. E., Howell, D. C., Ledoux, N., Phares, V., & Williams, R. A. (1989). Parent and child stress and symptoms: An integrative analysis. *Developmental Psychology, 25,* 550–559.

Compas, B. E., Malcarne, V. L., & Fondacaro, K. M. (1988). Coping with stressful events in older children and young adolescents. *Journal of Consulting and Clinical Psychology, 56,* 405–411.

Compas, B. E., Wagner, B. M., Slavin, L. A., & Vannatta, K. (1986). A prospective study of life events, social support, and psychological symptomatology during the transition from high school to college. *American Journal of Community Psychology, 14,* 241–257.

Cox, D. J., Taylor, A. G., Nowacek, G., Holley-Wilcox, P., Pohl, S. L., & Guthrow, E. (1984). The relationship between psychological stress and insulin-dependent diabetic blood glucose control: Preliminary investigations. *Health Psychology, 3,* 63–75.

Csikszentmihalyi, M., & Larson, R. (1984). *Being adolescent: Conflict and growth in the teenage years.* New York: Basic Books.

Danowski, T. S., Ohlsen, P., & Fisher, E. R. (1980). Diabetic complications and their prevention and reversal. *Diabetes Care, 3*, 94-99.

Dunn, J., & Kendrick, C. (1982). Siblings and their mothers: Developing relationships within the family. In M. E. Lamb & B. Sutton-Smith (Eds.), *Sibling relationships: Their nature and significance across the lifespan* (pp. 39-60). Hillsdale, NJ: Erlbaum.

Emery, R. E. (1988). *Marriage, divorce, and children's adjustment.* Newbury Park, CA: Sage.

Engel, G. I. (1977). The need for a new medical model: A challenge for biomedicine. *Science, 196*, 129-136.

Feingold, K. R., & Elias, P. M. (1990). Dermatologic complications: Associations with diabetes. *Diabetes Spectrum, 3*, 282-287.

Gavin, J. R., & Goodwin, N. (Guest Eds.). (1990). Diabetes in black populations: Current state of knowledge. *Diabetes Care, 13*(Suppl. 4), 1139-1208.

Glasgow, R. E. (1991). Compliance to diabetes regimens: Conceptualization, complexity, and determinants. In J. A. Cramer & B. Spilker (Eds.), *Patient compliance in medical practice and clinical trials* (pp. 209-224). New York: Raven Press.

Glasgow, R. E., McCaul, K. D., & Schafer, L. C. (1987). Self-care behaviors and glycemic control in Type 1 diabetes. *Journal of Chronic Disease, 40*, 399-412.

Halford, W. K., Cuddihy, S., & Mortimer, R. H. (1990). Psychological stress and blood glucose regulation in Type 1 diabetic patients. *Health Psychology, 9*, 516-528.

Hamburg, B. A., & Inoff, G. E. (1983). Coping with predictable crises of diabetes. *Diabetes Care, 6*, 409-415.

Hanson, C. L. (1989). *Cardiovascular and metabolic health in high risk youth.* National Institute of Diabetes, Digestive, and Kidney Diseases Grant No. DK41969.

Hanson, C. L. (1990). Understanding insulin-dependent diabetes mellitus (IDDM) and treating children with IDDM and their families. In S. W. Henggeler & C. M. Borduin (Eds.), *Family therapy and beyond: A multisystemic approach to treating the behavior problems of children and adolescents* (pp. 278-323). Pacific Grove, CA: Brooks/Cole.

Hanson, C. L., Cigrang, J. A., Harris, M. A., Carle, D. L., Relyea, G., & Burghen, G. A. (1989). Coping styles in youths with insulin-dependent diabetes mellitus. *Journal of Consulting and Clinical Psychology, 57*, 644-651.

Hanson, C. L., & Henggeler, S. W. (1984). Metabolic control in adolescents with diabetes: An examination of systemic variables. *Family Systems Medicine, 12*, 5-16.

Hanson, C. L., Harris, M. A., Rodrigue, J. R., Cigrang, J. A., & McKee, E. (1989). *Negative family interactions related to treatment regimen behaviors in diabetic children: Does it indicate more pervasive problems in child and family functioning?* Paper presented at the Second Florida Conference on Child Health Psychology, Gainesville.

Hanson, C. L., Henggeler, S. W., & Burghen, G. A. (1987a). Model of associations between psychosocial variables and health outcome measures in adolescents with IDDM. *Diabetes Care, 10,* 752–758.

Hanson, C. L., Henggeler, S. W., & Burghen, G. A. (1987b). Race and sex differences in metabolic control of adolescents with IDDM: A function of psychosocial variables? *Diabetes Care, 10,* 313–318.

Hanson, C. L., Henggeler, S. W., & Burghen, G. A. (1987c). Social competence and parental support as mediators of the link between stress and metabolic control in adolescents with insulin-dependent diabetes mellitus. *Journal of Consulting and Clinical Psychology, 55,* 529–533.

Hanson, C. L., Henggeler, S. W., Harris, M. A., Burghen, G. A., & Moore, M. (1989). Family system variables and the health status of adolescents with IDDM. *Health Psychology, 8,* 239–253.

Hanson, C. L., Henggeler, S. W., Harris, M. A., Mitchell, K. A., Carle, D. L., & Burghen, G. A. (1988). Associations between family members' perceptions of the health care system and the health of youths with insulin-dependent diabetes mellitus. *Journal of Pediatric Psychology, 13,* 543–554.

Hanson, C. L., Henggeler, S. W., Harris, M. A., Cigrang, J. A., Schinkel, A. M., Rodrigue, J. R., & Klesges, R. C. (in press). Contributions of sibling relations to the adaptation of youths with insulin-dependent diabetes mellitus. *Journal of Consulting and Clinical Psychology.*

Hanson, C. L., Henggeler, S. W., Rodrigue, J. R., Burghen, G. A., & Murphy, W. D. (1988). Father-absent adolescents with insulin-dependent diabetes mellitus: A population at risk? *Journal of Applied Developmental Psychology, 9,* 243–252.

Hanson, C. L., & Onikul-Ross, S. R. (1990). Developmental issues in the lives of youths with insulin-dependent diabetes mellitus. In S. B. Morgan & T. M. Okwumabua (Eds.), *Child and adolescent disorders: Developmental and health psychology perspectives* (pp. 201–240). Hillsdale, NJ: Erlbaum.

Hanson, C. L., Rodrigue, J. R., Henggeler, S. W., Harris, M. A., Klesges, R. C., & Carle, D. L. (1990). The perceived self-competence of adolescents with insulin-dependent diabetes mellitus: Deficit or strength? *Journal of Pediatric Psychology, 15,* 605–618.

Hanson, S. L., & Pichert, J. W. (1986). Perceived stress and diabetes control in adolescents. *Health Psychology, 5,* 439–452.

Harter, S. (1983). Developmental perspectives on the self-system. In E. M. Hetherington (Vol. Ed.), *Handbook of child psychology (4th ed.): Vol. 4. Socialization, personality, and social development* (pp. 275–385). New York: Wiley.

Harter, S. (1987). The determinants and mediational role of global self-worth in children. In N. Eisenberg (Ed.), *Contemporary topics in developmental psychology* (pp. 219–242). New York: Wiley.

Harter, S. (1988). Developmental processes in the construction of the self. In T. D. Yawkey & J. E. Johnson (Eds.), *Integrative processes and socialization: Early to middle childhood* (pp. 45–78). Hillsdale, NJ: Erlbaum.

Harter, S. (1989). Causes, correlates, and the functional role of global self-worth: A life-span perspective. In J. Kolligian & R. Sternberg (Eds.), *Competence considered: Perceptions of competence and incompetence across the life-span* (pp. 67–97). New Haven, CT: Yale University Press.

Harter, S. (1990). Processes underlying adolescent self-concept formation. In R. Montemayor, G. R. Adams, & T. P. Gullotta (Eds.), *From childhood to adolescence: A transitional period?* (pp. 205–239). Newbury Park, CA: Sage.

Hartup, W. W. (1983). Peer relations. In E. M. Hetherington (Vol. Ed.), *Handbook of child psychology (4th ed.): Vol. 4. Socialization, personality, and social development* (pp. 103–196). New York: Wiley.

Hauser, S. T., Jacobson, A. M., Lavori, P., Wolfsdorf, J. I., Herskowitz, R. D., Milley, J. E., Bliss, R., Wertlieb, D., & Stein, J. (1990). Adherence among children and adolescents with insulin-dependent diabetes mellitus over a four-year longitudinal follow-up: II. Immediate and long-term linkages with the family milieu. *Journal of Pediatric Psychology, 15,* 527–542.

Henggeler, S. W., & Borduin, C. M. (Eds.). (1990). *Family therapy and beyond: A multisystemic approach to treating the behavior problems of children and adolescents.* Pacific Grove, CA: Brooks/Cole.

Jacobson, A. M., Hauser, S. T., Lavori, P., Wolfsdorf, J. I., Herskowitz, R. D., Milley, J. E., Bliss, R., Wertlieb, D., & Stein, J. (1990). Adherence among children and adolescents with insulin-dependent diabetes mellitus over a four-year longitudinal follow-up: I. The influence of patient coping and adjustment. *Journal of Pediatric Psychology, 15,* 511–526.

Johnson, J. H. (1986). *Life events as stressors in childhood and adolesence.* Newbury Park, CA: Sage.

Johnson, S. B. (1987). Childhood diabetes: The role of the pediatric psychologist. *Newsletter of the Society for Pediatric Psychology, 11,* 7–12.

Johnson, S. B., Freund, A., Silverstein, J., Hansen, C. A., & Malone, J. (1990). Adherence–health status relationships in childhood diabetes. *Health Psychology, 9,* 606–631.

Johnson, S. B., Pollak, R. T., Silverstein, J. H., Rosenbloom, A. L., Spillar, R., McCallum, M., & Harkavy, J. (1982). Cognitive and behavioral knowledge about insulin-dependent diabetes among children and parents. *Pediatrics, 69,* 708–713.

Johnson, S. B., Silverstein, J., Rosenbloom, A., Carter, R., & Cunningham, W. (1986). Assessing daily management in childhood diabetes. *Health Psychology, 5,* 545–564.

Kaplan, R. M. (1990). Behavior as the central outcome in health care. *American Psychologist, 45,* 1211–1220.

Kazak, A. E. (1989). Families of chronically ill children: A systems and social-ecological model of adaptation and challenge. *Journal of Consulting and Clinical Psychology, 57,* 25–30.

Klemp, S. B., & La Greca, A. M. (1987). Adolescents with IDDM: The role of family cohesion and conflict. *Diabetes, 36,* 18A. (Abstract).

Kovacs, M., Brent, D., Steinberg, T. F., Paulauskas, S., & Reid, J. (1986). Children's self-reports of psychologic adjustment and coping strategies during the first year of insulin-dependent diabetes mellitus. *Diabetes Care, 9*, 472–479.

Kovacs, M., Feinberg, T. L., Paulauskas, S., Finkelstein, R., Pollack, M., & Crouse-Novak, M. (1985). Initial coping responses and psychosocial characteristics of children with insulin-dependent diabetes mellitus. *Journal of Pediatrics, 106*, 827–834.

Kovacs, M., Finkelstein, R., Feinberg, T. L., Crouse-Novak, M., Paulauskas, S., & Pollock, M. (1985). Initial psychologic responses of parents to the diagnosis of insulin-dependent diabetes mellitus in their children. *Diabetes Care, 8*, 568–575.

Kurdek, L. A. (1981). An integrative perspective on children's divorce adjustment. *American Psychologist, 36*, 856–866.

La Greca, A. M. (1987). Diabetes in adolescence: Issues in coping and management. *Newsletter of the Society for Pediatric Psychology, 11*, 13–18.

La Greca, A. M. (1988). Children with diabetes and their families: Coping and disease management. In T. M. Field, P. M. McCabe, & N. Schneiderman (Eds.), *Stress and coping across development* (pp. 139–159). Hillsdale, NJ: Erlbaum.

La Greca, A. M. (1990a). Issues in adherence with pediatric regimens. *Journal of Pediatric Psychology, 15*, 423–436.

La Greca, A. M. (1990b). Social consequences of pediatric conditions: Fertile area for future investigation and intervention? *Journal of Pediatric Psychology, 15*, 285–307.

LaPorte, R. E., & Tajima, N. (1985, August). Prevalence of insulin-dependent diabetes. In National Diabetes Data Group, *Diabetes in America* (DHHS Publication No. NIH 85-1468, pp. V 1–8). Washington, DC: U.S. Government Printing Office.

Lawrence, D. B., & Russ, S. W. (1985). *Mediating variables between life stress and symptoms among young adolescents.* Paper presented at the annual meeting of the American Psychological Association, Los Angeles.

Lerner, R. M. (1989). Individual development and the family system: A life-span perspective. In K. Kreppner & R. M. Lerner (Eds.), *Family systems and life-span development* (pp. 15–31). Hillsdale, NJ: Erlbaum.

Lerner, R. M., & Foch, T. T. (1987). Biological-psychosocial interactions in early adolescence: An overview of the issues. In R. M. Lerner & T. T. Foch (Eds.), *Biological-psychosocial interactions in early adolescence* (pp. 1–6). Hillsdale, NJ: Erlbaum.

Maccoby, E. E., & Martin, J. A. (1983). Socialization in the context of the family: Parent–child interactions. In E. M. Hetherington (Vol. Ed.), *Handbook of child psychology* (4th ed.): Vol. 4. *Socialization, personality, and social development* (pp. 1–101). New York: Wiley.

Mash, E. J. (1989). Treatment of child and family disturbances: A behavioral-systems perspective. In E. J. Mash & R. A. Barkley (Eds.), *Treatment of childhood disorders* (pp. 3–36). New York: Guilford Press.

Montemayor, R. (1982). The relationship between parent–adolescent conflict and the amount of time adolescents spend alone and with parents and peers. *Child Development, 53*, 1512–1519.

Montemayor, R., & Flannery, D. J. (1990). Making the transition from childhood to early adolescence. In R. Montemayor, G. R. Adams, & T. P. Gullotta (Eds.), *From childhood to adolescence: A transitional period?* (pp. 291–301). Newbury Park, CA: Sage.

Montemayor, R., & Hanson, E. (1985). A naturalistic view of conflict between adolescents and their parents and siblings. *Journal of Early Adolescence, 5,* 23–30.

Newbrough, J. R., Simpkins, C. G., & Maurer, H. (1985). A family development approach to studying factors in the management and control of childhood diabetes. *Diabetes Care, 8,* 83–92.

O'Leary, A. (1990). Stress, emotion, and human immune function. *Psychological Bulletin, 108,* 363–382.

Orchard, T. J., Dorman, J. S., Maser, R. E., Becker, D. J., Ellis, D., LaPorte, R. E., Kuller, L. H., Wolfson, S. K., & Drash, A. L. (1990). Factors associated with avoidance of severe complications after 25 yr of IDDM: Pittsburgh Epidemiology of Diabetes Complications, study I. *Diabetes Care, 13,* 741–747.

Patterson, G. R. (1986). Performance models for antisocial boys. *American Psychologist, 41,* 432–444.

Pirart, J. (1978). Diabetes mellitus and its degenerative complications: A prospective study of 4,400 patients observed between 1947 and 1973. *Diabetes Care, 1,* 168–188.

Procidano, M. E., & Heller, K. (1983). Measures of perceived social support from friends and from family: Three validation studies. *American Journal of Community Psychology, 11,* 1–24.

Rohrlich, J. A., Ranier, R., Berg-Cross, L., & Berg-Cross, G. (1977). The effects of divorce: A research review with a developmental perspective. *Journal of Clinical Child Psychology, 6,* 15–20.

Schafer, L. C., Glasgow, R. E., McCaul, K. D., & Dreher, M. (1983). Adherence to IDDM regimens: Relationship to psychosocial variables and metabolic control. *Diabetes Care, 6,* 493–498.

Schafer, L. C., McCaul, K. D., & Glasgow, R. E. (1986). Supportive and nonsupportive family behaviors: Relationships to adherence and metabolic control in persons with Type 1 diabetes. *Diabetes Care, 9,* 179–185.

Schwartz, G. E. (1982). Testing the biopsychosocial model: The ultimate challenge facing behavioral medicine? *Journal of Consulting and Clinical Psychology, 50,* 1040–1053.

Siegel, J. M., & Brown, J. D. (1988). A prospective study of stressful circumstances, illness symptoms, and depressed mood among adolescents. *Developmental Psychology, 24,* 715–721.

Simmons, R. G. (1987). Social transitions and adolescent development. In C. E. Irwin, Jr. (Ed.), *New directions for child development: No. 37. Adolescent social behavior and health* (pp. 33–61). San Francisco: Jossey-Bass.

Tarnow, J. D., & Silverman, S. W. (1981–1982). The psychophysiologic aspects of stress in juvenile diabetes mellitus. *International Journal of Psychiatry in Medicine, 11,* 25–44.

Wallander, J. L. (Chair). (1991). *Family, sibling, and peer issues in pediatric psychology*. Symposium presented at the Third Florida ⬛ference on Child Health Psychology, Gainesville.

Wallander, J. L., Varni, J. W., Babani, L., Banis, H. T., & Wilcox, K. T. (1989). Family resources as resistance factors for psychological maladjustment in chronically ill and handicapped children. *Journal of Pediatric Psychology, 14,* 157–173.

Weiss, R. S. (1979). Growing up a little faster: The experience of growing up in a single-parent household. *Journal of Social Issues, 35,* 97–111.

Wrubel, J., Benner, P., & Lazarus, R. S. (1981). Social competence from the perspective of stress and coping. In J. D. Wine & M. D. Smye (Eds.), *Social competence* (pp. 61–99). New York: Guilford Press.

CHAPTER 11

Long-Term Family Coping with Acute Lymphoblastic Leukemia in Childhood

MARY JO KUPST
Medical College of Wisconsin

Over the past 20 years, dramatic changes have taken place in the treatment and prognosis of many forms of pediatric cancer. This chapter describes a research project that was designed to study long-term coping with pediatric leukemia. Its development and progress reflect many of the changes that have occurred in the field. In 1975, when the planning for this study began, there was increasing interest in the psychosocial aspects of pediatric cancer, but much confusion in terms of the assumptions underlying the psychological functioning of these patients and families.

Early work (e.g., Bozeman, Orbach, & Sutherland, 1955; Grobstein, & Smith, 1976) established the importance of psychosocial factors in pediatric cancer, and indicated the need for psychological intervention, usually to help parents prepare for the death of a child. Most of the early studies were based upon retrospective accounts, anecdotal information, or observations during a single occasion (e.g., diagnosis, remission, or the period after the death of a child). Different types of cancer were frequently combined in these studies, although the prognosis, treatment, and coping demands might vary greatly. On the basis of these clinical observations, which focused primarily on the grieving process, investigators concluded that many of these patients and families had serious psychological problems. An assumption frequently held by mental health professionals was that the diagnosis of pediatric cancer led to individual and family dysfunction, and that family members needed intensive psychological intervention.

Despite the generally poor prognosis, a few researchers found that many parents and patients failed to develop serious problems (e.g., Futterman & Hoffman, 1973; Schulman, 1976); in fact, many family members coped surprisingly well. Later studies using more standardized measurements (e.g., Kellerman, 1980, Spinetta & Deasy-Spinetta, 1981) indicated that although patients and families underwent a series of intense stressful encounters, most of them were able to adjust adequately to the illness and treatment, with few instances of serious psychological dysfunction. In our clinical experiences with children who had cancer and their families, my colleagues and I found few who became dysfunctional: indeed, we were struck with their adaptation and growth. Psychosocial intervention was seen as helpful to alleviate stresses connected with the illness and treatment, but what type of and how much intervention these families needed were still unclear.

As treatment protocols became more effective and survival rates increased, the primary coping task for families shifted from preparing for death to learning how to cope with a potentially life-threatening illness and its treatment. The child and adolescent patient, who had been largely ignored in early years, became a focus of increased attention. In particular, Spinetta and colleagues (Spinetta & Deasy-Spinetta, 1981) studied children's reactions to hospitalization, diagnosis, and possible death; encouraged open communication within the family; and developed programs to help with school re-entry. Koocher and O'Malley's (1981) comprehensive study emphasized the issues involved in long-term survival, and suggested that survivors encountered problems that had not been addressed previously. These studies underscored the need to address coping with the chronicity of the illness, coping with the aftermath of treatment, and coping with life as a long-term survivor.

Given these considerations, an interest in coping with pediatric disease, and the potential availability of research funding, Jerome L. Schulman and I embarked in 1975 upon a study of family coping with pediatric cancer. Originally, all types of cancer were to be included. However, cancer is really many different diseases, which differ in terms of prognosis, treatment, and severity of treatment effects, and which place different coping demands upon patients and families. Acute lymphoblastic leukemia (ALL) was chosen because it is the most common type of cancer in children (it constitutes one-third of all pediatric cancer diagnoses). Since this was a single-site study, ALL represented the largest sample size (20–25 new cases per year over a 3-year accrual period). At that time, the 5-year survival rate for ALL was about 60%, which would allow follow-up of a reasonable number of patients and families over a 5-year period. In addition, variability of treatment was fairly well controlled, because there were uniform treatment protocols for ALL patients.

COPING: DEFINITIONS AND ASSUMPTIONS

From a review of existing literature and from consultation with several coping theorists, it was clear that no single "gold standard" definition of coping existed. (Compas, Worsham, & Ey, Chapter 1, this volume, discuss this problem in greater detail.) Although there was general agreement that coping implies more than the absence of problems in response to stress, there were more differences than similarities among various views of coping. To some (Vaillant, 1977; White, 1974), coping meant a general dispositional style of adaptation, and most of the early measures of "coping" were really measures of personality or general adjustment (i.e., how one typically copes). The assumption was that the way one is disposed to behave should predict how one will cope with a specific crisis. Others (Lazarus, Averill, & Opton, 1974), however, argued that such measures were not necessarily predictive of coping behavior in specific situations. They saw coping as a process involving thoughts and behaviors exhibited within a specific context (e.g., what one actually does when presented with a diagnosis of cancer). Lazarus et al. considered coping to involve "problem-solving efforts made by an individual when the demands he faces are highly relevant to his welfare (that is, a situation of considerable jeopardy or promise) and when these demands tax his adaptive resources" (1974, p. 251). Haan (1977) distinguished coping as the highest form of adaptation, as opposed to defense and fragmentation. She felt that evaluation of coping (e.g., how well one deals with treatment) is unavoidable. Lazarus et al. (1974), however, admitted all efforts or strategies as part of the coping process, without evaluating them in terms of "good" or "poor" coping.

Thus, coping was variously seen as a disposition, a style, a strategy, a state, a trait, a set of behaviors and cognitions, the same as defense, different from defense, a process, and an outcome. We decided to include as many aspects of coping in our study as possible, with the following assumptions: (1) that what people actually said and did in the specific context of the diagnosis and treatment of pediatric ALL was important (the "what" of coping); (2) that although the specific behaviors might not be good or bad in themselves, certain criteria could be established to evaluate coping behaviors and strategies in terms of outcome (how well one copes, coping as outcome); (3) that the process of coping necessitated a prospective, longitudinal perspective (coping as process); and (4) that because coping was a multidimensional construct, multiple sources and measures should be used to assess areas of convergence and divergence.

The goals of the proposed study were (1) to describe how patients with ALL and their families coped at the time of diagnosis, during treatment, and after treatment; (2) to discover what variables were related to healthy coping; and (3) to assess the impact of a psychosocial intervention designed to promote healthy coping with the diagnosis and treatment of pediatric ALL. In this chapter, I focus primarily upon the first two goals.

METHOD

Variables and Measures

Measures were to be chosen on the basis of acceptable reliability and validity, as well as allowance for both positive and negative functioning. They also had to be easily administered, relatively nonthreatening, and nonintrusive, and they had to tap specific aspects of coping with pediatric cancer rather than simple general adjustment. At that time, few measures were available that could be said to be true measures of coping. Personality measures were well validated and normed; however, they were dispositional measures at best, were more appropriate for clinical populations, and really did not measure coping with a serious illness. Rating scales might be more relevant to the actual situation of coping with the illness and treatment, and could provide a measure of how well a person was coping, but they were subjective and frequently had little reliability or validity data. Systematic observations of behaviors might provide more objective data on what people actually did, but were labor-intensive and frequently narrow in perspective. Interviews were a rich source of information, but were difficult to quantify. Several of the scales selected for this study were not widely used or were adapted to include issues specific to this population. Despite these limitations, it was decided to use all of these approaches in an attempt to obtain a more comprehensive picture of family coping.

What People Did: Coping Behaviors

The Mood and Behavior Scale (Bunney & Hamburg, 1963) was designed for longitudinal observation in the hospital. Although not widely used, it offered a simple, brief way for oncologists and nursing staff members to note their observations of emotional reactions and behaviors of children and parents during inpatient stays and clinic visits over the first 2 years of treatment. Direct observations of behaviors in the hospital were made by means of the Observation Scale, which was developed for this study by observing children in the oncology clinic and in the inpatient unit. The most frequently exhibited behaviors were coded into these categories: Nonverbal Interaction, Verbal Interaction, Passive, Positive, and Negative/ Avoidant behaviors. Average interobserver agreement was 97.73% at the beginning of the study and 86.40% 1 year later.

What People Did: Coping Reactions, Modes, and Strategies

At each phase, data from all indicators, especially from taped interviews and from written reports of the medical, nursing, and psychosocial staffs were examined to determine the prevalence of coping strategy categories drawn from a combination of classifications (e.g., Haan, 1977; Lazarus et al., 1974). These included information seeking; intrapsychic strategies (e.g., denial, intellectualization, search for meaning, focusing on the present); direct action (e.g., seeking support, activity, treating children normally, open communication about the disease and treatment); and inhibition of action (e.g., avoidance, withdrawal). Family members were rated on these strategies on a 3-point scale (not, somewhat, or usually characteristic of this person or family).

How Well People Coped

Children and parents were rated by oncologists, nurses, and psychosocial staff members on the Family Coping Scale (FCS), which was adapted from a scale by Hurwitz, Kaplan, and Kaiser (1962). This scale tapped cognitive, affective, and behavioral responses of family members to a crisis, and specific criteria related to coping with pediatric cancer were added. The cancer-specific criteria were as follows: (1) The family works toward a cognitive understanding of the realities and implications of the disease and its treatment; (2) family members are able to manage the emotional aspects of the disease; and (3) family members cope behaviorally by participating in the medical care of the child, dealing with other family and outside responsibilities, and providing support and communication within the family. For each criterion, scores ranged from 10 (not at all constructive or appropriate) to 40 (very constructive or appropriate).

A second evaluative measure, the Current Adjustment Rating Scale (CARS), was completed by parents at all measurement occasions and by older children at the 6-year assessment. A 12-item self-report scale, it has correlated significantly with other standard adjustment measures (Berzins, Bednarm, & Severy, 1975). Areas of adjustment included personal, social, family, work, leisure, and (included for this study) adjustment to the hospital and treatment. Item scores ranged from 1 (very poor adjustment) to 9 (very high adjustment).

Parents of children who had died were also rated by project staff members on the Post-Death Adaptation Scale (Spinetta, Swarner & Sheposh, 1981) which specifies 10 criteria for successful adaptation (e.g., return to normal activities, ability to make future plans, learning of new coping skills).

In addition, at the later (2-, 5-, and 10-year) assessments, families and family members were divided into those who coped well and those who coped poorly (composite coping score). Criteria were as follows: total FCS score of less than 30 (a difference of two standard deviations in this sample); CARS scores less than a mean of 6.0; or Post-Death Adaptation Scale scores of less than 25.

Personality/Dispositional Measures

During the early outpatient phase of treatment, each parent was asked to complete the California Psychological Inventory (CPI; Gough, 1964), which was selected because it was widely used with normal nonpsychiatric patients and involves positive and negative aspects of personality. In addition to the 18 subscales scored, the Summed Coping scale was factored from the CPI on the basis of Haan's classification of 10 coping processes (Joffe & Naditch, 1977). This scale was again given to parents at 2 years after diagnosis.

During the first month of the study, children over age 5 were given the Missouri Children's Picture Series (MCPS; Sines, Pauker, & Sines, 1974), which was selected over other tests on the basis of ease of administration during a time when many children felt sick or fatigued. Children also completed the Nowicki–Strickland Locus of Control Scale for Children (Nowicki & Strickland, 1973), to enable us to assess internal and external attribution of control and how it might relate to coping.

Hypothesized Correlates

Antecedent variables such as age and sex of the child, parental educational and occupational levels, mothers' and fathers' CPI subscale scores and Summed Coping scores, children's MCPS subscale scores and Locus of Control Scale scores, and previous FCS and CARS scores were correlated with FCS and CARS scores over time. Variables such as good marital relationship of parents, adequacy of family and social (nonfamily) support, and degree of other concurrent stresses were given global ratings by members of the project staff (0 — absent; 1 = sometimes; 3 = usually true) and were correlated with composite family ratings (chi-square analyses). In addition, medically related variables, such as medical status and previous course of the illness, were also included.

Table 11.1 shows the primary variables and measures used in this study. For a more thorough description, see Kupst et al., (1982).

Setting

The data collection took place primarily in the inpatient unit and Hematology/Oncology Division of the Children's Memorial Hospital, Chicago, Illinois, which is a teaching hospital, housing the Department of Pediat-

Table 11.1. Primary Measures Used in the Coping Project

Variable	Instrument	Source	Time
Parent adjustment	Current Adjustment Rating Scale (CARS)	Parents	I, OP, Y
Personality	California Psychological Inventory (CPI)	Parents	OP
Personality	Missouri Children's Picture Series (MCPS)	Child	OP
Coping style	CPI Summed Coping Scale	Parents	I, 2Yr
Clinic behaviors	Observation Scale	Observers	I, OP
Mood/behavior	Mood and Behavior Scale	MD, RN	I, OP
Locus of control	Nowicki–Strickland Locus of Control Scale	Child	I, 1Yr
Family coping	Family Coping Scale (FCS)	MD, RN, PS	I, OP, Y
Postdeath coping	Post-Death Adaptation Scale	PS	After death of a child

Note. MD, primary hematologist/oncologist; RN, clinical nurse specialist; PS, psychosocial staff; I, initial week; OP, outpatient; Y, yearly; 1Yr, 1-year assessment; 2Yr, 2-year assessment.

rics of the Northwestern University Medical School. The Hematology/ Oncology Division was a member of the Children's Cancer Study Group (a multi-institutional group of children's cancer centers, which provides uniform treatment protocols for many types of children's cancer), and most of the patients in this project participated in this group's treatment protocols. The 1-, 2-, and 6-year assessments usually involved visits to each family's home. The Coping Project team was multidisciplinary, and the strong collaborative relationship among the medical, nursing, and psychosocial staffs was essential for the success of the study.

Subjects

Between January 1977 and March 1979, all new admissions with diagnoses of pediatric ALL were potential subjects for this study. Excluded were patients who had been previously treated elsewhere, who had multiple diagnoses, or for whom language translation was necessary ($n = 6$). Four eligible families refused participation initially, and three dropped out shortly after the beginning of the study. Thus, 64 patients and their families remained as subjects.

The mean patient age at diagnosis was 6.5 years ($SD = 4.5$ years). Twenty-one were 3 years of age or younger (11 males, 10 females); 16 were 4–5 years of age (6 females, 10 males); 12 were 6–10 years of age (8 males, 4 females); and 15 were 11 years of age or older (9 females, 6 males). Fifty-seven of the children were Caucasian, four were Hispanic, and three were African-American. Based on Deasy's (1960) classification of socioeconomic status (SES), 18 families (28.1%) were in the high-SES category; 32 (50%) were middle-SES; and 14 (21.9%) were low-SES.

At 2 years after diagnosis, 60 families of children with ALL (94%) remained in the study. Forty-four (73%) of the children were in first remission and doing well medically at this time. At the 6-year assessment, 43 families remained in the study (67% of the original sample). Of the children in these families, 27 were still in remission, 1 had relapsed, and 15 had died. Of the original sample, 24 children (37.5%) had died, which was similar to the overall death rate from ALL at that time.

A comparison group of 28 patients with bacterial meningitis and their families was also followed from diagnosis for 2 years, and results based on this sample are described elsewhere (Kupst, Schulman, Davis, & Richardson, 1983). At 2 years, 19 (68%) families remained in the study.

Procedure

Assessments were done at diagnosis, early outpatient treatment (1–3 months after diagnosis), later outpatient treatment (4–6 months after diagnosis), early remission (6 months), and 1 and 2 years after diagnosis. Later, 5- and 10-year points would be added for the ALL sample. Sources included the patients, their parents, and the medical, nursing, and psychosocial staffs at each of these points.

Families were seen within 48 hours of diagnosis, and usually within the first 24 hours. Parents and children over 7 years of age provided their written consent to participate. Families were randomly assigned to one of three groups: total intervention (an intensive, outreach approach); moderate intervention (a more parent-initiated, contact-as-needed approach); and a no-project-intervention control group. All families received an initial interview, and they were observed by research assistants each day during hospitalization and at each clinic visit for the first 6 months of treatment. In the intervention groups, taped interviews were conducted at diagnosis, early and later outpatient treatment, early remission, and 1, 2, and 6 years after diagnosis; these were rated by Coping Project staff members. Taped interviews were conducted with the control group at 1, 2, and 6 years after diagnosis.

RESULTS

The study encompassed over 6 years for these families, and results have been discussed in several articles. This chapter highlights the main findings which are presented in summary form. Readers are referred to other sources for specific results on the following phases and aspects of the study: diagnosis and initial phase (Kupst & Schulman, 1980); first 6 months (Kupst, Schulman, Maurer, et al., 1983); 1 year (Kupst et al., 1982); 2 years (Kupst et al., 1984); 6 years (Kupst & Schulman, 1988); intervention strategies (Kupst, Tylke et al., 1983); and sibling coping (Kupst, 1986).

Parental Coping

Coping Behaviors and Strategies

Results on the Mood and Behavior Scale suggest that anxiety, sadness, and information seeking were common behaviors after diagnosis of ALL, but there were no significant indications of severe grief reactions. Most of the families were seen as cooperative with treatment and communicating well with staff members. They tended to show intellectual, if not emotional, acceptance of the illness and treatment. For the first year, about one-third of the mothers tended to exhibit anxiety. Parents showed considerable fluctuation of mood from one occasion to the next, and they exhibited a wide variety of behaviors. Based on classifications of coping strategies described previously, in terms of behaviors hypothesized to be related to coping at 1 year, most of the families showed open communication (72%), employed a "one-day-at-a-time" orientation (84%), relied on their religious or philosophical beliefs for support (91%), affirmed an optimistic outlook (99%) and tried to treat their children as normally as possible (97%).

At 2 years after diagnosis, parents' coping behaviors varied widely. For example, 16% of the mothers and fathers openly discussed problems as a coping strategy, but nearly an equal number avoided discussion of problems. Other predominant strategies included focusing on positive aspects, searching for meaning, keeping active, and seeking help. By 6 years, most (95%) of the parents continued to treat their children as normally as possible, to live one day at a time (79%) and to have an optimistic outlook (77%). The lower percentage of parents who endorsed the last two strategies may reflect a decreased need to use these strategies to cope with leukemia survival and a return to normal perspectives in daily life.

How Well Parents Coped

On their FCS ratings, physicians and nurses showed significant agreement that parents generally coped well from diagnosis through treatment up to 2 years. The Coping Project team rated taped interviews of the families at the same times with similar results. Significant agreement with physicians and nurses was found initially and again at 2 years after diagnosis.

Although parents exhibited diverse coping behaviors over time, coping scores tended to be stable (within the constructive range) across occasions from diagnosis to 2 years, although mean FCS scores for both parents were significantly higher from the 2-year to the 6-year point. For example, the mean FCS score for mothers increased from 31.9 at diagnosis to 33.08 at 2 years and 37.65 at 6 years. Fathers' mean score was 30.56 at diagnosis, 31.52 at 2 years, and 37.04 at 6 years. On the CARS, parents tended to score toward the positive end of the scale (for mothers, a mean of 6.24 at diagnosis, 7.01 at 1 year, and 7.55 at 6 years; for fathers, a mean of 6.60 at diagnosis and 7.33 at 6 years); the scores indicated significant improvements over time.

Mothers' and fathers' ratings of their own adjustment were significantly correlated in the initial phase and at 2 years. Interestingly, from the initial phase through all subsequent assessments, parents' CARS ratings did not correlate with FCS ratings by the medical, nursing, and psychosocial staffs. One hypothesis is that the lack of relationship was due to the restricted range of responses, since most parents tended to score toward the upper end of both measures. Another speculation was that parents and staff members interpreted parents' reactions differently. Whereas emotional upsets to crises during the illness and treatment were frequently viewed by staff members as appropriate under the circumstances, parents frequently interpreted their stress-related reactions as evidence that they were not coping very well.

Personality/Dispositional Measures

Similar to the results of other studies of personality in cancer patients (see review by Cella, 1987), the means of the 18 CPI subscales were within the normal range for both parents, but were not correlated with FCS, CARS, or composite coping ratings. This indicated that personality measures are not necessarily related to measures of situational coping. Mothers' and fathers' scores on the Summed Coping scale were not significantly different from those of the normative sample. Summed Coping scores were correlated with early outpatient staff FCS ratings for fathers and again at 2 years. Mothers' Summed Coping scores were also correlated with staff FCS ratings at two years, indicating that this coping disposition measure does have some relationship to situational coping. By 2 years after diagnosis, the coping demands related to treatment are considerably fewer, and the FCS ratings at this time may have been more reflective of more generalized parental coping.

Other Coping Issues for Parents

At 2 years, most parents (95%) reported that they had experienced significant changes in their functioning since diagnosis. Over half reported that they had a more positive attitude. About a third reported closer family relationships; however, 10% said that their relationships were less close and that they were less able to plan for the future. Four families had experienced separation or divorce, and two parents had remarried. Ten families had experienced the birth of another child. Some families (40%) remained involved in leukemia-related activities, such as volunteering and fund raising.

Based on interview results at 2 and 6 years, the most difficult times for parents were diagnosis (over half) and treatment, especially painful procedures (nearly a third). Common areas of difficulty included the following: uncertainty of prognosis; having to deal with other people's reactions; changes in a child's appearance; other medical complications; relapse; and, in all cases it was applicable, the death of the child. What parents found most helpful were support of family and friends, quality of the medical and nursing care, support from the Coping Project, talking to other patients and families, and taking things one day at a time. Common advice that parents would give others included: seeking support and talking about their feelings, being optimistic and focusing on positives, and treating their children as normally as possible.

Coping with the Death of a Child

Although the type and degree of stress were certainly much greater for them, parents of children who had died did not generally exhibit significantly more psychological problems than did parents of survivors, nor was the level of their coping significantly different. However, parents of children who had died by 2 years after diagnosis ($n = 10$) were more likely to show residual anger than were survivors' families. It should also be noted that of the six families who refused the 6-year assessment, five were families of children who had died. Interpretation of these findings in terms of coping is difficult. Might it not be appropriate to have more anger because a child has died? And is not wanting to discuss how one is coping with the death of a child evidence of poor coping?

The Post-Death Adaptation Scale indicated that by 6 years after diagnosis, most of these families were able to return to normal activities, to make plans for the future, to talk comfortably about the children, and to have learned new coping skills through this experience.

Child Coping

Coping Behaviors

Time-sampling observations of the children in the outpatient clinic showed significant differences across age groups. Children 6–10 years of age were significantly higher in both Verbal and Nonverbal Interaction, whereas older children and adolescents (ages 11 and up) were higher in Passive behavior. Those who were higher on Negative/Avoidant behavior were also higher in Inhibition on the MCPS, whereas those who were higher on Nonverbal Interaction were higher in Maturity on the MCPS. The Mood and Behavior Scale data and the staff observations indicated that children's behaviors were characterized by many individual differences, and it was not possible to categorize them as had been done with parents.

Personality/Dispositional Measures

Mean subscale scores of the MCPS were within normal ranges, with the exception of Inhibition and Activity Level, which were significantly higher than the norms for this instrument. Of note was the finding that children and adolescents 11 years of age or older tended to be more conforming, less mature, and more predisposed to be active than the normative sample. At 1 year, Activity Level remained higher than the norms. The finding of a higher level of activity is difficult to interpret, but has been seen before in a study of children with chronic illness (Tavormina, Kastner, Slater, & Watt, 1976). It is not clear, however, whether a high activity level preceded the diagnosis and treatment, or whether it resulted from some aspects of the illness and treatment. In this population, there is some evidence that central nervous system (CNS) irradiation (a treatment that all of these children underwent) produces changes in neuropsychological functions, including attention deficits and distractibility (e.g., Brouwers & Poplack, 1990; Fletcher & Copeland, 1988); perhaps these changes include alterations in activity level as well. Because this study did not include measures of attention deficits and distractibility however, the point must be left to other investigators to determine. It must also be remembered that the MCPS is a dispositional measure and may not reflect actual behavior. Nowicki-Strickland Locus of Control Scale scores for children with ALL were not significantly different from norms.

How Well Children Coped

Like parental coping, child coping was consistently within the constructive range and tended to improve over time. On the FCS, mean scores showed a significant rise (from 29.5 at diagnosis to 31.9 at 2 years and 37.2 at 6 years). Coping scores were not related to any of the MCPS scores or to Locus of Control Scale scores. Children's coping was significantly related to the adequacy of their parents' coping (as assessed by FCS ratings at all measurement occasions). Other behavioral indicators of adjustment included the time to return to school and academic functioning. In the first 3 months of treatment, 28 of 31 school-age children had returned to school. By 6 years, 75% were in school and doing well, but one-fourth of the survivors were reported to have poor grades, to be in a special class, or to have been diagnosed with a learning disability.

Differences Among Groups

With regard to the comparison between the ALL and meninigitis groups, no significant differences were found for FCS, CARS, or Mood and Behavior Scale scores at any of the assessment points for mothers, fathers, or children. Since the meningitis sample was considerably younger, no meaningful comparisons of MCPS scores or Observation Scale categories were possible. With regard to the comparisons based on intervention groups, a significant difference was found in the early outpatient treatment phase for the ALL sample. Mothers in the two intervention groups, although not significantly different from one another, were given significantly higher FCS scores by physicians than were mothers in the control group. This would suggest that early treatment, with its many stresses, is an optimal time for intervention. No such differences among intervention groups were found at other measurement occasions, nor were there differences based on other measures.

Correlates of Family Coping

Table 11.2 shows the variables that were found to correlate significantly with coping over time. Coping outcomes measured by FCS and CARS scores were correlated by means of Pearson product–moment correlations. Composite scores differentiated "good" copers from "poor" copers on the basis of previously mentioned criteria. During the early phases of treatment, good copers were those who had coped well at diagnosis, who were (or were parents of) older children, who had good family and outside support, and who were in families where other family members coped well and where other concurrent stresses were absent. The coping picture was similar at 1 year, with the addition of higher occupational level of fathers. Having sufficient financial resources may have helped to mitigate stress at a time when numerous medical bills had accumulated. The quality of the marital relationship also became more important at this

Table 11.2. Correlates of Coping Over Time

Variable	Outpatient	1 year	2 years	6 years
Antecedent variables				
Parent personality (CPI)				
Child personality (MCPS)				
CPI Summed Coping scale			M,F	F
Past coping (FCS, CARS)		M,F	A	A
Age of child	M	M,F		
Occupational level (father)		F		X
Concurrent variables				
Family support	X	X	X	X
Marital relationship		F	M	X
Coping, other family members	A	A	A	A
Concurrent stresses	X	X	X	X
Outside support	X	M	X	X
Medical status				
Psychological intervention	M			
Living in present			M	
Open communication			X	X
Low Negative/Avoidant behavior on Observation Scale			C	

Note. ✕, composite family scores; A, mother, father, and child together; M, F, and C, mother, father, and child, respectively.

stage, as a family moved toward achieving some level of stability during treatment. Open communication about the disease and treatment within the family, and an attitude of living from day to day, were apparent in good copers at 2 and 6 years. Although data on children did not yield many significant correlations with coping, children who had exhibited more Negative/Avoidant behavior in the later outpatient phase tended to cope more poorly at 2 years than did those with lower Negative/Avoidant scores.

Psychosocial intervention appeared to be helpful to mothers in the early stages of treatment. Those who had received intervention were significantly better able to live day to day than those who did not, a strategy correlated with positive coping. Although these were not formally tested, the elements of the intervention that families reported to be most helpful to them were intervenors' (1) providing concrete information and direction during the early months of treatment, (2) being readily available to provide support and to act as a liaison with the medical staff, and (3) helping the families to mobilize their own resources to deal with stress.

DISCUSSION

The results indicate that pediatric patients with ALL and their family members tended to cope well with the diagnosis, treatment, and survival, despite the upsets and upheavals surrounding the illness and treatment, and despite widely disparate styles of coping. Although certain strategies, (e.g., open communication, living in the present, and interactive behavior in patients) were found to be characteristic of healthy functioning at follow-up assessments, common coping styles were not readily identifiable across earlier phases. Rather, these were characterized by many individual differences. Examination of the coping process indicated much fluctuation within individuals as well.

This point challenges some commonly held assumptions about healthy coping behaviors—for example, that those who actively seek information about leukemia and its treatment should cope better than those who use distraction or denial, or that people who are more verbal about their feelings should do better than those who are more quiet and reserved. In this study, these opposite styles could be equally effective, depending upon the person, time, and situation.

Thus, when the definition and measurement of coping included positive, health-oriented indicators, and when a longitudinal, situation-specific perspective was adopted, very little significant pathology was found. Perhaps we can lay to rest the search for prevalence of serious psychiatric diagnoses in this population, and can view most of these children and parents as relatively normal people who are undergoing the stresses surrounding the diagnosis and treatment of a life-threatening illness. Temporary intense emotional reactions or behaviors may be viewed as part of the process of learning to cope with the illness.

Although the results support our views regarding the lack of psychopathology in this population, they should not be interpreted to mean that no one needs help; rather, these results indicate that we should discover those who may be at risk for development of problems and should concentrate our initial intervention efforts on avoiding future problems. In the early years of this study, correlates of coping were not very clear. This study and other recent studies have found that those particularly at risk are those who have little family or outside support; who have other concurrent stresses, particularly financial; who have younger children; poor communication; and other family members who appear to be coping poorly with the illness. Certain times, such as diagnosis, relapse, development of medical complications, and death of a child, are also particularly stressful for most patients and families.

This study paralleled in time an evolution of philosophy and treatment in pediatric cancer; some aspects of this process had begun prior to the research, but others had been unforeseen. By the beginning of the study, the psychological focus had shifted from coping with impending death to coping with a potentially life-threatening illness. The emphasis was still on survival as an endpoint, however, and this study did not focus on reactions to specific procedures or on side effects of treatment. In recent years, survival has become a necessary but not sufficient outcome for these patients; this change is reflected by the increased interest in quality of life during and after treatment. For example, recent work (e.g., Jacobsen et al., 1990; Zeltzer, Jay & Fisher, 1989) has focused on finding ways to alleviate or lessen pain, procedural distress, and nausea and vomiting. Pediatric psychologists working with childhood cancer now have an impressive array of techniques and strategies to deal with these very real problems.

Another quality-of-life issue has to do with late effects of treatment. When this study began, we knew very little about the impact of chemotherapy and CNS irradiation on cognitive functioning of pediatric ALL patients. Because the goal of treatment was disease-free survival, little attention was paid to this issue until some late effects began to emerge. Although there have been conflicting results with regard to the effects on overall IQ, it is becoming evident that a significant minority of long-term survivors exhibit cognitive and academic problems, and sometimes social adjustment problems. Recent work done by others (e.g., F. D. Armstrong, personal communication, August 14, 1990; H. Huszti, personal communication, August 14, 1990) and preliminary results of our longitudinal studies at the Midwest Children's Cancer Center, Medical College of Wisconsin, indicate that these problems include difficulties in memory, attention, concentration, visual-motor-spatial abilities, and mathematical ability. The prevalence reported in this recent work appears to be similar to the proportion of survivors who reported cognitive or academic problems in the study described in this chapter. Such patients require additional assessment, intervention, and consultation with schools and other providers of care. Because the early identification of these problems requires more precise measurement than simply the use of intelligence tests, inter-institutional collaborative studies are in progress to determine more precisely the extent and severity of these problems.

A positive recent development has been the emergence of improved coping measures. As mentioned earlier, the Coping Project used what we felt were the best measures at the time, but they were not as precise or as specifically coping-related as we would have liked. Since then, several measures, such as the Ways of Coping Questionnaire, the Kidcope (see Spirito, Stark, & Knapp, chapter 15, this volume), the Family Coping Inventory, and the Questionnaire on Resources and Stress, have been developed. These tap more specific aspects of coping and adjustment, and have been used with medical and pediatric patients and their families. Although they were not available earlier, we have incorporated some of them into a 10-year follow-up study. In addition to these self-report measures, excellent progress has been made in more precise behavioral assessment of children who experience procedural distress. With increased interest in late effects, there is also more emphasis on quality-of-life assessment, and several measures have been developed for adults (see review by Cella & Tulsky, 1990); however, pediatric measures of quality of life are still in development.

Another development has been the recognition of the need for longitudinal studies of pediatric cancer patients and of their families. Because of the lack of funding available for individual studies, and the need to achieve adequate sample sizes in a timely manner, this is best accomplished by collaborative interinstitutional projects. Currently, several large-scale projects are in progress, and these should provide important longitudinal data over the next 10 years regarding cognitive and behavioral functioning of pediatric cancer patients.

To turn to recommendations for those who work with this population, the importance of comprehensive psychosocial assessment cannot be stressed enough. In pediatric cancer centers that are part of collaborative study groups, psychological evaluation of patients on treatment protocols is increasingly becoming standard procedure. Together with social assessments and interviews with family members, an assessment of current functioning and risk factors can be made shortly after diagnosis. Special attention should be paid to patients and families during the first months of treatment, because of the stresses connected with the reality of a life-threatening diagnosis, the need to assimilate a vast amount of information, the beginning of frequently painful or uncomfortable treatment procedures, and the general disruption that inevitably occurs in the patients' and families' lives. Most centers would probably agree that a team approach works well, not only to provide adequate mental health coverage to these patients and families, but to prevent staff stress and burnout.

It is also important to conduct follow-up cognitive and psychological assessment of patients, preferably at 1 year after diagnosis, and at the end of treatment, which generally occurs 2–3 years after diagnosis. Parental reports of school functioning should also be obtained, along with school records where possible. Consultation with the school should be provided as well, because many schools do not have experience in dealing with the academic and psychological issues of children with cancer.

With the spate of studies that have been completed in this area, it may appear that we have exhausted the psychosocial area of pediatric cancer. However, we still do not know what happens to these same patients as their survival lengthens. Several centers have inaugurated late-effects and long-term-survivor clinics, which in time will yield more data on this subject. The patients and families in the Coping Project are also being seen in a 10 year postdiagnosis follow-up study, as noted earlier. Although it is true that much has been studied about pediatric leukemia, other types of cancer are less predictable and more problematic in terms of sequelae, but have been understudied. It is suggested while there are some psychological similarities across all pediatric cancers, but that many issues differ, depending upon the diagnosis, severity, and treatment of the disease. Studies of different types of cancer can help to delineate specific issues and areas for intervention. We have learned a great deal over the past 20 years, but there is still a great deal to accomplish in achieving a better quality of life for children with cancer and their families.

Acknowledgments

I gratefully acknowledge the help and support of the Hematology/Oncology Division of the Children's Memorial Hospital, Chicago; the Pediatric Hematology/Oncology Section of the Medical College of Wisconsin; and the Midwest Athletes against Childhood Cancer (MACC) Fund. Thanks are also due to Bettie Lyles for her help in preparation of the manuscript. Most of all, I wish to thank the children and their families for their participation in the study described in this chapter.

REFERENCES

Berzins, J. I., Bednarz, R. L., & Severy, L. J. (1975). The problem of intersource consensus in measuring therapeutic outcomes: New data and multivariate perspectives. *Journal of Abnormal Psychology, 84*, 10–19.

Bozeman, M. F., Orbach, C. E., & Sutherland, A. M. (1955). The adaptation of mothers to the threatened loss of their children through leukemia. *Cancer, 8*, 1–33.

Brouwers, P. & Poplack, D. (1990). Memory and learning sequelae in long-term survivors of acute lymphoblastic leukemia: Association with attention deficits. *American Journal of Pediatric Hematology/Oncology, 12*, 174–181.

Bunney, W. E., & Hamburg, D. A. (1963). Methods for reliable longitudinal observation of behavior. *Archives of General Psychiatry, 9*, 280–284.

Cella, D. F. (1987). Cancer survival: Psychosocial and public issues. *Cancer Investigation, 5*, 59–67.

Cella, D. F., & Tulsky, D. S. (1990). Measuring quality of life today: Methodological aspects. *Oncology, 4*, 29–37.

Deasy, L. C. (1960). Socio-economic status and participation in the poliomyelitis vaccine trial. In D. Apple (Ed.), *Sociological studies of health and sickness* (pp. 15–25). New York: McGraw-Hill.

Fletcher, J. M., & Copeland, D. R. (1988). Neurobehavioral effects of central nervous system prophylactic treatment of cancer in children. *Journal of Clinical Experimental Neuropsychology, 10,* 495–538.

Futterman, E. H., & Hoffman, I. (1973). Crisis and adaptation in families of fatally ill children. In E. J. Anthony & C. Koupernik (Eds.), *The child in his family: The impact of disease and death.* (pp. 127–143). New York: Wiley.

Gough, H. (1964). *The California Psychological Inventory manual* (rev. ed.). Palo Alto, CA: Consulting Psychologists Press.

Haan, N. (Ed.). (1977). *Coping and defending: Processes of self-environment Organization.* New York: Academic Press.

Hurwitz, J. I., Kaplan, D. M., & Kaiser, E. (1962). Designing an instrument to assess parental coping mechanisms. *Social Casework, 10,* 527–532.

Jacobsen, P. B., Manne, S. L., Gorfinkle, K., Schorr, O., Rapkin, B., & Redd, W. H. (1990). Analysis of child and parent behavior during painful medical procedures. *Health Psychology, 9,* 599–576.

Joffe, P., & Naditch, M. P. (1977). Paper and pencil measures of coping and defense processes. In N. Haan (Ed.), *Coping and defending: Processes of self-environment organization* (pp. 280–298). New York: Academic Press.

Kaplan, D.M., Grobstein, R., & Smith, A. (1976). Predicting the impact of severe illness in families. *Health and Social Work, 1,* 71–82.

Kellerman, J. (Ed.) (1980). *Psychological aspects of childhood cancer.* Springfield, IL: Charles C Thomas.

Koocher, G. P., & O'Malley, J. E. (Eds.). (1981). *The Damocles syndrome: Psychological consequences of surviving childhood cancer.* New York: McGraw-Hill.

Kupst, M. J. (1986). Coping in siblings of children with serious illness. In S. M. Auerbach & A. L. Stolberg (Eds.), *Crisis intervention with children and families* (pp. 173–188). Washington, DC: Hemisphere.

Kupst, M. J., Mudd, M. E., & Schulman, J. L. (1990, August). *Predictors of coping and adjustment in long-term pediatric leukemia survivors.* Paper presented at the meeting of the American Psychological Association, Boston.

Kupst, M. J., Schulman, J. L. (1980). Family coping with leukemia in a child: Initial reactions. In J. L. Schulman & M. J. Kupst (Eds.), *The child with cancer: Clinical approaches to psychosocial care—Research in psychosocial aspects* (pp. 111–128). Springfield, IL: Charles C Thomas.

Kupst, M. J. & Schulman, J. L. (1988).Long-term coping with pediatric leukemia. *Journal of Pediatric Psychology, 13,* 7–22.

Kupst, M. J., Schulman, J. L., Davis, A. T., & Richardson, C. C. (1983). The psychological impact of bacterial meningitis on the family. *Pediatric Infectious Disease, 2,* 12–17.

Kupst, M. J., Schulman, J. L., Honig, G., Maurer, H., Morgan, E., & Fochtman, D. (1982). Family coping with childhood leukemia: One year after diagnosis. *Journal of Pediatric Psychology, 7,* 157–174.

Kupst, M. J., Schulman, J. L., Maurer, H., Honig, G., Morgan, E., & Fochtman, D. (1983). Family coping with pediatric leukemia: The first six months. *Medical and Pediatric Oncology, 11,* 269–278.

Kupst, M. J., Schulman, J. L., Maurer, H., Morgan, E. Honig, G., & Fochtman D.

(1984). Coping with pediatric leukemia: A two-year followup. *Journal of Pediatric Psychology, 9,* 149-163.

Kupst, M. J., Tylke, L., Thomas, L., Mudd, M. E., Richardson, C. C., & Schulman, J. L. (1983) Strategies of intervention with pediatric cancer patients. *Social Work in Health Care, 8,* 31-47.

Lazarus, R. S., Averill, J. R., & Opton, E. M. Jr. (1974).The psychology of coping: Issues of research and assessment. In G. V. Coelho, D. A. Hamburg, & J. E. Adams, (Eds.), *Coping and adaptation* (pp. 249-315). New York: Basic Books.

Lazarus, R. S., & Folkman, S. (1984). *Stress, appraisal, and coping.* New York: Springer.

Nowicki, S., Jr., & Strickland, B. R. (1973). A locus of control scale for children. *Journal of Consulting and Clinical Psychology, 40,* 148-155.

Schulman, J. L. (1976). Coping with tragedy: Successfully facing the problem of a seriously ill child. Chicago: Follett.

Sines, T. O., Pauker, T. D., & Sines, L. K. (1974). *Missouri Children's Picture Series manual.* Iowa city, IA: Psychological Assessment Services.

Spinetta, J. J., & Deasy-Spinetta, P. (Eds.). (1981). *Living with childhood cancer.* St. Louis: C. V. Mosby.

Spinetta, J. J., Swarner, J. A. & Sheposh, J. P. (1981). Effective parental coping following the death of a child from cancer. *Journal of Pediatric Psychology, 6,* 251-264.

Tavormina, J. B., Kastner, L. S., Slater, F. M., & Watt, S. L. (1976). Chronically ill children: A psychologically and emotionally deviant population? *Journal of Abnormal Child Psychology, 4,* 99-110.

Vaillant, G. E. (1977). *Adaptation to life.* Boston: Little, Brown.

White, R. W. (1974) Strategies of adaptation: An attempt at systematic description. In G. V. Coelho, D. A. Hamburg, & J. E. Adams (Eds.), *Coping and adaptation* (pp. 47-48). New York: Basic Books.

Zeltzer, L. K., Jay, S. M., & Fisher, D. M. (1989). The management of pain associated with pediatric procedures. *Pediatric Clinics of North America, 36,* 941-964.

CHAPTER 12

The Social Context of Coping with Childhood Chronic Illness: Family Systems and Social Support

ANNE E. KAZAK
University of Pennsylvania School of Medicine
Children's Hospital of Philadelphia

This chapter presents a program of research on family adaptation to chronic childhood illness and disability—one that integrates family systems theory and social ecology (Kazak, 1989a). The onset of serious childhood illness or disability, whether gradual or sudden, is a distressing experience, requiring coping and adaptation to multiple stressors over the family's life cycle. An organizing premise of this chapter is that the *social* context of the child and family is of critical importance in understanding the long-term adjustment to pediatric illness, and coping processes related to such illness, for all family members. "Social context" includes the immediate and extended family and larger environments. The model addresses the issue of social isolation of individuals and families, and the associated risk status.

The underlying theories and methods for this model include diverse sources within the social sciences, including sociology, family therapy, developmental psychology, and community psychology. The scope of the present chapter precludes a thorough review of all pertinent literature and related research. It is, rather, an overview and focuses upon select papers that assist in clarifying the approach. Besides providing a review and summary of completed studies, the chapter includes suggestions regarding future research and applications for practice.

SOCIAL ECOLOGY THEORY

"Social ecology" is the study of the relation between the developing human being and the settings and contexts in which the person is actively involved (Bronfenbrenner, 1979). The child is considered to be at the center of a series of concentric rings, with the nested circles representing increasingly larger environments with which the child interacts.

Of primary emphasis in families with ill children has been the "microsystem"—the ring that represents a child's most immediate setting, the family. The growing literature on family adaptation to an ill or disabled child has primarily addressed the microsystem of the family, examining, for example, resources, interactions, and adaptations in coping with stressful life events related to the illness or disability (Wallander, Varni, Babani, Banis, & Wilcox, 1989). The next ring is the "mesosystem," which encompasses the interactive relationships of smaller settings in which the person participates (e.g., schools, hospitals, neighborhoods, and agencies). Research on children with handicaps and chronic illness has focused upon individual settings in isolation, instead of exploring the interfaces between systems and the implications of these interfaces for ongoing care (Kazak & Rostain, 1989).

More peripheral is the "exosystem," defined as including settings that do not involve the child directly, but that have an indirect impact (e.g., parents' work environments, parental networks, and schools attended by other siblings). Cochran and Brassard (1979) provide insightful examples of potential research that could address the exosystemic level, although attention to this level has remained largely theoretical. Most distant from the child is the "macrosystem," consisting of large environments that have an impact upon the child, including culture and policy. Some macrosystemic issues affect ill children and their families directly and quickly, such as the enactment of Public Law 99-457, providing access to educational services for preschool handicapped children. Others (e.g., societal beliefs and stigmas, ethnic and racial diversity) are more difficult to assess and integrate into clinical interventions.

As a developmental psychologist, Bronfenbrenner ultimately addresses the development of the individual child in his work. In contrast, the focus of the present research is upon the family system, and upon the stressors and coping responses of significant adults and siblings (as well as the patients themselves) over the course of illness. Several tenets are important in bridging social ecology, family functioning, and social support.

Interactions among persons are characterized by their *nonlinear* character and by their *reciprocity*. The chronically ill or handicapped child is not a passive recipient of unidirectional actions of other people and environments, but rather an active contributor in multidimensional inter-actions. Direct parallels exist between social ecology and family systems with respect to the importance of dyads and other subsystems within families; both approaches also maintain that a change experienced by one member of a system will affect others. Research from developmental psychology in general contributes a very strong background for under-standing dyadic interactions and their long-term implications, and can facilitate our understanding of competence in infancy and throughout childhood (Bell, 1979, Sroufe, Egeland, & Kreutzer, 1990). As a develop-mental theory, social ecology focuses on the importance of *transition* and the natural processes of change and transition inherent in growth.

As conceptualized in the present chapter, the social context of coping with childhood disability and chronic illness includes the struc-ture, functioning, and resources of the microsystem (the family), the mesosystem (schools, hospitals), and the exosystem (parental social sup-port networks), as each of these affects the coping of the ill child and family. My colleagues' and my empirical research on microsystem and exosystem variables is presented.

THE MICROSYSTEM: COPING AND DISTRESS IN FAMILIES WITH CHRONICALLY ILL CHILDREN

The diagnosis of a disabling or chronic health problem in a child is understandably a time of emotional distress, upheaval, and uncertainty for parents, and the beginning of a long-term process of reorganization and accommodation within a family. Research on adjustment has looked at ill children, parents, siblings, and families. The results are contradictory and methodologically complicated. Although it is beyond the scope of the present chapter to summarize all relevant findings and methodological constraints, some general findings have emerged.

Child Functioning

Higher incidences of psychiatric problems have been reported in chil-dren with chronic diseases (Cadman, Boyle, Szatmari, & Offord, 1987). Although psychological distress is not inevitably associated with chronic illness, chronically ill children are "at risk" and often show elevation of emotional behaviors, both negative and positive (Nelms, 1989). Research that addresses risk and examines ways in which family distress and resources can affect child outcome suggests the importance of evaluating parental mental health, family processes, and social support (Hampson, Hulgus, Beavers, & Beavers, 1988). There is less research examining other children in the family. Results regarding sibling outcome are mixed, with studies usually not integrating sibling data with that of other members of the system.

Marital and Family Functioning

Although having a chronically ill child can be stressful for a marital relationship, the research points quite clearly to normative levels of marital satisfaction and distress (Sabbeth & Leventhal, 1984). Research on families with chronically ill or handicapped children has been relatively sparse and complicated by general conceptual and method-ological concerns. Reviews and critiques of the difficulties and needs in conducting research on families and health can be found elsewhere (Kazak & Nachman, 1991). A few issues particularly salient to under-standing families from a systems and social-ecological perspective are discussed here.

One problem is understanding the characteristics and demands of particular medical conditions in terms of child and family outcome. Rolland (1984) suggests psychosocial elements of illnesses that may affect the family's responses to and beliefs about the condition and its meaning. Others suggest a noncategorical approach to childhood illness (Stein & Jessop, 1982). Much research combines children with diverse conditions, or compares different illness groups, without a clear theoretical organiza-tion for these comparisons. Research suggests that different conditions may have some elements in common, but that they also have specific characteristics and demands, which may be associated with differential family responses.

Another question is that of how diversity can be included in re-search. One type of diversity is developmental. Much research includes children across a wide age range without including pertinent develop-mental concerns. Another example of how diversity is neglected is the scant attention given to normality in families. In most research, underly-ing models and instrument norms are assumed to be of relevance to all families; the suitability of the construct and measure for heterogeneous groups of families is not called into question. In a study comparing perceptions of normality in four samples (college students, families with young children, grandmothers, and therapists), perceptions of normality did not correspond to instrument norms and varied developmentally and ethnically (Kazak, McCannell, Adkins, Himmelberg, & Grace, 1989). At a broader level, the ways in which ethnic and racial differences may affect the relationship among patient, family, and the medical system, as well as compliance with treatment, remains unexplored (Kazak & Rostain, 1989).

Empirical Studies

In three studies, my colleagues and I focused on understanding differences in family subsystems (affected children, parents, siblings, marriages, families, social networks) between families with children with a physical handicap or chronic illness and those without such children. The samples were as follows: in study I, families of children with spina bifida, ages 1–16 ($n = 56$); Kazak & Clark, 1986; Kazak & Marvin, 1984; Kazak & Wilcox, 1984); in study II, families of children with early-treated phenylketonuria (PKU), ages 1–8 ($n = 43$; Kazak, Reber, & Carter, 1988; Kazak, Reber, & Snitzer, 1988; Reber, Kazak, & Himmelberg, 1987); and in study III, families of institutionalized young adults with mental retardation (MR) ($n = 36$; Kazak, 1988, 1989b). In each study, families with disabled children were compared with control group families (matched for child age and demographic characteristics) on measures of distress within the family and of social support network characteristics. Both fathers and mothers were included in all studies. Results of the multivariate and univariate analyses for the family stress variables in these three studies follow (Kazak, 1987).

The data have helped to dismantle the notion of pervasive levels of distress in families with handicapped children, and to identify specific areas of concern. In Study I, mothers and fathers of children with spina bifida were found to have higher incidences of anxiety and depression than the comparison families, although this difference was more striking for mothers. Marital satisfaction differences between the groups provided some evidence that the families of handicapped children actually perceived themselves as having somewhat higher levels of marital cohesion. Although the marital relationship did not seem to be an area of distress, parenting stress levels were significantly higher for the spina bifida group. The children with spina bifida reported lower self-concepts, but no differences were found for siblings.

Somewhat different results emerged in Study II. Parents of children with PKU did not differ from the comparison group in terms of parental distress, marital satisfaction, or parenting stress. Parents of children with PKU perceived their families to be less cohesive and adaptable than the comparison families, and children with PKU were found to have lower levels of social competence than matched comparison children. These results not only underscore the lack of group differences, but also suggest that differences between the two groups of families are understandable, given the demands of the medical condition.

Study III focused upon a quite different group; parents of older institutionalized offspring with MR. In this study, remarkable comparability between the target and comparison groups was also found. The families with offspring with MR were found to be more cohesive than the comparison families, and there was evidence that family adaptability was linked to parental coping.

When the samples of Studies I–III were combined, multivariate analyses indicated that maternal distress and marital satisfaction, in combination, differentiated the groups, and that the strongest group difference was that in maternal distress. Data from these three studies showed relatively few differences between families with disabled or ill children and comparison families. However, the vulnerability of mothers is significant and merits further investigation. Presumably, mothers assume a very large caretaking burden, and hence become more vulnerable to anxiety and depression. The generally normative levels of marital satisfaction and higher levels of parenting stress suggest that much of the distress stems from the demands of parenting. Systemically, more information is needed on how families cope and adjust, and on how they can be helped to provide needed support for all members of the system. It is also important to consider extrafamilial variables (e.g., mothers' employment outside the home) that have been found to be related to general satisfaction and child behavior problems in families with handicapped or ill children (Walker, Ortiz-Valdes, & Newbrough, 1989).

As evidence accumulates supporting the positive adaptation made by many families with disabled children, the "deficit" orientation toward these families has lessened. However, it is important that the reaction of professionals and the public not swing too widely in the opposite direction. Although comparison groups are generally preferred in research design, the limitations of comparison groups must also be considered, particularly with respect to this population. Historically, research on families with ill children has been based upon the premise that these families should differ from matched controls, or that the null hypothesis of no differences between the groups should be rejected. If repeated studies indicate no differences, investigations might focus upon what differentiates better and worse adjustment and adaptation within groups, instead of examining gross group differences (Kazak & Meadows, 1989). This is particularly important when general difficulties in identifying family comparison groups are considered and the complexity of identifying a meaningful "control" for serious childhood illness or physical handicap is acknowledged.

In recent and ongoing studies, the approach described above has been utilized with families of children with cancer in a developmentally focused manner. One project has followed 70 long-term survivors of childhood cancer (ages 10–15 years at the beginning of the study) and their families over 3 years during adolescence (Kazak & Meadows, 1989). With respect to overall functioning, the data are consistent with the results of other studies in supporting normative levels of adjustment (Greenberg, Kazak, & Meadows, 1989). Among the more interesting results were the following (Kazak & Meadows, 1989): Relative to a comparison group, the cancer survivors reported somewhat less support from friends, and over the course of the prospective study they showed declines in perceived social support from family, friends, and teachers. Learning problems in cancer survivors predicted family distress; however, those long-term survivors with learning problems who received special services in school reported higher levels of social support. These findings suggest that cognitive sequelae of treatment affect emotional, social, and family functioning, as well as learning ability and achievement.

Another study focused upon 25 siblings (ages 3–5) of children in treatment, investigating differences between these children and a comparison group on developmentally relevant variables, including prosocial behavior and behavior problems (Horwitz & Kazak, 1990). As a link among siblings as individuals, the sibling subsystem, and family functioning, data were collected on parental perceptions of similarities and differences between the siblings and on family adaptability and cohesion. The results indicated positive prosocial behaviors in preschool siblings. More extreme family configurations were also seen in these families compared to normative standards.

THE MESOSYSTEM: PEERS, SCHOOLS, HOSPITALS, COMMUNITIES

Some literature exists on children with chronic illnesses or physical handicaps in peer groups, schools, hospitals, and their communities. These systems are extensions of a child's world and part of the reciprocal, changing environment in which the child and family exist, rather than static settings in which the child is considered in isolation. Thus, instead of looking at whether children are accepted by peers or not, research guided by a social-ecological model would ask how the child's experiences of interactions with peers shape the social world of the child and the ways in which the child adapts to illness and disability.

How children with chronic illness or physical handicaps interact with peers is an important and often neglected area of concern. In a study that carefully matched children with cancer with peers and utilized teacher ratings, children with cancer were found to be more isolated and were perceived as having less leadership potential than peers (Noll, Bukowski, Rogosch, LeRoy, & Kulkarni, 1990). The peer group parallels the family system as an environment. In both, children learn about interpersonal relationships and social strengths and weaknesses, and establish templates for personal and work relationships.

The school is a critical system for chronically ill and disabled children. A vast pool of knowledge exists regarding the educational needs of these children; less well understood are the ways in which schools become part of a child's social environment, and the implications of these for coping and adaptation. Power and Bartholomew (1987) describe five theoretical interaction styles between schools and families (avoidant, competitive, merged, one-way, and collaborative), and Schwartzman and Kneifel (1985) discuss ways in which families and other systems replicate or complement one another in their interrelationships. In discussing reasons for a lower-than-expected utilization of mental health services by chronically ill children and their families Sabbeth and Stein (1990) identify attitudes and behaviors from families, hospital staff, and mental health providers as important. These theoretical papers provide useful and provocative areas for research. For example, identifying characteristics of hospital and school systems and ways of measuring them could lead to research testing "goodness-of-fit" hypotheses among families and other systems.

THE EXOSYSTEM: PARENTAL SOCIAL SUPPORT AND SOCIAL SUPPORT NETWORKS

Examining social support represents an alternative to examining social isolation. Whereas isolation is associated with health risk and psychopathology, social support is seen as a strong protective factor (Cassel, 1976; Cobb, 1976). A striking statement in support of social support affecting health and life quality comes from House, Landis, and Umberson (1988): "The evidence regarding social relationships and health increasingly approximates the evidence in the 1964 Surgeon General's report that established cigarette smoking as a cause or risk factor for mortality and morbidity from a range of diseases" (p. 543).

The study of social support is complicated and requires methodological rigor. Indeed, "social support" is a broad construct and includes many potentially helpful components (e.g., emotional support, tangible assistance). One important complication concerns the appropriateness of general measures of social support for particular populations. Although it is likely that there may be a general positive effect of social support, it may also be that the types and amounts of support that are optimal for coping depend on life circumstances (e.g., parenting, divorce, college life). Studies of social support relevant to families of handicapped or chronically ill children follow. The general premise is that social support can be operationalized and integrated in a meaningful way into research, and that it also holds immense potential for preventive and therapeutic intervention.

Social Networks

One of the ways in which social support can be measured is by analysis of social support networks. Barnes (1954) initially defined social networks as a set of points which are joined by lines; the points of the image are people, or sometimes groups and the lines indicate which people interact with each other" (p. 43). Several important structural and functional aspects of social networks related to family coping are defined and reviewed here.

"Network size," or the number of people identified, is the simplest and most straightforward dimension. In general, larger networks are associated with more positive adjustment, although some research indicates that having just one confidant has a significant impact on mental health. "Network density" is the extent to which members of the social network know and interact with one another, independently of the focal person (Bott, 1971). Generally, less dense networks have been found to be associated with more positive adjustment in divorced women, college students, and widows. "Boundary density" is the proportion of possible interconnections existing between two different networks or two segments within a network, and has been conceptualized as a way in which microsystem linkages can be explored (Hirsch & Reischl, 1985).

Besides these structural components, social network assessment also includes qualitative or evaluative aspects, including types of network members, types of help, perceived helpfulness, dimensionality, and reciprocity. Even within the subsets of family and friendship networks, examination of the roles and involvements of different types of relatives and friends is useful in understanding the ways in which grandparents and work associates, for example, function in the broader network. Assessing multiple types of help provided by network members is also important, in order to determine what gaps may exist.

"Dimensionality" is the number of functions served by a relationship (Mitchell & Trickett, 1980), and provides an indication of the extent to which persons are providing several types of help, or assist in one specific area. "Reciprocity" is defined as the degree to which aid is given and received (Mitchell & Trickett, 1980). This balance is important in understanding the nature of a family's interaction with its broader environment. Imbalance may occur when more help is received than given, particularly over time. A network that is "drained" of its resources is one related to higher incidences of child abuse (Garbarino & Sherman, 1980).

Measuring Social Networks in Families

Instrument

A semistructured interview measure adapted from Hirsch (1980), the Social Network Reciprocity and Dimensionality Assessment Tool (SNRDAT; Kazak, 1984), was developed to assess social networks in families with chronically ill children. Network size is determined by asking parents to name up to 10 family members, 10 friends, and 5 professionals. Parents are asked to indicate types of help received (emotional, informational, tangible, service-related) from each person, how helpful each person is, and how often help is provided (from once a day to once a month). They also indicate the types and frequency of help they themselves provide. These questions allow for determination of dimensionality, helpfulness, and reciprocity. Density is measured quantitatively by a grid that asks whether each two network members know each other. Boundary density is calculated by comparing membership overlap among subnetworks.

Results

In Study I (the study of families of children with spina bifida; see "Empirical Studies," above), mothers and fathers had significantly smaller total networks than comparison parents, although the difference was accounted for by size of the friendship network, not by size of the family network (Kazak & Wilcox, 1984). These differences were not demonstrated in Studies II and III (the studies of families of offspring with PKU and MR, respectively) (Kazak, Reber, & Carter 1988; Kazak, 1988). In Studies I and III, higher-density networks were found in the families with disabled children. Higher density was associated with higher levels of maternal distress in Study I. In Study II, the interaction between level of distress and social network characteristics was examined. Main effects for distress were found for network size and density, with an interaction between group and distress for mothers' friendship network density (Kazak, Reber, & Carter, 1988). Analysis of qualitative data in Study II indicated that parents of children with PKU perceived less support from immediate family members than comparison parents did.

Multivariate analyses combining data from the three samples supported overall differences with respect to network size and density. Differences in network structure among the three groups were also intriguing. When the children's age was controlled for, there were significant difference among the groups with respect to mothers' and fathers' total network size, family network size and density, and fathers' friendship network size. These data suggest that differences in medical condition or other untested parameters of the disease, its treatment, or the family may be interacting with network structure. Different network structures may be equally adaptive, under different family and health circumstances.

Implications

Contrary to the commonly held belief that families with handicapped or ill children are socially isolated, the overall analysis of network size suggests that they are not. The differences in social network size between families with disabled children and comparison families are not striking. Of concern are the subset of families who are more isolated, and hence are at greater risk. A comprehensive social-ecological approach must also include consideration of aspects of individuals that may influence their perceptions of networks and inclinations to seek help. Hobfoll and Lerman (1988) investigated mothers of well, acutely ill and chronically ill children; their data indicated that mothers' emotional distress and mastery affected their perceptions of social networks. They also presented intriguing data showing that the timing of social support and the balance of support received from spouse and others, at different times during the illness, had a differential impact on adjustment. Other stress and coping paradigms, such as "goodness-of-fit" models, may provide useful frameworks for understanding the role of social support and networks in adaptation to childhood illness (Forsythe & Compas, 1987).

These data suggest the importance of close examination of the type of memberships in the network. In an independent study of families of young hearing-impaired children (Quittner, Glueckauf, & Jackson, 1990), smaller networks were found among these families than among families in a comparison group. It was also noted that the networks of the disabled children's families had a large membership of professionals. My colleagues and I also found that professionals were often considered integral members of the network. The benefits and difficulties of this network composition have not been explored. They provide, however, a natural link among studying the family, the network, and the larger systems to which the professionals belong.

The results with respect to network density indicate a tendency for the networks of parents of disabled children to be more dense than those of comparison children, and show consistency with previous research in terms of linking higher levels of density to distress. Networks with high levels of density may be akin to family systems characterized by "enmeshment," a well-known family construct often associated with less adaptive functioning. This may help explain the higher levels of distress associated with dense networks. More dense networks lack what Granovetter (1973) termed "weak links," or persons outside the immediate, highly connected network. High-density networks may reduce individuals' ability to act independently and may thus result in conflict avoidance. Some of the potentially negative implications of social support reported in other papers (e.g., Brenner, Norvell, & Limacher, 1989) may be related to high density—a possibility that has not been tested in other work. Within the professional network, high density may approximate the type of coordinated care that is usually considered ideal. Investigations of the density of the professional network could be explored in more detail with regard to reciprocal impact on families, as well as impact upon treatment goals.

A related point concerns the need to determine the meaning of different levels of density. Density is a relative concept, and specifying levels of involvement among network members that are associated with levels of distress will be important. In an interesting study of "successful" families with young disabled children, which employed measures comparable to ours, Trute and Hauch (1988) found that high-density networks were characteristic of well-functioning families. A small, interconnected, rich network, with involvement from both sides of the child's extended family, may be optimal. These data point to the need to explore the texture of network interactions in more detail, as well as to the ongoing importance of understanding and evaluating competent responses to chronic stressors.

FUTURE DIRECTIONS

The topics covered in the present chapter are broad. What follows is a brief discussion of some of the research needs that, if met, could help expand a social-ecological approach to understanding families of handicapped and chronically ill children.

The research reported in this chapter has shown quite clearly the relative strengths of families with ill children, and the lack of group differences between families with and without affected children. The undoing of a "deficit" orientation toward these families is welcome. However, we need to maintain a keen interest in the potential *vulnerability* of some of these families.

The vulnerability of chronically ill and disabled children is apparent in the largely unanswered question of what happens to these children as they grow older. Existing research suggests a mixed picture, particularly with respect to mental health (Pless, Cripps, Davies, & Wadsworth, 1989). The risk status of mothers is also of great concern, as is the need to attend to gender in coping with childhood illness. Stressors can become compounded, and the way in which this process affects adjustment over time warrants investigation. Although recent epidemiological evidence suggests that abuse among disabled children is less than suspected (Benedict, White, Wulff, & Hall, 1990), the association between domestic violence and depleted social resources is a strong one and should not be ignored in this population (Garbarino & Sherman, 1980).

At the level of the family, research methodologies are still in early stages of development, and many needs remain (Kazak & Nachman, 1991). Of note is the need to understand which coping mechanisms and risk factors are general across different diseases and which may be specific to different medical conditions. For example, although asthma, muscular dystrophy, and spina bifida are all chronic and probably require similar family reorganizations, they differ with respect to the course of the illness. These differences in illness course may affect the structure and function of the social network, which in turn may have an impact upon family functioning.

One important unanswered question in this field is as follows: How can we predict different levels of psychological risk and study families prospectively to assess the strength of our predictor variables? Such studies would have important implications for providing psychosocial services to handicapped and chronically ill children. Besides the disease-specific concerns noted above, three other issues that have been addressed throughout the chapter merit consideration.

The first issue is the need for meaningful integration of child and family diversity into studies. As noted earlier, neglect of developmental concerns of children and families provides biased data on family functioning. And ethnic and racial variation in families coping with illness needs to be considered as an integral part of the coping process, rather than as a variable to be "controlled for." The second, related point is that points of transition may be valuable opportunities for studying processes of coping and change. Developmentally, the transitions to adolescence or to young adulthood are points at which ill or handicapped persons and their families must reorganize to face new challenges. Treatment teams and educational systems must also change with transitions in individuals and families. The third issue is the need to develop models for identifying interactional variables that can be assessed over time.

A family systems/social-ecological model, combined with knowledge on family coping with childhood illness, suggests that several types of bridges need to be built in systematic research. The first series of bridges consists of research that connects different levels of the social-ecological model. For example, we need to understand the ways in which parental social networks and their utilization affect ill children and their siblings. We also need to understand how individual differences in help seeking, and the types of personality variables that influence seeking and being satisfied with help, are related to social networks.

A second series of bridges are those that must be built within treatment centers and among treatment systems. In addition to the obvious collaboration necessary among treatment team members from different disciplines (e.g., medicine, nursing, education), a social-ecological approach argues that interdisciplinary boundaries can be stretched among mental health professionals. For example, rather than maintaining rigid distinctions among psychiatrists, psychologists, and social workers as treating biological, individual, and social concerns, respectively, the likelihood that a child's needs may span several different systems supports an integrated plan of action.

The final set of bridges consists of those that must be built across institutions for research. To address the multiple factors presented, the number of variables involved precludes data collection at one site. Although multisite studies are more difficult to organize and complete, they can foster creative research and overcome many of the shortcomings of earlier studies.

REFERENCES

Barnes, J. (1954). Class and communities in a Norwegian island parish. *Human Relations, 7*, 39-58.

Bell, R. (1979). Parent, child, and reciprocal influences. *American Psychologist, 34*, 821-826.

Benedict, M., White, R., Wulff, L., & Hall, B. (1990). Reported maltreatment in children with multiple disabilities. *Child Abuse and Neglect, 14*, 207-217.

Bott, E. (1971). *Family and social network: Norms and external relationships in ordinary urban families.* London: Tavistock.

Brenner, G., Norvell, N., & Limacher, M. (1989). Supportive and problematic social interactions: A social network analysis. *American Journal of Community Psychology, 17*, 831-836.

Bronfenbrenner, U. (1979). *The ecology of human development.* Cambridge, MA: Harvard University Press.

Cadman, D., Boyle, M., Szatmari, P., & Offord, D. (1987). Chronic illness, disabilities and mental and social well-being: Findings of the Ontario Child Health Study. *Pediatrics, 79*, 805-813.

Cassel, J. (1976). The contribution of the social environment to host resistance. *American Journal of Epidemiology, 104*, 107-123.

Cobb, S. (1976). Social support as a mediator of life stress. *Psychosomatic Medicine, 38*, 300-314.

Cochran, M., & Brassard, J. (1979). Child development and personal social networks. *Child Development, 50*, 601-616.

Forsythe, C., & Compas, B. (1987). Interaction of cognitive appraisals of stressful events and coping: Testing the goodness of fit hypothesis. *Cognitive Therapy and Research, 11*, 473-485.

Garbarino, J., & Sherman, D. (1980). High risk neighborhoods and high risk families: The human ecology of child maltreatment. *Child Development, 51*, 188-198.

Granovetter, M. (1973). The strength of weak ties. *American Journal of Sociology, 78*, 1360-1380.

Greenberg, H., Kazak, A., & Meadows, A. (1989). Psychological adjustment in 8 to 16 year old cancer survivors and their parents. *Journal of Pediatrics, 114*, 488-493.

Hampson, R., Hulgus, Y., Beavers, W., & Beavers, J. (1988). Competence in families with a retarded child. *Journal of Family Psychology, 2*, 32-53.

Hirsch, B. (1980). Natural support systems and coping with major life changes. *American Journal of Community Psychology, 8,* 159–172.

Hirsch, B., & Reischl, T. (1985). Social networks and developmental psychopathology: A comparison of adolescent children of a depressed, arthritic or normal parent. *Journal of Abnormal Psychology, 94,* 272–281.

Hobfoll, S., & Lerman, M. (1988). Personal relationships, personal attributes, and stress resilience: Mothers' reactions to their child's illness. *American Journal of Community Psychology, 16,* 565–589.

Horwitz, W., & Kazak, A. (1990). Family adaptation to childhood cancer: Sibling and family systems variables. *Journal of Clinical Child Psychology, 19,* 221–228.

House, J., Landis, K., & Umberson, D. (1988). Social relationships and health. *Science, 241,* 540–545.

Kazak, A. (1984). *The Social Network Reciprocity and Dimensionality Assessment Tool (SNRDAT).* Unpublished manuscript, Children's Hospital of Philadelphia.

Kazak, A. (1987). Families with disabled children: Stress and social networks in three samples. *Journal of Abnormal Child Psychology, 15,* 137–146.

Kazak, A. (1988). Stress and social networks in families with older institutionalized retarded children. *Journal of Social and Clinical Psychology, 6,* 448–461.

Kazak, A. (1989a). Families of chronically ill children: A systems and social ecological model of adaptation and challenge. *Journal of Consulting and Clinical Psychology, 57,* 25–30.

Kazak, A. (1989b). Family functioning in families with older institutionalized retarded offspring. *Journal of Autism and Developmental Disabilities, 19,* 501–509.

Kazak, A., & Clark, M. (1986). Stress in families of children with myelomeningocele. *Developmental Medicine and Child Neurology, 28,* 220–228.

Kazak, A., & Marvin, R. (1984). Differences, difficulties, and adaptation: Stress and social networks in families with a handicapped child. *Family Relations, 33,* 67–77.

Kazak, A., McCannell, K., Adkins, E., Himmelberg, P. & Grace, J. (1989). Perceptions of normality in families: Four groups. *Journal of Family Psychology, 2,* 277–291.

Kazak, A., & Meadows, A. (1989). Families of young adolescents who have survived cancer: Social–emotional adjustment, adaptability, and social support. *Journal of Pediatric Psychology, 14,* 175–191.

Kazak, A., & Nachman, G. (1991). Family research on childhood chronic illness: Pediatric oncology as an example. *Journal of Family Psychology, 4,* 462–483.

Kazak, A., Reber, M., & Carter, A. (1988). Structural and qualitative aspects of social networks in families with young chronically ill children. *Journal of Pediatric Psychology, 13,* 171–182.

Kazak, A., Reber, M., & Snitzer, L. (1988). Childhood chronic disease and family functioning: A study of phenylketonuria. *Pediatrics, 81,* 224-230.

Kazak, A. & Rostain, A. (1989). Systemic aspects of family noncompliance. *Newsletter of the Society of Pediatric Psychology, 13,* 12-17.

Kazak, A. & Wilcox, B. (1984). The structure and function of social networks in families with handicapped children. *American Journal of Community Psychology, 12,* 645-661.

Mitchell, R., & Trickett, E. (1980). Social networks as mediators of social support: An analysis of the effects and determinants of social networks. *Community Mental Health Journal, 15,* 27-44.

Nelms, B. (1989). Emotional behaviors in chronically ill children. *Journal of Pediatric Psychology, 17,* 657-668.

Noll, R., Bukowski, W., Rogosch, F., LeRoy, S., & Kulkarni, R. (1990). Social interactions between children and their peers: Teacher ratings. *Journal of Pediatric Psychology, 15,* 43-56.

Pless, I., Cripps, H., Davies, J., & Wadsworth, M. (1989). Chronic physical illness in childhood: Psychological and social effects in adolescence and adult life. *Developmental Medicine and Child Neurology, 31,* 746-755.

Power, T., & Bartholomew, K. (1987). Family-school relationship patterns: An ecological assessment. *School Psychology Review, 16,* 498-512.

Quittner, A., Glueckauf, R., & Jackson, D. (1990). Chronic parenting stress: Moderating versus mediating effects of social support. *Journal of Personality and Social Psychology, 59,* 1266-1278.

Reber, M., Kazak, A., & Himmelberg, P. (1987). Outcome in early treated phenylketonuria: Family psychosocial and metabolic variables. *Journal of Developmental and Behavioral Pediatrics, 8,* 311-317.

Rolland, J. (1984). Towards a psychosocial typology of chronic and life threatening illness. *Family Systems Medicine, 2,* 245-262.

Sabbeth, B., & Leventhal, J. (1984). Marital adjustment to chronic childhood illness. *Pediatrics, 73,* 762-768.

Sabbeth, B., & Stein, R. (1990). Mental health referral: A weak link in comprehensive care of children with chronic physical illness. *Journal of Developmental and Behavioral Pediatrics, 11,* 73-78.

Schwartzman, H., & Kneifel, A. (1985). Familiar institutions: How the childcare system replicates family patterns. In J. Schwartzman (Ed.), *Families and other systems* (pp. 87-107). New York: Guilford Press.

Sroufe, L., Egeland, B., & Kreutzer, T. (1990). The fate of early experience following developmental change: Longitudinal approaches to individual adaptation in childhood. *Child Development, 61,* 1363-1373.

Stein, R., & Jessop, D. (1982). A noncategorical approach to childhood chronic illness. *Public Health Reports, 97,* 354-362.

Trute, B., & Hauch, C. (1988). Social network attributes of families with positive adaptation to the birth of a developmentally disabled child. *Canadian Journal of Community Mental Health, 7,* 5-16.

Walker, L., Ortiz-Valdes, J., & Newbrough, J. (1989). The role of maternal employ-

278 • CURRENT RESEARCH PERSPECTIVES

ment and depression in the psychological adjustment of chronically ill, mentally retarded, and well children. *Journal of Pediatric Psychology, 14,* 357–370.

Wallander, J., Varni, J., Babani, L., Banis, H., & Wilcox, K. (1989). Family resources as resistance factors for psychological maladjustment in chronically ill and handicapped children. *Journal of Pediatric Psychology, 14,* 157–174.

CHAPTER 13

Adjustment in Children with Chronic Physical Disorders: Programmatic Research on a Disability-Stress-Coping Model

JAN L. WALLANDER
University of Alabama at Birmingham

JAMES W. VARNI
Orthopaedic Hospital, Los Angeles
University of Southern California

Advances in biomedical sciences over the past several decades have resulted in dramatic improvements in the mortality and physical functioning of children with chronic physical illness or disability. As their mortality and morbidity has improved, increased attention has been paid to the psychological functioning of these children. It is a desirable goal that the psychosocial development of children with chronic physical disorders is largely indistinguishable from that of their healthy peers. However, large epidemiological surveys conducted in the late 1960s (see review by Pless & Roghmann, 1971) found quite consistently that the proportion of chronically ill and disabled children who were deemed maladjusted was about twice that of physically healthy children. In contrast, studies conducted in the late 1970s found less of a difference, if any at all, between children with specific chronic physical disorders and controls (e.g., Drotar et al., 1981; Gayton, Friedman, Tavormina, & Tucker, 1977).

Our own findings are more consistent with those reviewed by Pless and Roughman (1971) than with the findings of the more recent reports.

For example, when the Child Behavior Checklist (CBCL; Achenbach & Edelbrock, 1983) was administered to the mothers of 270 chronically ill or disabled children, we found that they perceived their chronically ill or disabled children as displaying on the average more behavior and social problems than children in the general norm sample (Wallander, Varni, Babani, Banis, & Thompson, 1988). However, their adjustment was reported as better than that of a normative sample of children referred to mental health clinics. These findings, we feel are most consistent with the view that they constitute a group *at risk* for psychosocial maladjustment. This means that, on the average, they may display more psychosocial problems than expected in healthy peers; however, few will evidence clinically significant problems or psychopathology. Nonetheless, we feel that their at-risk status must be viewed seriously.

Research is needed to identify those children who are at particular risk for developing adjustment problems. Research is also needed to identify risk and protective factors, in order to prevent these children from becoming maladjusted, as well as to intervene with those who already evidence problems. Our research programs aim to meet these needs by identifying factors that may play a role in the development and maintenance of adjustment problems in this population and studying processes by which this may happen. This research has employed an expanded stress and coping theoretical framework. The conceptual emphasis has been on the stress these children experience and on the coping resources that may be available to them in dealing with this stress. We will first discuss the theoretical basis for our work and the general methodology we have used; this discussion is followed by a review of our research conducted thus far.

CONCEPTUAL MODEL
Disability-Stress-Coping Model

In embarking on these programs of research, we had to develop an a priori conceptual model that would identify the variables we needed to investigate and indicate how they were related to one another and to adjustment. On the basis of prior research on adjustment in chronically ill or disabled children, children in general, and the theoretical developments put forth by Pless and Pinkerton (1975), we have proposed an integrative, multivariate model of adjustment to guide our efforts. First introduced elsewhere (Wallander, Varni, Babani, Banis, & Wilcox, 1989), and presented in Figure 13.1 here, the various factors hypothesized in this model to play a role in the adjustment of children with chronic physical disorders are organized into a risk-and-resistance framework. Disease/disability parameters, functional independence, and psychosocial stress are considered categories of factors

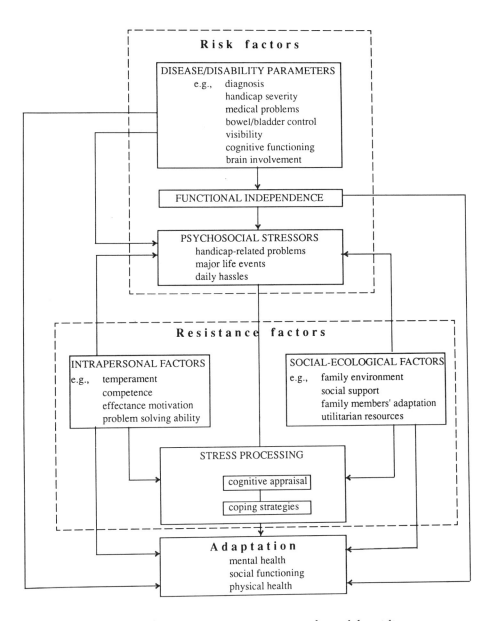

Figure 13.1. Disability-stress-coping conceptual model guiding our research programs. From "Family Resources as Resistance Factors for Psychological Maladjustment in Chronically Ill and Handicapped Children" by J. L. Wallander, J. W. Varni, L. V. Babani, H. T. Banis, and K. T. Wilcox, 1989, *Journal of Pediatric Psychology, 14,* 157–173. Copyright 1989 by Plenum Publishing Corp. Reprinted by permission.

primarily responsible for causing adjustment problems in children with chronic physical conditions. However, since children with similar risk factors (e.g., identical physical status, similar exposure to negative life events) obviously display wide differences in adjustment, this relationship is not a simple one. Therefore, resistance factors are thought to influence the risk-adjustment relationship, both through a moderation process and via direct influence on adjustment (see Fig. 13.1). We distinguish among intrapersonal factors, social-ecological factors, and stress processing as categories of resistance factors in our model.

Risk Factors

As noted in Figure 13.1, a host of disease/disability parameters have been proposed to put children at risk for adjustment problems. Simply having a chronic physical condition puts children at risk (e.g., Wallander, Varni, et al., 1988). It has also been proposed that adjustment covaries with, for example, the severity of the physical condition, the visibility of the condition, presence of bladder or bowel control problems, or presence of brain damage. These specific parameters may exert a direct and/or indirect influence on adjustment. For example, brain damage that causes a motor disability, such as is the case in cerebral palsy, may also affect those parts of the brain involved in the modulation of affect and behavior. In contrast, a visible condition may primarily cause social stressors, which in turn may affect adjustment.

A closely associated yet conceptually distinct risk factor is the functional independence displayed by the child in relation to age expectations. A chronic physical condition will to varying degrees impair the child's ability to function independently, such as in activities of daily living, communication, and involvement with the community. According to Pless and Pinkerton (1975), this represents the prototypical chronic strain for the child with a disability.

Our own conceptual emphasis has been on the psychosocial stress resulting from a chronic physical condition. We hypothesize that children with chronic physical conditions face additional stressful events not typically experienced by healthy peers (e.g., surgeries, cumbersome transportation needs). Furthermore, stressors experienced by most children and which are not in and of themselves related to the physical condition (e.g., start of junior high school) may be harder to confront for these children because of existing disability-related stressors.

Resistance Factors

The impact of the above-described risk factors on adjustment should be influenced by personal characteristics of the child—that is, his or her intrapersonal style. It is difficult, however, to identify *a priori* which characteristics may play a role. From research on adjustment in children in general, we hypothesize that temperament (Thomas & Chess, 1984), effectance motivation (Harter, 1987), and social problem-solving ability (Spivack & Shure, 1974) play a primary role. Similarly, among many potentially relevant characteristics of the social environment in which the child lives, we have emphasized the psychosocial environment or relationship within the family, adjustment of family members, utilitarian or practical resources available to the family, and social support as especially important for the child's adjustment. We acknowledge that the choice of specific intrapersonal and social-ecological variables is somewhat arbitrary.

Consistent with the central role of psychosocial stress in our conceptual model, and following the theory and research of Lazarus and Folkman (1984), we also put considerable emphasis on the role of cognitive appraisal of and coping with the stress in attempting to explain differences in adjustment. These processes together are labeled "stress processing" in our model. Both intrapersonal and social-ecological factors are thought in part to influence adjustment indirectly, by influencing children's appraisal of stress and their management of that stress.

Noncategorical Application

We hold that the process influencing adjustment contains many similarities across different handicapping conditions. In general, disability/disease parameters, functional independence, and psychosocial stress are considered risk factors, and the child's personal style, social ecology, and stress processing are considered resistance factors for adjustment, regardless of specific diagnosis. The specific constitution of these general risk and resistance factors, however, may in part be specific to a diagnostic group. Thus we have adopted an explicitly noncategorical approach (Pless & Perrin, 1985) in our research. Consequently, we are investigating the applicability of our conceptual model to a variety of conditions.

GENERAL RESEARCH METHODOLOGY

Disorders and Sample Descriptions

Most of the research to be reviewed here has been conducted on one of three samples. These are described only briefly below, as further details are available in published reports. In addition to these, we have used this conceptual model as the basis for research on children with cancer (Katz & Varni, 1988), emotional disturbance (Mellins & Wallander, 1991), diabetes (e.g., Keith & Wallander, 1989), and mental retardation (Wallander, 1991), as well as mothers of children with physical disabilities (e.g., Wallander, Pitt, & Mellins, 1990).

Spina Bifida and Cerebral Palsy

We discuss several studies in which 50 children who had either spina bifida or cerebral palsy and who were between the ages of 6 and 11 participated (Wallander, Hubert, & Varni, 1988; Wallander & Varni, 1991; Wallander, Varni, Babani, Banis, DeHaan, & Wilcox, 1989). The commonality in these disorders is the children's impaired gross motor functioning. Spina bifida is a congenital spinal cord defect resulting in various orthopedic, central nervous system, and functional impairments (e.g., bladder and bowel control problems) necessitating a multimodal therapeutic regimen (e.g., exercise and hygiene behaviors). Cerebral palsy is a motor coordination dysfunction of varying degrees resulting from a brain lesion. This lesion can cause concomitant mental and sensory impairments, which necessitates multimodal therapies (e.g., physical, medical, educational). This sample was formed by inviting (via telephone) parents of children who were patients in relevant clinics to participate, of whom 63% did.

Limb Deficiency

As part of an ongoing project designed to assess children's and their families' psychological and social needs, different samples of up to 54 children ages 8–13 with limb deficiencies were investigated (Varni, Rubenfeld, Talbot, & Setoguchi, 1989a, 1989b, 1989c; Varni & Setoguchi, 1991; Varni, Setoguchi, Rappaport, & Talbot, 1991). Limb deficiencies in children are the result of trauma, disease, and congenital causes. All patients in a specialty clinic at a medical school who were in the appropriate age range were invited to participate, of whom the vast majority did.

General Physical and Sensory Disability

A general sample of 118 children ages 2–18, with varying physical or sensory disabilities has been investigated (Wallander & Bachanas, 1991; Wallander et al., 1990). Each had some degree of handicapped motor and/or sensory functioning, which had begun prior to the child's second birthday. The most common conditions were hearing problems, orthopedic impairments (e.g., spina bifida, cerebral palsy), cognitive impairments (e.g., mental retardation), and brain damage (e.g., epilepsy). Many in fact had multiple handicaps.

General Methodology

The specific methodology used in each of the studies has been described in the referenced papers; several general methodological themes, however, should be noted. First, all samples were volunteer samples. Because of restrictions enforced by the clinics, or the recruitment strategies we used (e.g., newspaper notices), we were not able to ascertain the representativeness of our samples. In all cases, however, a broad representation of various demographic backgrounds was obtained.

Second, we have relied to a great extent on paper-and-pencil instruments in measuring variables in each study. Exceptions included, for example, archival data on physical status, test performance for intellectual functioning, and teacher reports for some variables. Depending on the age of the children, self-reports were also obtained in some studies. Nonetheless, we frequently obtained parental (typically maternal) reports about the target children and their environments. This approach was necessitated, we felt, by the limited resources we had for conducting most of the studies, as well as logistical constraints on what could realistically be done with the participants. Of course, some variables are most appropriately assessed via parental report. For example, a parent's perspective on the child's adjustment is important. However, it will be beneficial to obtain more objective assessments in future work.

A final theme that warrants note is the correlational nature of all our research. Obviously, correlation does not prove causation. At the same time, it is difficult to envision experimental studies of the model we have proposed. Although the limitations of correlational research must be acknowledged, it is a bona fide research strategy for many problems. If such research has a strong conceptual basis and takes the form of model testing, it is acceptable to speak about obtaining support for causal hypotheses on the basis of correlational findings. If the research can also be conducted longitudinally, stronger statements can be made about causal priority, since the temporal ordering of the variables is addressed. Unfortunately, we have only lately been able to study some aspects of our model using a prospective time-line design.

Multidimensional Aspect of Adjustment

Adjustment in children is not unidimensional. We have considered behavioral adjustment, self-esteem, and social integration as important dimensions. Of the various dimensions of children's adjustment, behavioral adjustment may be of paramount importance. Distinctions are often made between "externalizing" behavior problems, which are directed toward others or the environment, and "internalizing" behavioral problems, which are manifested as affective expressions. Self-esteem reflects a child's cognitive appraisal of both his or her competence and adequacy in areas that are important to the child and society, and the support and regard the child receives from significant others in his or her environment (Harter, 1987). The child's social integration and activity also need to be considered. Included here are peer relationships and contacts, as well as involvement in social and recreational activities appropriate for the child's age. Given concerns about stigmatization of children with a chronic physical disorder or disability (Richardson, 1970), these children's social functioning is an important dimension of adjustment.

Demographic Factors

As noted, our samples have represented broad demographic characteristics. Because we have not hypothesized that demographic characteristics exert a direct causal influence, demographic differences in adjustment in children with chronic physical disorders are not of theoretical importance to us. Whenever we have tested these relationships, we have found that demographic factors by and large do not explain significant amounts of the variance in the children's adjustment (e.g., Varni et al., 1989a; Wallander, Varni, Babani, Banis, DeHaan, & Wilcox, 1989). Consequently, it is not possible to predict adjustment in children with chronic physical disorders by considering their demographic status.

PHYSICAL PARAMETERS

Disease/Disability and Functional Parameters

We have generally not found a relationship between medical parameters, disability status, or functional ability and behavioral adjustment in investigations of children with a range of chronic physical disorders, as we discuss in more detail below. Social adjustment, in contrast, is significantly related to some of these hypothesized risk factors. For example, maternal reports of the adjustment of 270 children with either juvenile diabetes, spina bifida, hemophilia, chronic obesity, juvenile rheumatoid arthritis (JRA), or cerebral palsy were compared in one study (Wallander, Varni, et al., 1988). There were generally no differences in externalizing or internalizing behavior problems or in social functioning for children with different disorders. Only the externalizing behavior problems for children with JRA were significantly lower than those of children with the other disorders. Similarly, only the social functioning of the children with cerebral palsy was significantly lower than that of children with other disorders.

The medical charts of 61 children ages 4-16 with spina bifida were reviewed with regard to several medical parameters (Wallander, Feldman,

& Varni, 1989). There were no differences in maternal reports of adjustment between children who differed in terms of lesion level, number of surgeries for shunt replacement, number of surgeries for ulcer below the waist, number of overall surgeries, ambulation status, or bladder function. Similarly, there was no association between these children's adjustment and a composite index formed from the aforementioned medical parameters.

Degree of limb loss was assessed in the children with limb deficiencies by means of a specially developed scale (Varni et al., 1989a, 1989b, 1989c). Separate ratings were completed for a child's upper and lower body limb loss, from which a total limb loss score was calculated. However, degree of limb loss was not correlated with children's general self-esteem, depressive symptoms, or behavior problems.

Broader measures of physical, disability, and functional status were obtained in the sample of children with spina bifida and cerebral palsy (Wallander, Varni, Babani, Banis, DeHaan, & Wilcox, 1989). Severity of physical handicap was measured with a global rating made by an independent evaluator, based on observation of the child and interview information from the parent. Intellectual functioning was estimated via several methods, including a brief intelligence test. Functional independence was measured by each child's primary teacher, who completed a standardized adaptive behavior scale. Combining these variables into a multiple regression system did not predict a significant portion of the variance in behavioral adjustment. However, almost 50% of the variance in social adjustment was related to these variables. Intellectual functioning, community self-sufficiency, and personal–social responsibility contributed positively and independently to the children's social adjustment.

The relationship between functional status and adjustment has also been investigated longitudinally in the children with general physical or sensory disabilities (Wallander & Bachanas, 1991). The mothers completed an adaptive behavior scale, from which a composite score (reflecting both daily living skills and communication ability relative to age norms) was computed. They then completed the CBCL 10–12 months later. Consistent with our previous findings, there was no relationship between the children's functional independence and report of behavior problems, but a small significant positive relationship was manifested between the children's functional independence and social adjustment.

Perceived Physical Appearance

It appears from the described work above that objective representations of medical, physical, and functional status are not highly predictive of children's adjustment. Yet we know that having a chronic physical disorder puts children at risk for adjustment problems. Varni has raised the possibility that the child's *perception* of his or her physical appearance influences his or her adjustment (Varni & Setoguchi, 1991). This notion was not initially represented in our conceptual model, but can be integrated into it. Perceived physical appearance is thus thought to be a psychosocial representation of the disease/disability parameters risk factor. Many, but not all, children with chronic physical disorders appear physically different from healthy peers. Others may simply feel physically different, without a visible difference. Widespread cultural values concerning physical appearance may influence the social behavior of others toward individuals with visible physical defects.

Perceived physical appearance has consequently been hypothesized as a predictor of adjustment. Moreover, this construct is thought to mediate the influence of some social-ecological processes, such as social support, on affective adjustment. Consistent with this notion, Varni and Setoguchi (1991) showed that although demographic variables and degree of limb loss were not related to perceived physical appearance, social support from classmates, parents, and teachers and family discord did explain a significant amount of the variance in perceived physical appearance in children with limb deficiencies. Further consistent with our model, Varni, and Setoguchi (1991) showed that negatively perceived physical appearance was related to higher levels of daily microstress, a dimension of the psychosocial stress risk factor. Finally, perceived physical appearance was a significant predictor of psychosocial adjustment, with positively perceived physical appearance being associated with lower depressive and anxious symptoms and higher self-esteem. Varni's work indicates the need for more investigation of perceived physical appearance as a risk factor for maladjustment in children with chronic physical disorder.

PSYCHOLOGICAL STRESS

As noted earlier, we put major emphasis on stress as a risk factor for adjustment problems in children with chronic physical disorders. We think that a child with a chronic physical disorder experiences more stressful life events than a child who is healthy. These stressful events may happen directly to the child (e.g., missing school because of complications, being teased) or indirectly, via effects on his or her family (e.g., marital discord in parents, financial difficulties). Life events may be major (e.g., surgery) or minor (e.g., going to the clinic frequently); the latter events are often called "daily hassles" or "microstressors." Given our findings of a lack of a relationship between adjustment and medical, physical, and functional parameters, we hypothesize that the heightened psychological stress is the proximal or direct cause of adjustment problems. Of course, there is much research establishing a link between life events and adjustment problems in children (see Johnson, 1988), but very little of this has dealt directly with children with chronic physical disorders. Even though we are intrigued by the possibilities of studying stress in this population, we have only begun this investigation.

Varni et al. (1989b, 1989c) reported significant bivariate relationships in children with limb deficiencies between self-reported daily and both depressive symptoms and self-esteem. The children rated the impact of daily hassles that had occurred recently. The sum of these negative ratings constituted the score for daily microstress. Consistent with our thinking that perceived physical appearance is a psychological representation of the child's physical status and that medical or physical parameters should influence psychological stress, Varni and Setoguchi (1991) found a relationship between perceived physical appearance and daily microstress. Higher levels of daily microstress were associated with lower perceived physical appearance in the children with limb deficiencies.

As noted earlier, concurrent relationships between stress and different dimensions of adjustment of the type obtained in these studies (Varni et al, 1989b, 1989c; Varni & Setoguchi, 1991) can be interpreted to support causal influences in either direction. Obtaining prospective longitudinal relationships diminishes this possibility, because the measurements of stress and adjustment have been separated temporally. However, the hypothesized directional influence is not unequivocally supported even then. It is difficult to remove influences from chronic adjustment problems in the occurrence of stressful events in the first place. Nonetheless, longitudinal data do strengthen the argument that stress may have a casual influence on adjustment.

Using data obtained on children with general physical or sensory disabilities, Wallander and Bachanas (1991) found significant relationships between mothers' reports of both major life events and daily microstressors that had occurred to them and their children's behavioral adjustment 10–12 months later. Over 15% of the variance in children's behavior problem could be predicted jointly from the mothers' rated impact of negative major life events and daily microstressors, even when differences in children's functional independence were controlled. It is noteworthy that stress was measured from the mothers' perspective. It can be argued that these stress reports reflected both generally occurring stressful life events that directly affected all family members, and stress experienced indirectly by the children because it created problems for the mothers. These potential mechanisms ought to be teased apart in further research.

Wallander, Keith, and Shay (1991) are currently developing a procedure for the measurement of stress in adolescents with a physical disability. A behavior-analytic procedure was used to interview people in a critical position to note what problematic situations physically disabled adolescents may encounter. These people included parents, teachers, physicians, social workers, and therapists, in addition to disabled adolescents themselves. Over 300 nonredundant problem situations were then categorized, resulting in a two-level hierarchical system describing the types of problem situations encountered by adolescents with a physical disability. The categories at this most general level were as follows: physical limitations and health, health care and therapies, activity restrictions, school, social, future concerns, family, and general negative feelings.

Over 90 specific situations, distributed over all categories, were then generated and presented in written form to 50 adolescents who had a physical disability. They were asked how often each occurred and how difficult each was to deal with. Although problems related directly to the adolescents' physical limitations and health (e.g., going to the clinic/ doctor) occurred most frequently, problems dealing with future concerns (e.g., worry about getting a good job), parents (e.g., parents' not encouraging independence), and social implications (e.g., not having many friends) were rated as most difficult to handle. Higher total frequency of handicap-related problems and difficulty, as reported by the adolescents, significantly predicted parental reports of behavior problems (Wallander et al., 1991).

SOCIAL-ECOLOGICAL FACTORS

Parental Adjustment and Marital Satisfaction

Much research supports a link between parental and child psychosocial functioning (see Hetherington & Martin, 1986). For these reasons, we have hypothesized relationships between parental mental health and marital satisfaction and adjustment in children with chronic physical disorders. Varni et al. (1991) investigated maternal and paternal depression, anxiety, and marital discord as predictors of depression, anxiety, and self-esteem in the children with limb deficiencies. Parents and children reported independently on their mental status. Higher paternal depression and anxiety predicted higher child depression and anxiety; higher paternal anxiety also predicted lower self-esteem in the children. Higher marital discord predicted higher child depression and anxiety and lower child self-esteem. Notably, maternal depression and anxiety did not predict any dimension of child adjustment.

Moreover, Wallander and Bachanas (1991) have addressed some of these relationships in the longitudinal study of children with general physical or sensory disabilities. Mothers who reported more depression, anxiety, and general psychological distress also reported more behavior problems in their children 10–12 months later. Maternal mental health did not predict child social functioning, however. Although the longitudinal feature is an advancement over the Varni et al. (1991), Wallander and Bachanas did not obtain independent measures of maternal and child adjustment, which may account for the differences in their results. Previous research suggests that distressed mothers over-report behavior problems in their children (e.g., Brody & Forehand, 1986). Whether this relationship is apparent over a 1-year period is less clear; some mothers may remain distressed through the year and continue to misrepresent the children's adjustment. A longitudinal study with independent measures would be highly desirable.

Family Environment and Resources

The family psychosocial environment was evaluated in 42 of the children with limb deficiencies (Varni et al. 1989a). Various dimensions of the family environment, considered jointly, predicted over 39% of the variance in these children's behavioral adjustment and 25% in their social adjustment. The specific dimensions of family cohesion and moral/religious emphasis were consistently predictive of better adjustment.

The family psychosocial environment can be considered as one of several resources available to a family in protecting a child from the risk associated with having a chronic physical condition. Family resources were investigated broadly in 153 children ages 4–16, who had either juvenile diabetes, JRA, chronic obesity, spina bifida, or cerebral palsy (Wallander, Varni, Babani, Banis, & Wilcox, 1989). A distinction was made between the psychosocial resources in the family, such as its internal relationships and organization, and the utilitarian resources available to the family to deal with acute and chronic problems. Family income and maternal education level were considered as utilitarian resources in this particular study. These may be indicators of practical resources generally available to a family—namely, financial problem-solving ability. Both psychological and utilitarian family resources were significantly and about equally related to maternal reports of the children's adjustment. However, psychological resources added significantly to the variance in child adjustment, beyond that already contributed by utilitarian resources. These two aspects of the family ecology accounted for about 17% of the variance in the children's behavioral adjustment and 44% in their social adjustment.

Similar analysis have been conducted on data from the children with general physical or sensory disabilities (Wallander & Bachanas, 1991). In a longitudinal analysis, mothers' reports of the psychological family resources were not predictive of the children's behavioral or social adjustment 10–12 months later. However, reports of family mastery and health (which we think of as utilitarian resources) were significantly positively related to children's behavioral, but not social, adjustment.

Finally, we (Wallander & Varni, 1991) investigated a broader set of family ecological factors in the sample of children with either spina bifida or cerebral palsy. Several specific measures of psychosocial and utilitarian family resources were obtained from mothers of these children. Psychological family resources in this study included: family dynamics, marital relationship quality, and maternal social support. Family utilitarian resources included family income, maternal educational level, family size, presence of an older sibling, duration of the marital relationship, and maternal age. Preliminary analysis identified a subset of these as adequate representations of each domain of the family ecology. Psychosocial and utilitarian family resources accounted together for significant proportions of the variance in children's externalizing, but not internalizing, behavior problems. Over 30% of the variance in externalizing behavior problems could be predicted jointly by psychosocial and utilitarian family resources. Further, over 70% of the variance in the children's social functioning could be similarly predicted.

Social Support

There is a long history of studying the role of social support in various health outcomes in adults, but relatively little work has been done on children thus far. In an initial study, mothers of over 150 children with one of several chronic diseases (e.g., juvenile diabetes) or disabling conditions (e.g., spina bifida) reported on the children's family support, peer support, and behavior problems (Wallander & Varni, 1989). Children reported as having high social support from both family and peers showed significantly better adjustment than those with high social support from only one of these sources. Chronically ill or physically disabled children without high support from both sources were reported to have significantly more behavior problems than children in general. Both family and peer support contributed negatively and independently to the variance in externalizing behavior problems, whereas only peer support did so for internalizing behavior problems.

A drawback in the above-described study was the reliance on mothers' reports of children's social support. This led Varni et al. (1989b, 1989c) to study social support as perceived by the child. First, classmate, parent, and teacher social support were significant negative predictors of depressive symptoms (Varni et al., 1989c). Over 70% of the variance in self-reported depressive symptoms could be accounted for by perceived social support. Although higher parent and teacher social support were associated with lower depressive symptomology, the most powerful predictor was classmate social support, followed by teacher social support. Higher levels of classmate, parent, teacher, and friend social support were also associated with higher levels of self-esteem (Varni et al, 1989c). Once again, there was a particularly strong association between classmate social support and self-esteem. The strong association between classmate social support and both fewer depressive symptoms and better self-esteem may reflect the negative values healthy children hold about visible physical handicaps. This in turn may influence classmates' behavior and attitudes toward children with limb deficiencies.

There also appears to be linkages between perceived social support and perceived physical appearance, as noted earlier. Higher levels of social support were associated with better perceived physical appearance (Varni & Setoguchi, 1991). This may suggest an additional indirect path of influence from perceived social support to adjustment, because better perceived physical appearance was also associated with lower depressive and anxious symptoms and higher general self-esteem (Varni & Setoguchi, 1991).

STABLE INTRAPERSONAL FACTORS

Because of our theoretical bias, we have not focused much attention on the role of stable intrapersonal factors in adjustment in children who have a chronic physical disorder. We feel that identifying predictors that are potentially modifiable has priority, given our stated objective to facilitate prevention and intervention efforts. Nonetheless, both for theoretical reasons and for enhanced identification of high-risk children, research is needed addressing the role of personal style in the adjustment of these children.

Thus far we have results pertaining only to the role of temperament in adjustment of children for two of our samples. First, the mothers of children with either spina bifida or cerebral palsy completed questionnaires to assess separately their children's and their own temperaments along several dimensions (Wallander, Hubert, & Varni, 1988). Between 17% and 27% of the variance in the different dimensions of child adjustment could be accounted for by considering the five temperament dimensions jointly. Maternal temperament generally did not predict child adjustment. However, specific knowledge of maternal rhythmicity (i.e., the extent to which a mother prefers a predictable day-to-day pattern) enhanced prediction of some child adjustment dimensions beyond that afforded by child temperament. The "goodness-of-fit" model, which is common in temperament theory and in which temperament characteristics of the child are purported to interact with characteristics in the environment to influence adjustment, was not supported in this study. That is, child and maternal temperament did not interact to predict child adjustment.

Second, mothers of 42 children with limb deficiencies reported on the children's temperament (Varni et al., 1989a). The specific temperament dimension of child emotionality was predictive of both behavioral and social adjustment in the children. Goodness of fit was also evaluated in this study, but this time the family psychosocial environment was considered as the environmental context. Child emotionality interacted with family cohesion in accounting for significant additional variance in behavioral (but not social) adjustment, beyond demographic characteristics, family psychosocial environment, and child temperament. More specifically, children's emotionality was unrelated to behavior problems in families with high cohesion, unlike the relationship existing in families with low cohesion; this finding suggests that family cohesion serves as a protective factor.

STRESS PROCESSING

Lazarus and Folkman (1984) argue that for a full understanding of the role of stress in adjustment, individuals' cognitive appraisals of stressful occurrences and attempts at coping or managing those stressors have to be considered. Although we have incorporated these notions in our conceptual model, we do not yet have data addressing them. However, Wallander and Hardy (1991) are in the process of developing and evaluating a behavioral inventory for assessing coping responses to disability-related stressors displayed by adolescents with a physical disability. The development of an inventory for assessing stress in this population (Wallander et al., 1991) has served as the basis for the development of this behavioral coping inventory. About 25 of the stressful situations that were considered most difficult to handle by the previous sample were identified. More elaborate vignettes were then developed for each stressful situation and recorded on audiotape. We have now played these vignettes to over 70 adolescents with a physical disability, and obtained their impromptu responses as to how they handled each problem situation. Trained coders are in the process of coding all responses. Validity and reliability evaluations will then be completed. Finally, associations of coping behaviors to adjustment will be investigated. We think that this methodology is promising because it prompts the adolescents for more immediate (and perhaps more honest) answers than a paper-and-pencil procedure. A better representation of the adolescents' real-life coping behavior may therefore possibly be obtained with this procedure.

CONCLUSIONS

We have presented here a "snapshot" of our research programs investigating the adjustment of children with chronic physical disorders, in order to illustrate a conceptually based effort at addressing a complex problem. It is important to note that our work is still in progress. Consequently, we are hard pressed to state very many conclusions at present, but we would like to offer a few comments at this point.

First, we think that our work demonstrates the applicability and utility of adopting a noncategorical approach to address our basic research questions. It is applicable, we feel, because our findings are quite consistent across varied disorders. It is a useful approach because it allows investigators to combine samples of relatively low-incidence disorders to achieve, in many cases, the sample sizes needed for more powerful research.

Second, we are fairly firmly convinced that medical or physical status, in whatever form either is expressed, is not very helpful in explaining these children's adjustment. It appears, rather, that psychosocial processes are the primary influences on this psychosocial outcome. Preliminary evidence suggests, we feel, that perceived physical appearance and psychological stress may be significant risk factors for adjustment problems in children with chronic physical disorders.

Third, it is hard to pinpoint powerful resistance factors. Findings regarding these are less consistent across our studies. However, we feel that family resources probably play an important role, but we are not sure of the specific types of resources. We need more longitudinal research to be in a better position to identify these. At present, both psychological and utilitarian resources appear important.

Fourth, social support also appears to be an important resistance factor. We are more certain here that peer support may be especially important. This is not to say that family support is unimportant, but it probably does not stand out in our analysis because there is less variability in family support among children with chronic physical disorders. However, children's peer support is quite variable. Having peer support may also be crucial in protecting them from the negative impact of their special status.

Clearly, much more work is needed, with better methodologies than we have been able to employ thus far. In particular, (1) larger sample sizes that can support analysis of complex multivariate relationships (e.g., through structural equation analysis); (2) prospective longitudinal designs that can better address the causal priority of the theoretical constructs; and (3) independent and objective measurements that avoid the potential for source confounds are all needed in future research. Alternative conceptual models should also be entertained. Nevertheless, we feel that future work must follow from a conceptual model.

REFERENCES

Achenbach, T. M., & Edelbrock, C. (1983). *Manual for the Child Behavior Checklist and Revised Behavior Profile*. Burlington, VT: Thomas M. Achenbach.

Brody, G. M., & Forehand, R. (1986). Maternal perceptions of child maladjustment as a function of the combined influences of child behavior and maternal depression. *Journal of Counseling and Clinical Psychology, 54*, 237–240.

Drotar, D., Doershuk, C. F., Stern, R. C., Boat, C. F., Boyer, W., & Matthews, L. (1981). Psychosocial functioning of children with cystic fibrosis. *Pediatrics, 67*, 338–343.

Gayton, W. F., Friedman, S. B., Tavormina, J. F., & Tucker, F. (1977). Children with cystic fibrosis: I. Psychological test findings of patients, siblings, and parents. *Pediatrics, 59*, 888–894.

Harter, S. (1987). The determinants and mediational role of global self-worth in children. In N. Gisenberg (Ed.), *Contemporary topics in developmental psychology* (pp. 219–242). New York: Wiley.

Hetherington, E. M., & Martin, B. (1986). Family factors and psychopathology in children. In H. C. Quay & J. S. Werry (Eds.), *Psychopathological disorders of childhood* (3rd ed., pp. 332–389). New York: Wiley.

Katz, E. R., & Varni, T. W. (1988). *The impact of social skills training on cognitions and adjustment in newly diagnosed children with cancer*. (Grant funded by the American Cancer Society). Long Beach, CA: Long Beach Memorial Hospital.

Johnson, J. H. (1988). *Life events as stressors in childhood and adolescence*. Newbury Park, CA: Sage.

Keith, B. R., & Wallander, J. L. (1989, August). A cognitive–social model of regimen adherence in adolescent diabetes. In J. L. Wallander (Chair), *Conceptual programmatic research in child health: Diabetes as exemplar*. Symposium conducted at the annual convention of the American Psychological Association, New Orleans.

Lazarus, R. S., & Folkman, S. (1984). *Stress, appraisal, and coping*. New York: Springer.

Mellins, C. A., & Wallander, J. L. (1991). *Emotionally disturbed children's adjustment to a new environment as a function of prior stress and coping abilities*. Manuscript submitted for publication.

Pless, I. B., & Perrin, J. M. (1985). Issues common to a variety of illnesses. In N. Hobbs & J. M. Perrin (Eds.), *Issues in the case of children with chronic illnesses* (pp. 41–60). San Francisco: Jossey-Bass.

Pless, I. B., & Pinkerton, P. (1975). *Chronic childhood disorders: Promoting patterns of adjustments*. Chicago: Year Book Medical.

Pless, I. B., & Roghmann, K. J. (1971). Chronic illness and its consequences: Observations based on three epidemiological surveys. *Journal of Pediatrics, 79*, 351–359.

Richardson, S. A. (1970). Age and sex differences in values toward physical handicaps. *Journal of Health and Social Behavior, 11*, 207–214.

Spivack, G., & Shure, M. B. (1974). *Social adjustment of young children: A cognitive approach to solving real-life problems.* San Francisco: Jossey-Bass.

Thomas, A., & Chess, S. (1984). Genesis and evolution of behavioral disorders: From infancy to early adult life. *American Journal of Psychiatry, 141,* 1-9.

Varni, J. W., Rubenfeld, L. A., Talbot, D., & Setoguchi, Y. (1989a). Family functioning, temperament, and psychological adaptation in children with congenital or acquired limb deficiencies. *Pediatrics, 84,* 323-330.

Varni, J. W., Rubenfeld, L. A., Talbot, D., & Setoguchi, Y. (1989b). Stress, social support, and self-esteem effect on depressive symptomatology in children with congenital/acquired limb deficiencies. *Journal of Pediatric Psychology, 14,* 515-530.

Varni, J. W., Rubenfeld, L. A., Talbot, D., & Setoguchi, Y. (1989c). Determination of self-esteem in children with congenital/acquired limb deficiencies. *Journal of Developmental and Behavioral Pediatrics, 10,* 13-16.

Varni, J. W., & Setoguchi (1991). Correlates of perceived physical appearance in children with congenital/acquired limb deficiences. *Journal of Developmental and Behavioral Pediatrics, 12,* 171-176.

Varni, J. W., Setoguchi, Y., Rappaport, L. R., & Talbot, D. (1991). *Effects of parental adjustment on the adaptation of children with congenital/acquired limb deficiencies.* Manuscript submitted for publication.

Wallander, J. L. (1991). *Mentally retarded adolescents' stress and coping.* (Grant funded by the National Institute of Child Health and Human Development. Birmingham: University of Alabama at Birmingham.

Wallander, J. L., & Bachanas, P. (1991). *Stressful life events and adjustment one year later in children with a chronic physical disability: The role of maternal adjustment and family environment.* Manuscript in preparation, University of Alabama at Birmingham.

Wallander, J. L., Feldman, W. S., & Varni, J. W. (1989). Physical status and psychosocial adjustment in children with spina bifida. *Journal of Pediatric Psychology, 14,* 89-102.

Wallander, J. L., & Hardy, D. (1991). [Physically disabled adolescents' coping with disability-related psychosocial problems]. Unpublished raw data, University of Alabama at Birmingham.

Wallander, J. L., Hubert, N. C., & Varni, J. W. (1988). Child and maternal temperament characteristics, goodness of fit and adjustment in physically handicapped children. *Journal of Clinical Psychology, 17,* 336-344.

Wallander, J. L., Keith, B. R., & Shay, K. A. (1991). *Disability-related problematic psychosocial situations and adjustment in adolescent with a chronic physical disability.* Manuscript in preparation, University of Alabama at Birmingham.

Wallander, J. L., Pitt, L. C., & Mellins, C. A. (1990). Child functional independence and maternal psychosocial stress as risk factors threatening adaptation in mothers of physically or sensorially handicapped children. *Journal of Counseling and Clinical Psychology, 58,* 818-824.

Wallander, J. L., & Varni, J. W. (1989). Social support and adjustment in chronically ill and handicapped children. *American Journal of Community Psychology, 17,* 185–201.

Wallander, J. L., & Varni, J. W. (1991). Social-ecological factors in the adjustment of physically handicapped children. In S. R. Boggs & C. M. Rodriquez (Eds.), *Advances in child health psychology: Abstracts.* Gainesville, FL: Clinical and Health Psychology Publishing.

Wallander, J. L., Varni, J. W., Babani, L. V., Banis, H. T., DeHaan, C. B., & Wilcox, K. T. (1989). Disability parameters, chronic strain, and adaptation of physically handicapped children and their mothers. *Journal of Pediatric Psychology, 14,* 23–42.

Wallander, J. L., Varni, J. W., Babani, L. V., Banis, H. T., & Wilcox, K. T. (1988). Children with chronic physical disorders: Maternal reports of their psychological adjustment. *Journal of Pediatric Psychology, 13,* 197–212.

Wallander, J. L., Varni, J. W., Babani, L. V., Banis, H. T., & Wilcox, K. T. (1989). Family resources as resistance factors for psychological maladjustment in chronically ill and handicapped children. *Journal of Pediatric Psychology, 14,* 157–173.

CURRENT PERSPECTIVES ON INTERVENTION

Overview

C. EUGENE WALKER
University of Oklahoma Health Sciences Center

This section deals with clinical perspectives on stress and coping in children. It is the last section, but by no means the least in importance. The present volume fittingly reflects the nature of pediatric psychology as a discipline. Earlier sections in this volume have carefully examined the conceptual and theoretical issues related to stress and coping in children, and have carefully reviewed the research literature pertaining to individual and family aspects of coping with a wide range of pediatric illnesses. This section contains four chapters that report procedures for clinical intervention with problems of this sort. These interventions are empirically based and are logical extensions and applications of material presented in the earlier chapters. The commitment of pediatric psychologists to the scientist/professional orientation is clearly evident in the coverage provided in this volume. The strong ties of pediatric psychology to behavioral medicine as well as to provision of health care are also abundantly clear in the present volume. Perceptive conceptualization, careful research, and effective intervention are the hallmarks of pediatric psychology in the health care system.

The range of intervention strategies presented in this section reflects the breadth of options open to pediatric psychologists in practice. In Chapter 14, Gagnon, Hudnall, and Andrasik review a number of biologically oriented procedures for coping with stress that have been found to be effective with children and adults. These procedures have a high degree of specificity, work within a relatively short period of time, and can be used with a wide range of subjects. In Chapter 15, Spirito, Stark, and Knapp describe the development of Kidcope, which assesses 10 cognitive and behavioral coping strategies used by children and adolescents in stressful situations related to chronic illness. The clinical use of this instrument and of similar procedures is carefully reviewed. Next, in Chapter 16, Dahlquist discusses her impressive research program on the use of a wide variety of cognitive, modeling, and environmental coping strategies that have been found to be highly effective with children undergoing acutely aversive medical procedures. Finally, Mullins, Gillman, and Harbeck remind us in Chapter 17 that our involvement with patients and interventions as pediatric psychologists take place within a context or system—actually, multiple systems or layers of systems. Therapeutic effectiveness depends not only on scientific sophistication, but also on a sophisticated understanding of the context within which an intervention will either succeed or be sabotaged. The importance of sensitivity to these issues should not be underestimated. The difference between successfully providing care that only the pediatric psychologist can provide and being ignored or rejected by colleagues in a major medical setting often hinges on these issues.

Biofeedback and Related Procedures in Coping with Stress

DOREEN J. GAGNON, LESLIE HUDNALL,
and FRANK ANDRASIK
University of West Florida

The stress response can be elicited by a number of sources in children. Stressors may include family relationships, school, friendships, physical handicaps, and chronic illnesses. Stress can also result from poverty, personal problems, religion, and other sources. The adjustments that children make to the stressors in their lives demonstrate their coping styles. A successful coping style is a way of behaving that reduces adverse stress or enhances healthy stress. An unsuccessful coping style leaves the child feeling incompetent, uncomfortable, frustrated, or disappointed, and may actually contribute to physical illness.

Psychological processes involved in the stress reaction include fear, anger, anxiety, and depression. Physiological processes involved in the stress reaction result from arousal of the sympathetic portion of the autonomic nervous system, which prepares the individual for the "fight-or-flight" response. Research has shown that children can learn to control these responses to stress, just as adults can (Lewis, 1989). The application of biofeedback and related procedures, such as relaxation, the "Quieting Reflex" (QR), guided imagery, meditation, hypnosis, and autogenics, to stress is based on these physiological responses and represents a way of learning self-control to cope with stress. It is important to remember that there is often a need to supplement self-regulatory training with individual and family counseling, in order to address the complexities of a child's presenting problems. Recently, attention to biofeedback has expanded to include cognitive aspects of human learning as well (Andrasik & Blanchard, 1983; Kater & Spires, 1975; Strider & Strider, 1979).

Cognitive or cognitive–behavioral therapy is an important component of any treatment package for stress and is discussed in more detail in another chapter. Much of the literature has examined multiple treatment packages that have included biofeedback and/or relaxation training as the primary behavioral component, with guided imagery, autogenics, hypnosis, and cognitive techniques introduced as adjunctive procedures.

BIOFEEDBACK AND RELATED PROCEDURES

Biofeedback

There are a number of definitions of "biofeedback," varying in their degree of complexity. However, two components are common to all these definitions: (1) a constant monitoring of one or more physiological processes via electronic equipment; and (2) external feedback of the processes and subsequent changes in them, which permits the person to learn strategies that enable control of these processes. As this definition implies, biofeedback extends primarily from an operant learning paradigm wherein feedback serves as the reinforcing stimulus, although other explanatory models have been advanced (Olson & Schwartz, 1987). Most research on biofeedback technology and its clinical applications for stress management has been carried out with adult populations. In light of the operant nature of biofeedback, there does not seem to be a clear theoretical basis for excluding children and adolescents from biofeedback research, particularly since other operant conditioning procedures have been so successful with this age group.

Although it was once assumed that children would have greater difficulty with biofeedback than adults, several research studies and anecdotal reports suggest that the opposite is true. Suter and Loughry-Machado (1981) taught both parents and children how to control peripheral skin temperature and found that, in just two biofeedback sessions, children's performance was superior to that of their parents. Hunter, Russell, Russell, and Zimmerman (1976) compared the performance of learning-disabled and "normal" children and found that when learning skin temperature control, younger children performed better than older children, and learning-disabled children outperformed non-learning-disabled children.

There are many hypotheses for why children may exhibit better performance than adults (Attanasio et al., 1985). First, children seem more enthusiastic about biofeedback procedures than adults; many find the instrumentation fascinating, especially in this age of video and computer games. This game-like quality of biofeedback may help to mobilize children's interest and motivation, and it may also create serendipitous opportunities for them to learn how to manage the simultaneous effects of excitement and competitiveness. Another advantage in working with children is their lessened skepticism about biofeedback procedures. Children more easily accept explanations of the purpose of physiological self-control and are more able to maintain a positive attitude about their performance; these attributes may combine with a positive attitude about biofeedback to enable them to learn the desired responses more quickly. Moreover, children have positive expectations about their abilities in general, and subsequently enter biofeedback treatment certain that they can produce the desired response. In fact, clinicians should be on the lookout for unrealistic expectations among children and should attempt to correct them early in the treatment. Children can set themselves up for failure at a task through faulty thinking about their own abilities.

Some disadvantages associated with the use of biofeedback in children need to be acknowledged. Learning to control physiological processes requires attention to feedback for a reasonably extended period of time. In general, children have briefer attention spans and are more distractible than adults. Some children are unable to concentrate on the feedback signals because they do not find them intrinsically reinforcing. Experimenting with a variety of feedback signals to find one reinforcing to a particular child, or adding tangible reinforcers contingent on achieving certain performance standards, may be helpful in enhancing and sustaining the child's attention. In general, it appears that a computer display holds a child's attention longer, and the variety of displays available (including game-like graphics) allows the therapist to change feedback displays when needed to maintain the child's interest.

Another difficulty in working with children is the fear and apprehension they may experience about the equipment and procedures. Attanasio et al. (1985) suggest a number of strategies that a clinician can use to reduce a child's apprehension. There is a need to explain the treatment procedures carefully and demonstrate all the equipment to both children and parents; to provide reassurance frequently; to discourage "humorous" references to electric chairs and electric shock; and to refer to electrodes as "sensors" or "pickups." It is often desirable to have parents participate in all assessment procedures first, while the child observes and becomes accustomed to the procedures. Alternately, one parent may "sit in" on treatment sessions to ensure that the parent has a complete understanding of the treatment procedures and has been allowed the opportunity to question or comment on them.

Developmental differences, in addition to brief attention span, may pose further complications. One issue is children's varying ability to comprehend the treatment rationale and procedures. Frequently, the clinician will need to spend a great deal of time and effort simplifying instructions and explanations, as well as reviewing them numerous times with a child in order to ensure adequate comprehension. To enhance a child's ability to understand and participate in the procedures, biofeed-back can be presented in a classroom-like context, with the therapist being introduced as a "biofeedback teacher" who likes to question and be questioned by students (Green, 1983). Other helpful suggestions and more detailed discussions of biofeedback in pediatrics may be found in Andrasik and Attanasio (1985) and Green (1983).

Relaxation

Although research has shown that relaxation training is a successful stress management technique for adults (Borkovec, Grayson, & Cooper, 1978; Lehrer, Woolfolk, Rooney, McCann, & Carrington, 1983), the results with children have been limited and inconclusive. Many of these studies have been plagued with methodological problems and have lacked adequate control groups. However, reviews (Masek & Fentress, 1984; Richter, 1984) of more recent rigorous studies indicate that relaxation procedures can be effective in helping children cope with various physiological and psychological stressors.

Most relaxation training programs include an abbreviated version of Jacobson's progressive relaxation (Jacobson, 1938). This technique gener-ally involves a child's systematically tensing and releasing various muscle groups on command of the therapist. The child learns to discriminate various tension states by concentrating on the feelings of tension and relaxation.

Cautela and Groden (1978) have developed progressive relaxation exercises that are appropriate for children. To modify the adult procedure for children, Cautela and Groden make the following suggestions: Children should be taught to tighten and relax gross motor areas first; more than one session is usually necessary to go through all of the muscle groups; instruc-tions should be simplified with more discrete steps; shorter sessions should be taught daily or, if possible, twice a day; concrete and social reinforcers, modeling, and special toys may be useful; more touching and manipulation may be necessary; and prerequisite skills (e.g., maintaining eye contact, sitting still, and imitating movements) may need to be taught.

With practice, children can learn to relax on demand (Walker, 1979). For optimal results, children should receive relaxation training for at least 6 weeks (Richter, 1984). Another important part of relaxation training for children should be learning relaxed breathing. The therapist can use different exercises and examples to teach children to use dia-phragmatic rather than thoracic breathing. In most cases, children may learn by modeling the therapist's taking slow, deep breaths and by saying "relax" as they exhale. In special cases, toys such as whistles, harmonicas, and party blowers help facilitate air flow. Cautela and Groden (1978) describe "blowing games" that may be useful.

A variation of progressive relaxation tailored for children is creative relaxation (Humphrey & Humphrey, 1981), which combines a form of imagery and muscle tensing and releasing. Contrasting creative movements are performed to tense and relax individual muscles, muscle groups, or the entire body. For example, the instructor may ask, "What is the main difference between a baseball bat and a jump rope?" Following a brief group discussion, the leader instructs the children to make their arms like a bat and then like a rope. Questions are raised after the movements to help the children reflect on the feelings of tension and relaxation. Other comparisons may include hard versus soft or heavy versus light. A creative leader can generate many different movement exercises and promote discussions that will increase an understanding of the relaxation phenomenon. However, despite the face validity of this particular technique, no rigorous research has tested its effectiveness in reducing stress and tension.

Another form of relaxation is meditative relaxation, combining meditation and relaxation training. Children are instructed to sit quietly with their eyes closed, relax their muscles deeply, and become aware of their breathing. Each time they exhale, they should say a word silently to themselves. Distracting thoughts should be acknowledged, and then attention should be returned to the breath. After 20 minutes, they should sit quietly for a few moments and then slowly open their eyes (Benson, 1975).

Guided imagery, autogenic phrases, and breathing exercises are often used in conjunction with relaxation training for children. Using guided imagery, the therapist instructs the child through a pleasant, imagined scene that focuses on warmth and/or peace. Examples of typical scenes include walking in the woods, going to the beach, and lying in the grass. It is often advantageous to ask the child about a personal pleasant and relaxing event to be incorporated into the scene. A variation of this approach, guided fantasy, may be more effective with younger children. The child imagines himself or herself in a relaxing fantasy situation, such as being a butterfly or bird. At the end of these scenes, it is important that the therapist suggest to the child that he or she can enjoy the same type of calmness at another time by closing his or her eyes and taking some deep breaths (Angus, 1989). Masters and Houston (1975), DeMille (1973), and Lupin (1977) provide other examples of scenes and fantasies that are appropriate for children.

Autogenic phrases are often used with relaxation and biofeedback procedures to treat psychosomatic and stress-related disorders (Strider, 1981). Autogenic therapy was developed by J. H. Schultz and was introduced to the United States through the work and writings of Wolfgang Luthe (e.g., Luthe, 1969). Autogenic phrases are verbal statements, such as "My right leg is heavy and warm," designed to induce sensations of heaviness and warmth in various parts of the body. Autogenic training appears to be associated with a variety of important physiological changes, including decreased respiration rate, heart rate, and blood pressure. Different autogenic phrases and procedures are recommended, depending on the presenting problem, and Luthe (1969) provides examples of these phrases.

Studies in the schools with "healthy" children have indicated that relaxation training may be effective in reducing general stress. Zaichkowsky and Zaichkowsky (1984) evaluated a 6-week relaxation program (including a didactic lesson, progressive relaxation, mental imagery, and breathing exercises) with fourth-graders. The experimental group experienced significant pre- to postintervention improvements on all measures (heart rate, skin temperature, respiration rate, and state anxiety) except trait anxiety. The control subjects showed only a significant increase in their ability to raise skin temperature. LaMontagne, Mason, and Hepworth (1985) examined the efficacy of a 2-week program of progressive relaxation and guided imagery presented by the teacher to second-grade children. Although the results were not statistically significant, the pattern suggested that the treatment group experienced less anxiety (as assessed by the Gillis Child Anxiety Scale; Gillis, 1980) than the control group.

Quieting Reflex

The QR is another form of biofeedback/relaxation; it was discovered in 1974 as an outgrowth of an attempt to use biofeedback to treat stress disorders in an outpatient clinic population ranging from 7 to 70 years of age (Stroebel, Ford, Strong, & Szarek, 1981). Stroebel and Stroebel (1984) postulate that the QR is a 6-second response that is incompatible with and interrupts the emergency fight-or-flight response. Children's physiological responses to stress are often identical to those of adults, except that children have fewer choices than adults in avoiding stress. Bodies of healthy children quickly recover normal balance after their initial reaction to stress. This is the body's inherent quieting reaction, or QR. Many youngsters have learned to override their own natural quieting response until constant tension, anxiety, and muscle tightness begin to seem normal to them. The QR involves the following components: (1) increased discrimination of arousal cues and dysponesis ("dysponesis" is the term used for a faulty muscle bracing or a physiological condition of shortened muscle fibers and constricted blood flow to the muscles); (2) easy abdominal breathing and elements of progressive relaxation; (3) autogenic training; and (4) rational–emotive therapy. All are directed to achieving an inner balance of the body called "adaptive homeostasis."

The original QR training integrated frontal electromyographic (EMG) and digital thermal feedback with deep breathing exercises, progressive relaxation, and autogenic techniques taught in eight sessions. Application of this program to 340 adult patients (whose disorders included headache, Raynaud's disease, hypertension, irritable colon, anxiety, and pain) revealed 55% overall success in minimizing subjective components of the disorders at the end of 2 years (Stroebel et al., 1981). The field-tested treatment incorporated both feedback and relaxation procedures. The marketed packages (Stroebel, 1978; Stroebel, Stroebel, & Holland, 1980) have omitted feedback training, because clinical observations suggested that with practice, QR was sufficient for improving a person's ability to avoid and lessen stress-related illnesses. Unfortunately, the modified program has not been compared to the original program in either adult or pediatric populations.

The QR program comes in three forms: QR for Adults, QR for Young People, and Kiddie QR (for elementary-school-age children). The adult and adolescent versions consist of eight sessions. The Kiddie QR program is divided into 16 experiential exercises lasting 4 to 7 minutes each, with mental imagery playing a more prominent role in the children's version. Mental imagery is the main tool used to develop skill at discriminating tension states and replacing them with feelings of relaxation. Through a series of guided imagery exercises, children are taught (1) to perceive rising tension in their bodies and (2) to initiate some procedure to counter tension. Initially, the Kiddie QR program was written to be used with normal, fairly healthy youngsters ages 3 to 8, who were exposed to typical stressful situations of everyday living. As the program grew in popularity, Kiddie QR was reportedly used with some success with a multitude of children, such as those with emotional problems and the physically handicapped (Stroebel & Stroebel, 1984). However, well-controlled studies have not been carried out with these populations. Some clinicians have incorporated QR in their clinical practice, but they often add thermal and EMG biofeedback components for optimal results (Curran, 1989).

Ragan and Hiebert (1987), in the only controlled study, investigated the efficacy of implementing Kiddie QR (Stroebel et al., 1980) with primary-grade students in a classroom setting. Four female teachers from a large suburban elementary school, situated in a predominantly middle-class area, volunteered to implement the program in their classrooms (kindergarten and grades 1, 2, and 3). The Kiddie QR exercises were introduced to the students as an integral part of the regular classroom activity. Two significant treatment effects were found. First, there was a reduction in trait anxiety scores as measured by the State–Trait Anxiety Inventory for Children (Spielberger, 1973) for the third-grade students, whose higher level of self-reported pretest anxiety allowed room for change. Also, the treatment group reported a higher level of school satisfaction as measured by the Student's Perception of Ability Scale

(Boersma & Chapman, 1979) than did the control group, although the difference was small in terms of practical significance.

Overall, the results of this study were not strongly supportive, but several factors may have operated to weaken effects. First, the students reported relatively low levels of anxiety at the onset of the study, leaving little room for improvement. Second, the teachers had difficulty adhering to the program. Although the developers of the Kiddie QR program state that the training is easily integrated into the daily school routine, Ragan and Hiebert (1987) did not find this to be true. All four teachers in this study stated that, because the program started during the last quarter of the year, competing curricular demands prevented them from spending as much time as they otherwise might have in practicing the exercises and generalizing the techniques to school settings outside the classroom. A method of promoting teacher adherence might involve scheduling QR exercises at regular times during the school day to prevent other activities from taking priority. The problem of teacher adherence to the program might also be rectified by more careful screening of teachers; those who feel a responsibility for fostering the nonacademic development of students, and who are able to step aside from an authoritarian demeanor to allow children to develop more self-responsibility, should be selected.

Hypnosis

Another behavioral technique useful in reducing children's stress is hypnotherapy. Olness and Gardner (1978) define therapeutic hypnosis as "an altered state of consciousness, usually involving relaxation, in which a person develops heightened concentration on a particular idea or image for the purpose of maximizing potential in one or more areas" (p. 228). Hypnotherapy is a treatment modality in which a hypnotized client experiences some therapeutic intervention (Olness & Gardner, 1988). Olness and Gardner (1978) suggest that children may be able to use hypnosis more readily than adults because children have fewer inhibitions about engaging in fantasy and imagery. Practitioners and researchers have suggested that hypnotherapy is effective in reducing distress related to medical problems and pain through mastery and relaxation (Olness & Gardner, 1988). Although hypnotherapy has been applied to a wide range of medical problems, most of the controlled, well-designed research with children has involved asthma (Aronoff, Aronoff, & Peck, 1975; Barbour, 1980; Kohen, 1986) and headaches (Olness, MacDonald, & Uden, 1987). Case studies of children have also reported favorable results with diabetes (Olness & Gardner, 1988), gastrointestinal disorders (Williams & Singh, 1976), juvenile rheumatoid arthritis (Cioppa & Thal, 1975), and seizures (Olness & Gardner, 1988).

PHYSIOLOGICAL AND MEDICAL STRESSORS
Asthma

Asthma is a bronchial disorder characterized by intermittent, variable, and reversible airway obstruction (Chai, 1975). Asthma has also been described as a chronic disorder that is a psychophysiological reaction to stress (Bieliauskas, 1982). It is estimated that between 5% and 10% of all children under the age of 12 experience asthma (Weinstein, 1987). Life stress has been found to relate to symptom severity, degree of control over illness, and recurrent symptoms in children with asthma (De Araujo, Van Arsdel, Holmes, & Dudley, 1973). There is a continuing debate over whether asthma is primarily medical or psychological, but most believe that emotional behaviors play a part in the precipitation of an attack (Viney, 1983; Viney & Westbrook, 1985). Psychological intervention follows one of three basic approaches. The first is traditional psychotherapy, but evidence of the utility of this approach is nonexistent (Creer, 1982). The remaining two approaches attempt to alter either the abnormal pulmonary functioning (via biofeedback and relaxation) or the maladaptive asthma-related behaviors (Alexander, 1983); treatments often use both.

Two biofeedback approaches have been attempted to modify pulmonary functioning—one through indirect means, the other more directly. EMG biofeedback from the forehead area seeks to modify respiratory events by indirect means, assuming that changes in muscle tone will lead to subsequent changes in asthma symptomatology (progressive muscle relaxation is based on the same reasoning). Early investigations of frontal EMG biofeedback combined with relaxation therapy found that this combination had some effect on the respiratory components of the disease in children (Davis, Saunders, Creer, & Chai, 1973; Scherr, Crawford, Sergent, & Scherr, 1975). Subsequent work (Kotses, Glaus, Bricel, Edwards, & Crawford, 1978; Kotses, Glaus, Crawford, Edwards, & Scherr, 1976) isolated and examined the effects on respiratory functions of frontal EMG biofeedback alone, with promising short-term results. Kotses and Glaus (1981) and Glaus and Kotses (1983) speculate that relaxing the forehead muscles leads to concomitant changes in pulmonary tone because of a neural reflex comprising trigeminal and vagal components. In their model, afferent trigeminal activity induced by facial muscle tension changes affects efferent vagal activity, a determinant of bronchomotor tone. A recent replication of the biofeedback-induced facial relaxation treatment revealed both short- and long-term (5-month) improvements in pulmonary functioning for child asthmatics (Kotses et al., 1991). Some traditional measures of asthma severity did not improve following treatment, however, leading Kotses et al. to point out appropriately that biofeedback cannot be considered a comprehensive treatment for this condition. Rather, it is to be viewed as an important component of an asthma self-management program.

Relaxation training alone has been examined as an adjunct therapy for the purpose of increasing airflow rates during an asthma attack. Alexander, Miklich, and Hershkoff (1972) compared peak expiratory flow rates in children trained in progressive relaxation versus children who rested quietly. They found significant mean increases in flow rate over sessions for the treatment group, while control subjects experienced a nonsignificant decrease. However, in a follow-up study, Alexander, Cropp, and Chai (1979) failed to replicate the previous results. Using children as their own controls, they found no differences between relaxation and resting on four measures of pulmonary functioning. Discouraging data for relaxation training have also been reported by Davis et al. (1973).

The second type of biofeedback involves direct feedback of airflow or airway resistance variables as a more straightforward means of controlling the symptoms of asthma. Two procedures have been developed to alter airflow resistance. The first procedure uses airflow biofeedback in a counterconditioning paradigm (Khan, 1977; Khan, Staerk, & Bonk, 1973). A child first receives biofeedback for the level of forced expiratory volume, in order to relax the bronchial tubes. Once this response is acquired, bronchoconstriction is induced by a variety of procedures (e.g., hyperventilation, recall of past attacks, or inhalation of a bronchoconstrictor) to the point of wheezing, at which time the child uses his or her biofeedback skills to abort the bronchospasms. The counterconditioning approach produced promising initial results, but subsequent attempts at replication have not been as successful (Danker, Miklich, Pratt, & Creer, 1975).

The second procedure, devised by Feldman (1976), employs an alternative airway biofeedback procedure that involves continuous monitoring of total respiratory resistance (TRR) by a forced-oscillation technique. In this procedure, a small-amplitude pressure of a known and well-calibrated quantity is directed into a subject's airway through a tightly sealed mouthpiece. TRR can be measured with each exhalation, and this information is then fed back to the child as a tone via an external speaker. A detailed study of this technique with four male asthmatics (ages 10–16) revealed that changes in certain parameters rivaled those occurring as a result of medication; this was the first biofeedback procedure for which this result was obtained. However, the elaborate nature of this treatment and the high associated equipment costs appear to be limiting further exploration of the treatment.

Hypnosis has also been investigated with promising results. A study of asthmatic children given direct hypnotic suggestions for chest relaxation, easy breathing, and reduction of wheezing (Aronoff et al., 1975) reported that in most cases the children experienced immediate improvement. Barbour (1980) found that adolescents employing self-hypnosis over a 5-month period experienced reductions in the severity and frequency of asthma attacks. Interesting results were reported by Kohen (1986): Although there were no differences between the self-hypnosis and control groups in pulmonary function tests during or immediately after intervention, at 1- and 2-year follow-up assessments improvements were noted in the experimental group. These studies lend credibility to the idea that hypnosis can have an effect, in both the short and the long term, on physiological components of asthma.

Efforts aimed at teaching asthmatics to better manage their condition and the behavioral responses to and consequences associated with asthma are beginning to be viewed as important, legitimate adjuncts to medical care. More research is needed to clarify the role of biofeedback and other techniques such as awareness, education, relaxation, and self-management skills in modifying behavioral excesses and deficits related to asthma. Common behavioral excesses targeted for treatment include anxiety-induced hyperventilation, "asthma panic," malingering, and inappropriate coughing (see Alexander, 1983, and Creer, 1979, 1991, for further details).

There is a paucity of studies examining biofeedback treatment of asthmatics in the past several years, with the only exception being the recent publication by Kotses et al. (1991). Attempts to aid in regulation of asthma through biofeedback are very encouraging, but by no means definitive (Andrasik, Kabela, & Blake, 1988). The data at hand do support EMG biofeedback as a very useful adjunct to treatment. Until the equipment costs and the technical requirements decrease, however, the other biofeedback treatments will probably remain experimental. Although initial research on the use of relaxation with asthmatic children looked promising, later studies did not support relaxation training alone as an effective treatment for asthma. Hypnosis has produced promising preliminary results for both short- and long-term effects on pulmonary functioning and warrants further investigation.

Headache

Headache has been described as one of the most common types of recurrent pain among children (Bush, 1987). Rothner (1978) reported that from 3% to 16% of children under the age of 16 suffer from significant headache problems. By the age of 15, the percentage of adolescents experiencing frequent, recurrent headache climbs to approximately 20% (Bille, 1962; Sillanpaa, 1983). Available longitudinal data suggest that headache continues into adulthood for the majority of children (Bille, 1981). Headache has both physiological and psychological components, with the most commonly reported precipitant being stress. Dalsgaard-Nielson (1965) observed that 68% of a group of chronic pediatric headache patients recognized that psychological stress due to school demands and conflict in the home accounted for over half of all migraines. An assessment study of young people with headaches (Leviton, Slack, Masek, Bana, & Graham, 1984) noted that the most commonly acknowledged contributor to headache in children up to age 16 was "an especially hard day," with "worrying a lot" and "unexpected excitement or pressure" following closely behind. Data collected on child headache sufferers, however, indicate that they are exposed to much the same levels of stress as are children who are headache-free (Andrasik, Kabela, Quinn, et al., 1988) Therefore, it appears that migraine and tension headaches are precipitated by typical everyday stresses to which the headache-prone child responds in a psychologically and biologically atypical and extreme manner. Unfortunately, most analyses of the link between stress and headache have been retrospective in nature; studies with repeated prospective assessments are needed to explicate more fully the role of stress as a trigger for pediatric headache.

The effectiveness of relaxation and biofeedback procedures for treatment of adult headaches is well documented (Andrasik, 1990; Holroyd, 1986; Holroyd & Penzien, 1986). Pediatric studies have lagged far behind. Numerous self-regulatory procedures (biofeedback, guided imagery, progressive muscle relaxation, meditation, hypnosis, and cognitive restructuring) have been used in an attempt to train children to regulate headaches. Most studies conducted in this area have focused on the use of biofeedback (EMG and thermal), relaxation, and autogenic approaches. Typical treatment effects for psychophysiological procedures in children fall within the range of 50–90% symptom improvement over the short run (see review by Andrasik, Blake, & McCarran, 1986).

Two forms of biofeedback treatment exist for management of migraine headache: thermal biofeedback and cephalic blood volume pulse (BVP) biofeedback. EMG biofeedback is used most often for treatment of tension headaches. Hoelscher and Lichstein (1984), in a review of self-regulatory methods for child migraine, reported that skin temperature biofeedback with autogenic training was associated with significant reductions in migraine headache activity. Only one study (Feuerstein & Adams, 1977) was found that looked at BVP biofeedback for pediatric migraine, and this single-subject experiment supported the effectiveness of the BVP procedure. A more recent review by Duckro and Cantwell-Simmons (1989) evaluated the effectiveness of EMG biofeedback for tension headaches, thermal biofeedback for migraine headaches, and relaxation for both. Overall outcome showed that 88% of the children met the criterion of 50% reduction in the combined change in frequency, duration, and intensity of headache when they used a combination of biofeedback and relaxation. In no study was the behavioral treatment found to be without positive benefit. Comparing biofeedback and relaxation was more difficult, since most treatments consisted of some combination of biofeedback and relaxation, and no comparable control group was used. Of the studies found that incorporated biofeedback into their treatment, only one study compared the biofeedback treatment to progressive relaxation (Fentress, Masek, Mehegan, & Benson, 1986), and that study also had both treatment groups using meditation. The researchers found no significant difference in treatment effects between temperature biofeedback and progressive relaxation in pediatric migraineurs.

In a study that examined relaxation training alone, Wisniewski, Genshaft, Mulick, Coury, and Hammer (1988) treated 10 chronic headache sufferers, ranging in age from 12 to 17 years, with progressive relaxation. Following treatment, subjects in the experimental group demonstrated significant decreases in global headache activity, compared to the subjects in the waiting-list control group. Limited follow-up data suggested that treatment effects were generally maintained. Larsson, Melin, Lamminen, and Ullstedt (1987) treated 34 adolescents having tension and/or combined headaches with either progressive muscle relaxation or general problem discussion. A control group was asked to keep headache diaries. The relaxation group reported greater decreases in frequency, intensity, and duration of their headaches than did the other two groups. A 5-month follow-up revealed that improvements in all areas of headache activity had increased. Richter et al. (1986) compared the efficacy of progressive relaxation and cognitive coping in treating migraines in 42 children and adolescents. The results showed no differences between the treatments; both treatments were superior to the nonspecific placebo control in reducing overall headache activity and frequency, but not duration or intensity. Both experimental groups continued to improve through a 16-week follow-up period. Other studies have demonstrated that relaxation groups experience greater decreases in global headache activity than do control groups (Larsson, Daleflod, Hakansson, & Melin, 1987; Larsson & Melin, 1986). Somewhat more equivocal results were reported by Emmen and Passchier (1987), who compared progressive relaxation with "concentration" exercises. In the adolescent relaxation group, frequency and duration of headaches decreased; however, intensity of headaches unexpectedly increased. Follow-up data were not collected, so it is not known whether this increase in intensity continued over time.

Olness et al. (1987) compared propranolol, placebo, and self-hypnosis in a within-subject study of juvenile classic migraine. They found a significant association between decrease in *frequency* of headaches and self-hypnosis training. However, the subjects did not experience significant changes in headache *severity* during any of the three treatment periods.

In general, the literature supports the conclusion that biofeedback combined with relaxation training is effective in managing headache among children and adolescents. Results are consistent with the observation that children respond well to relatively brief behavioral therapy with minimal follow-up. Long-term follow-up evaluations are very limited for relaxation-alone studies (from 0 to 6 months) at this time, but they seem to indicate that treatment effects are maintained. Follow-up evaluations for relaxation with biofeedback are more extensive: follow-up data from 6 months to 3 years reveal that improvement in headache persists over time. Few studies have looked at younger children. Future studies need to examine the efficacy of relaxation techniques with younger children and to report follow-up data collected at longer time intervals. Studies directly comparing various stress management approaches have revealed no differences in group outcome. Such studies, however, have not incorporated methodologies suitable for characterizing individual patient responses. Results from crossover (partial) designs with adult patients suggest that biofeedback may offer a treatment advantage over relaxation for certain individuals. Similar research strategies may be helpful in illuminating differential treatment responses with pediatric headache patients (see Andrasik, 1989, for a more complete discussion).

Nearly all investigations of biofeedback and relaxation treatment for headache involve the administration of treatment in the traditional one-to-one, in-office delivery mode. Burke and Andrasik (1989) tested two reduced-therapist-contact biofeedback treatments (one administered by children, the other by parents), and 1-year follow-up revealed a similar effectiveness for both home-based treatments when compared to standard, office-based procedures. Larsson and Melin (1986) administered relaxation training to groups of three to four adolescents in a school setting. Relaxation therapy led to significant improvements in headache activity when compared to an information-contact condition or a self-registration group. The majority of the students in the relaxation training attained more than 50% reduction in headache activity. The results from these investigations of ways to deliver relaxation-based treatments in a more economical, time-efficient manner are encouraging and warrant further research attention.

Insomnia

Reports of the effectiveness of relaxation training as a treatment for childhood insomnia are very limited and mainly anecdotal. No studies were found that utilized biofeedback for treatment of insomnia. Weil and Goldfried (1973) employed progressive relaxation in the treatment of insomnia in an 11-year-old girl. After 6 weeks of home practice with taped instructions used before bedtime, the girl had no difficulty falling asleep. At a 6-month follow-up, the girl still reported no sleep disturbances. Similarly, Anderson (1979) reported a successful case study of a 13-year-old boy with a 4-month history of insomnia. The treatment program involved progressive relaxation to reduce the level of arousal and a simple behavioral program to reduce the mother's attention to the problem.

These studies present suggestive evidence for the efficacy of relaxation training in the treatment of insomnia. However, controlled research is needed before stronger conclusions can be drawn.

Painful Medical Procedures

Stress reduction in young dental patients is an area of growing interest. Siegel and Peterson (1980) selected 42 preschool children from low-income families who had never visited the dentist. Children in the coping skills group were taught general body relaxation, deep and regular breathing, imagery, and calming self-talk. Children in the sensory information condition were presented with a description of the basic procedures and typical physical sensations, sights, and sounds that they would experience during the dental session. The results indicated that children in both treatment groups were less anxious and distressed and more cooperative than were children in the control procedure. This experiment, however, did not provide definitive information regarding which active component of the experimental treatments yielded beneficial experimental results. Future research is needed to assess the unique contributions of components of sensory information, coping skills, and preparation itself. Future investigations are also needed to examine the success of these procedures with older children who have had previous dental treatment, as well as the continuing success of the procedure with repeated dental treatments.

Relaxation combined with EMG biofeedback has been found useful in helping children cope with painful inpatient medical procedures (Campbell, Clark, & Kirkpatrick, 1986). Research has also provided suggestive evidence that hypnosis can help children cope with pain and anxiety. Researchers have examined the effects of hypnosis on pain control for child cancer patients who are required to receive painful medical treatments, such as chemotherapy, bone marrow aspirations, and lumbar punctures. Although most of the evidence is based on case studies, several investigations (Ellenberg, Kellerman, Dash, Higgins, & Zeltzer, 1980; Gardner, 1976; LaBaw, Holton, Tewell, & Eccles, 1975; Olness, 1981) indicate that hypnosis may reduce pain and anxiety in children with cancer. Hypnosis has also been successful in anecdotal reports of children with severe burns (Bernstein, 1965, 1972; Betcher, 1960; LaBaw, 1973). Other studies suggest that hypnosis may help children during dentistry procedures (Bernick, 1972; Crasilneck & Hall, 1975; Thompson, 1963).

Jay, Ozolins, Elliott, and Caldwell (1983) assessed levels of children's distress over such painful medical procedures as bone marrow aspiration. Clinical observation suggested that many older children might in fact be highly anxious about medical procedures, even though they often did not exhibit their distress behaviorally (by crying, screaming, flailing, etc.), as younger children often did. In this study, the need for intervention with older children was revealed more convincingly through self-report measures. This points out the necessity of using self-report measures of distress with older children; the additional use of physiological measures should contribute even more information in the assessment of anxiety, pain, and distress. Jay et al. (1983) also documented the relationship between parental anxiety and children's distress levels. Parents who were generally more anxious and who anticipated high levels of pain for their children had children who exhibited higher levels of behavioral distress during medical procedures. The direction of the causation is indeterminate. The authors' clinical observations suggested that children whose parents emphasized mastery over avoidance and who did not react in an overly anxious or overly indulgent manner had children who coped better, exhibited less anticipatory anxiety before a clinic visit, and accepted the medical procedure as a grim fact of life (despite their behavioral protests during the procedures). An alternative explanation, however, might be that some children are more vulnerable in stressful situations, and that parents of such children become more anxious and upset in reaction to their child's stress.

Jay, Elliott, Katz, and Siegel (1987) went on to evaluate the efficacy of a cognitive–behavioral intervention package and a low-risk pharmacological intervention (oral Valium) in reducing children's distress during bone marrow aspirations. The cognitive–behavioral therapy intervention consisted of five components: filmed modeling, breathing exercises, positive incentive, imagery/distraction, and behavioral rehearsal. This package was based on a stress inoculation model, incorporating education, skill acquisition, and rehearsal of coping skills (Turk, 1978). Results indicated that children in the cognitive–behavioral therapy condition had significantly lower behavioral distress, pain ratings, and pulse rates than those in an attention control group. Children in the Valium condition exhibited no significant differences from the children in the attention control condition except that they had lower diastolic blood pressure scores.

In summary, EMG biofeedback, relaxation, cognitive–behavioral therapy, imagery, and hypnosis show promise for reducing children's distress level when they are attempting to cope with painful medical procedures.

CONCLUSIONS

Studies have shown that children can easily learn self-regulatory techniques; in fact, they tend to learn more quickly and to have better results than adults. Biofeedback training and relaxation techniques have been shown to be beneficial in helping children cope with a variety of stressful conditions. The headache literature supports the use of biofeedback, relaxation, and stress coping training as effective methods in helping children deal with headache. EMG biofeedback and airway resistance biofeedback seem to be promising treatments for asthma, but there is a paucity of studies in the past several years to clarify these findings. Studies on relaxation as a treatment for asthma have had mixed results, whereas hypnosis has produced encouraging preliminary results for both short- and long-term improvement of asthma. There are very few studies on behavioral treatments for insomnia, but single-case studies have shown promising results with relaxation. Treatment packages to help children cope with painful medical procedures have utilized a wide variety of techniques, such as biofeedback, relaxation, cognitive–behavioral therapy, imagery, and hypnosis, and have obtained favorable results to date.

With the exception of the pediatric headache population, very little research has assessed the efficacy of biofeedback and related procedures in helping children to cope with stress. Also, only headache and asthma treatment studies have systematically collected long-term follow-up data. Much work is needed to help clarify the role of psychophysiological therapy in working with children.

REFERENCES

Alexander, A. B. (1983). The nature of asthma. In P. J. McGrath & P. Firestone (Eds.), *Pediatric and adolescent behavioral medicine: Issues in treatment* (pp. 28–66). New York: Springer.

Alexander, A. B., Cropp, H., & Chai, H. (1979). Effects of relaxation training on pulmonary mechanics in children with asthma. *Journal of Applied Behavior Analysis, 12,* 27–35.

Alexander, A. B., Miklich, D., & Hershkoff, H. (1972). The immediate effects of systematic relaxation training on peak expiratory flow rates in asthmatic children. *Psychosomatic Medicine, 34,* 388–394.

Anderson, D. (1979). Treatment of insomnia in a 13-year-old boy by relaxation training and reduction of parental attention. *Journal of Behavior Therapy and Experimental Psychiatry, 10,* 263–265.

Andrasik, F. (1989). Biofeedback applications for headache. In C. Bischoff, H. C. Traue, & H. Zenz (Eds.), *Clinical perspectives on headache and low back pain* (pp. 181–200). Lewiston, NY: Hogrefe.

Andrasik, F. (1990). Psychologic and behavioral aspects of chronic headache. *Neurologic Clinics, 8*, 961–976.

Andrasik, F., & Attanasio, V. (1985). Biofeedback in pediatrics: Current status and appraisal. In M. C. Wolraith & D. K. Routh (Eds.), *Advances in developmental and behavioral pediatrics* (Vol. 6, pp. 241–286). Greenwich, CT: JAI Press.

Andrasik, F., Blake, D. D., & McCarran, M. S. (1986). A biobehavioral analysis of pediatric headache. In N. A. Krasnegor, J. D. Arasteh, & M. F. Cataldo (Eds.), *Child health behavior: A behavioral pediatrics perspective* (pp. 394–434). New York: Wiley.

Andrasik, F., & Blanchard, E. B. (1983). Applications of biofeedback to therapy. In C. E. Walker (Ed.), *Handbook of clinical psychology: Theory, research and practice* (pp. 1123–1164). Homewood, IL: Dorsey Press.

Andrasik, F., Kabela, E., & Blake, D. D. (1988). Pediatrics: Psychological therapies. In J. L. Matson (Ed.), *Handbook of treatment approaches in childhood psychopathology* (pp. 429–463). New York: Plenum Press.

Andrasik, F., Kabela, E., Quinn, S., Attanasio, V., Blanchard, E. B., & Rosenblum, E. L. (1988). Psychological functioning of children who have recurrent migraine. *Pain, 34*, 43–52.

Angus, S. F. (1989). Three approaches to stress management for children. *Elementary School Guidance and Counseling, 23*, 228–232.

Aronoff, G., Aronoff, S., & Peck, L. (1975). Hypnotherapy in the treatment of bronchial asthma. *Annals of Allergy, 34*, 356–362.

Attanasio, V., Andrasik, F., Burke, E. J., Blake, D. D., Kabela, E., & McCarran, M. S. (1985). Clinical issues in utilizing biofeedback with children. *Clinical Biofeedback and Health, 8*, 134–141.

Barbour, J. (1980). Medigrams: Self hypnosis and asthma. *American Family Physician, 21*, 173.

Benson, H. (1975). *The relaxation response.* New York: Morrow.

Bernick, S. (1972). Relaxation, suggestion, and hypnosis in dentistry: What the pediatrician should know about children's dentistry. *Clinical Pediatrics, 11*, 72–75.

Bernstein, N. (1965). Observations on the use of hypnosis with burned children on a pediatric ward. *International Journal of Clinical and Experimental Hypnosis, 13*, 1–10.

Bernstein, N. (1972). Management of burned children with the aid of hypnosis. *Journal of Child Psychology and Psychiatry, 4*, 93–98.

Betcher, A. (1960). Hypnosis as an adjunct in anesthesiology. *New York State Journal of Medicine, 60*, 816–822.

Bieliauskas, L. A. (1982). *Stress and its relationship to health and illness.* Boulder, CO: Westview Press.

Bille, B. (1962). Migraine in school children. *Acta Paediatrica Scandinavica, 51*, 1–151.

Bille, B. (1981). Migraine in childhood and its prognosis. *Cephalalgia, 1*, 71–75.

Boersma, F. J., & Chapman, J. W. (1979). *Manual for the Student's Perception of Ability Scale*. Edmonton: University of Alberta Press.

Borkovec, T., Grayson, J., & Cooper, K. (1978). Treatment of general tension: Subjective and physiological effects of progressive relaxation. *Journal of Consulting and Clinical Psychology, 46,* 518–528.

Burke, E. J., & Andrasik, F. (1989). Home- versus clinic-based treatments for pediatric migraine headache: Results of treatment through one year follow-up. *Headache, 29,* 434–440.

Bush, J. (1987). Pain in children: A review of the literature from a developmental perspective. *Psychology and Health, 1,* 215–236.

Campbell, L., Clark, M., & Kirkpatrick, S. (1986). Stress management training for parents and their children undergoing cardiac catheterization. *American Journal of Orthopsychiatry, 56,* 234–243.

Cautela, J., & Groden, J. (1978). *Relaxation*. Champaign, IL: Research Press.

Chai, H. (1975). Management of severe chronic perennial asthma in children. *Advances in Asthma and Allergy, 2,* 1–12.

Cioppa, F., & Thal, A. (1975). Hypnotherapy in a case of juvenile rheumatoid arthritis. *American Journal of Clinical Hypnosis, 18,* 105–110.

Crasilneck, H., & Hall, J. (1975). *Clinical hypnosis: Principles and application.* New York: Grune & Stratton.

Creer, T. L. (1979). *Asthma therapy: A behavioral health care system for respiratory disorders.* New York: Springer.

Creer, T. L. (1982). Asthma. *Journal of Consulting and Clinical Psychology, 50,* 912–921.

Creer, T. L. (1991). The application of behavioral procedures to childhood asthma: Current and future perspectives. *Patient Education and Counseling, 17,* 9–22.

Curran, J. E. (1989, March). *Effective biofeedback techniques for working with children.* Workshop presented at the 23rd Annual Meeting of the Association for Applied Psychophysiology and Biofeedback, Washington, DC.

Danker, P. S., Miklich, D. R., Pratt, C., & Creer, T. L. (1975). An unsuccessful attempt to instrumentally condition peak expiratory flow rates in asthmatic children. *Journal of Psychosomatic Research, 19,* 209–213.

Dalsgaard-Nielson, T. (1965). Migraine and heredity. *Acta Neurologica Scandinavica, 41,* 287–300.

Davis, M., Saunders, D., Creer, T., & Chai, H. (1973). Relaxation training facilitated by biofeedback apparatus as a supplemental treatment in bronchial asthma. *Journal of Psychosomatic Research, 17,* 121–128.

de Araujo, G., Van Arsdel, P. O., Holmes, T. H., & Dudley, D. L. (1973). Life change, coping ability and chronic intrinsic asthma. *Journal of Psychosomatic Research, 17,* 359–363.

DeMille, R. (1973). *Put your mother on the ceiling.* New York: Viking Press.

Duckro, P. N., & Cantwell-Simmons, E. (1989). A review of studies evaluating biofeedback and relaxation training in the management of pediatric headache. *Headache, 29,* 428–433.

Ellenberg, L., Kellerman, J., Dash, J., Higgins, G., & Zeltzer, L. (1980). Use of hypnosis for multiple symptoms in an adolescent girl with leukemia. *Journal of Adolescent Health Care, 1,* 132–136.

Emmen, H., & Passchier, J. (1987). Treatment of headache among children by progressive relaxation. *Cephalalgia,* 7(Suppl. 6), 387–389.

Feldman, G. M. (1976). The effect of sham biofeedback training on respiratory resistance of asthmatic children. *Psychosomatic Medicine, 38,* 27–34.

Fentress, D. W., Masek, B. J., Mehegan, J. E., & Benson, H. (1986). Biofeedback and relaxation response training in the treatment of pediatric migraine. *Developmental Medicine and Child Neurology, 28,* 139–146.

Feuerstein, M., & Adams, H. E. (1977). Cephalic vasomotor feedback in the modification of migraine headache. *Biofeedback and Self-Regulation, 2,* 241–254.

Gardner, G. (1976). Childhood, death, and human dignity: Hypnotherapy for David. *International Journal of Clinical and Experimental Hypnosis, 24,* 122–139.

Gillis, J. S. (1980). *Child Anxiety Scale manual.* Champaign, IL: Institute for Personality and Ability Testing.

Glaus, K. D., & Kotses, H. (1983). Facial muscle tension influences lung airway resistance; limb muscle tension does not. *Biological Psychology, 17,* 105–120.

Green, J. A. (1983). Biofeedback therapy with children. In W. H. Rickles, J. H. Sandweiss, D. Jacobs, & R. N. Grove (Eds.), *Biofeedback and family practice medicine* (pp. 121–144). New York: Plenum Press.

Hoelscher, T. J., & Lichstein, K. L. (1984). Behavioral assessment and treatment of child migraine: Implications for clinical research and practice. *Headache, 24,* 94–103.

Holroyd, K. A. (1986). Recurrent headache. In K. Holroyd & T. Creer (Eds.), *Self-management of chronic disease: Handbook of clinical interventions and research* (pp. 373–413). New York: Academic Press.

Holroyd, K. A., & Penzien, D. B. (1986). Client variables and the behavioral treatment of recurrent tension headache: A meta-analytic review. *Journal of Behavioral Medicine, 9,* 515–536.

Humphrey, J. H., & Humphrey, J. (1981). *Reducing stress in children through creative relaxation.* Springfield, IL: Charles C Thomas.

Hunter, S. H., Russell, H. L., Russell, E. D., & Zimmerman, R. L. (1976). Control of fingertip temperature increases via biofeedback in learning disabled and normal children. *Perceptual and Motor Skills, 43,* 743–755.

Jacobson, E. (1938). *Progressive relaxation.* Chicago: University of Chicago Press.

Jay, S. M., Elliott, C. H., Katz, E., & Siegel, S. E. (1987). Cognitive-behavioral and pharmacologic intervention for children's distress during painful medical procedures. *Journal of Clinical and Counseling Psychology, 55*(6), 860–865.

Jay, S. M., Ozolins, M., Elliott, C. H., & Caldwell, S. (1983). Assessment of children's distress during painful medical procedures. *Health Psychology, 2*(2), 133–147.

Kater, D., & Spires, J. (1975). Biofeedback: The beat goes on. *School Counselor, 23,* 16–21.

Khan, A. U. (1977). Effectiveness of biofeedback and counterconditioning in the treatment of bronchial asthma. *Journal of Psychosomatic Research, 21,* 97–104.

Khan, A. U., Staerk, M., & Bonk, C. (1973). Role of counterconditioning in the treatment of asthma. *Journal of Psychosomatic Research, 17,* 389–392.

Kohen, D. (1986). Applications of relaxation/mental imagery (self-hypnosis) to the management of asthma in childhood: Report of behavioral outcomes of a prospective 2-year controlled study. *American Journal of Clinical Hypnosis, 28,* 196. (From *PsychLit,* Abstract)

Kotses, H., & Glaus, K. D. (1981). Applications of biofeedback to the treatment of asthma: A critical review. *Biofeedback and Self-Regulation, 6,* 573–593.

Kotses, H., Glaus, K. D., Bricel, S. K., Edwards, J. E., & Crawford, P. L. (1978). Operant muscular relaxation and peak expiratory flow rate in asthmatic children. *Journal of Psychosomatic Research, 22,* 17–23.

Kotses, H., Glaus, K. D., Crawford, P. L., Edwards, J. E., & Scherr, M. S. (1976). Operant reduction of frontalis EMG activity in the treatment of asthma in children. *Journal of Psychosomatic Research, 20,* 453–459.

Kotses, H., Harver, A., Segreto, J., Glaus, K. D., Creer, T. L., & Young, G. A. (1991). Long-term effects of biofeedback-induced facial relaxation on measures of asthma severity in children. *Biofeedback and Self-Regulation, 16,* 1–21.

LaBaw, W. (1973). Adjunctive trance therapy with severely burned children. *International Journal of Child Psychotherapy, 2,* 80–92.

LaBaw, W., Holton, C., Tewell, K., & Eccles, D. (1975). The use of self-hypnosis by children with cancer. *American Journal of Clinical Hypnosis, 17,* 233–238.

LaMontagne, L., Mason, K., & Hepworth, J. (1985). Effects of relaxation on anxiety in children: Implications for coping with stress. *Nursing Research, 34,* 289–292.

Larsson, B., Daleflod, B., Hakansson, L., & Melin, L. (1987). Chronic headaches in adolescents: Therapist-assisted versus self-help relaxation treatment of chronic headaches in adolescents. A school-based intervention. *Journal of Child Psychology, 28,* 127–136.

Larsson, B., & Melin, L. (1986). Chronic headaches in adolescents: Treatment in a school setting with relaxation training as compared with information-contact and self-registration. *Pain, 25,* 325–336.

Larsson, B., Melin, L., Lamminen, M., & Ullstedt, F. (1987). School-based treatment of chronic headaches in adolescents. *Journal of Pediatric Psychology*, 12, 553–566.

Lehrer, P., Woolfolk, R., Rooney, A., McCann, B., & Carrington, P. (1983). Progressive relaxation and meditation: A study of psychophysiological and therapeutic differences between techniques. *Behaviour Research and Therapy*, 21, 651–662.

Leviton, A., Slack, W. V., Masek, B., Bana, D., & Graham, J. R. (1984). A computerized behavioral assessment for children with headaches. *Headache*, 24, 36–44.

Lewis, S. (1989). Treating the whole child: A mind–body approach. *Mind–Body Health Digest*, 3, 1–2.

Lupin, M. (1977). *Peace, harmony, and awareness*. Austin, TX: Learning Concepts.

Luthe, W. (1969). *Autogenic therapy*. New York: Grune & Stratton.

Masek, B., & Fentress, D. (1984). Behavioral treatment of symptoms of childhood illness. *Clinical Psychology Review*, 4, 561–570.

Masters, R., & Houston, J. (1975). *Mind-games*. New York: Dell.

Olness, K. (1981). Imagery (self-hypnosis) as adjunct therapy in childhood cancer: Clinical experience with 25 patients. *American Journal of Pediatric Hematology/Oncology*, 3, 313–321.

Olness, K., & Gardner, G. (1978). Some guidelines for uses of hypnotherapy in pediatrics. *Pediatrics*, 62, 228–233.

Olness, K., & Gardner, G. (1988). *Hypnosis and hypnotherapy with children*. New York: Grune & Stratton.

Olness, K., MacDonald, J., & Uden, D. (1987). A prospective study comparing self-hypnosis, propranolol, and placebo in management of juvenile migraine. *Pediatrics*, 79, 593–597.

Olson, R. P., & Schwartz, M. S. (1987). An historical perspective on the biofeedback field. In M. S. Schwartz & Associates, *Biofeedback: A practitioner's guide* (pp. 3–16). New York: Guilford Press.

Ragan, L., & Hiebert, B. (1987, March). Kiddie QR (quieting reflex): Field testing a relaxation program for young children. *The School Counselor*, pp. 273–281.

Richter, I., McGrath, P., Humphreys, P., Goodman, J., Firestone, P., & Keene, D. (1986). Cognitive and relaxation treatment of paediatric migraine. *Pain*, 25, 195–203.

Richter, N. (1984). The efficacy of relaxation training with children. *Journal of Abnormal Child Psychology*, 12, 319–344.

Rothner, A. (1978). Headache in children: A review. *Headache*, 18, S169–S175.

Scherr, M. S., Crawford, P. L., Sergent, C. B., & Scherr, C. A. (1975). Effects of biofeedback techniques on chronic asthma in a summer camp environment. *Annals of Allergy*, 35, 289–295.

Siegel, L. J., & Peterson, L. (1980). Stress reduction in young dental patients through coping skills and sensory information. *Journal of Consulting and Clinical Psychology*, 48, 785–787.

Sillanpaa, M. (1983). Prevalence of headache in prepuberty. *Headache, 23,* 10-14.

Spielberger, C. D. (1973). *Manual for the State-Trait Anxiety Inventory for Children.* Palo Alto, CA: Consulting Psychologists Press.

Strider, F. D. (1981). Biofeedback and self-regulation therapies. In C. J. Golden, S. S. Alcaparras, F. D. Strider, & B. Graber (Eds.), *Applied techniques in behavioral medicine* (pp. 87-100). New York: Grune & Stratton.

Strider, F. D., & Strider, M. A. (1979). Current applications of biofeedback technology to the problems of children and youth. *Behavioral Disorders, 5,* 53-59.

Stroebel, C. F. (1978). *Quieting response training* [Audiocassettes]. New York: BMA.

Stroebel, C. F., Ford, M. R., Strong, P., & Szarek, B. L. (1981). Quieting response training: Five-year evaluation of a clinical biofeedback practice. In *Proceedings of the Twelfth Annual Meeting of the Biofeedback Society of America* (pp. 78-81). Wheatridge, CO: Biofeedback Society of America.

Stroebel, E., & Stroebel, C. F. (1984). The quieting reflex: A psychophysiologic approach for helping children deal with healthy and unhealthy stress. In J. H. Humphrey (Ed.), *Stress in childhood* (pp. 251-300). New York: AMS Press.

Stroebel, E., Stroebel, C. F., & Holland, M. (1980). *Kiddie QR.* Wetherfield, CT: QR Institute.

Suter, S., & Loughry-Machado, G. (1981). Skin temperature biofeedback in children and adults. *Journal of Experimental Child Psychology, 32,* 77-87.

Thompson, K. (1963). A rationale for suggestion in dentistry. *American Journal of Clinical Hypnosis, 5,* 181-186.

Turk, D. (1978). Cognitive behavioral techniques in the management of pain. In J. P. Foreyt & D. P. Rathjen (Eds.), *Cognitive behavior therapy* (pp. 199-227). New York: Plenum Press.

Viney, L. L. (1983). Assessing psychological states using content analysis. *Psychological Bulletin, 94,* 542-563.

Viney, L. L., & Westbrook, M. T. (1985). Patterns of psychological reaction to asthma in children. *Journal of Abnormal Child Psychology, 13,* 477-484.

Walker, C. (1979). Treatment of children's disorders by relaxation training: The poor man's biofeedback. *Journal of Clinical Child Psychology, 8,* 22-25.

Weinstein, A. M. (1987). *Asthma.* New York: McGraw-Hill.

Weil, G., & Goldfried, M. (1973). Treatment of insomnia in an eleven-year-old child through self-relaxation. *Behavior Therapy, 4,* 282-294.

Williams, D., & Singh, M. (1976). Hypnosis as a facilitating therapeutic adjunct in child psychiatry. *Journal of the American Academy of Child Psychiatry, 15,* 326-342.

Wisniewski, J., Genshaft, J., Mulick, J., Coury, D., & Hammer, D. (1988). Relaxation therapy and compliance in the treatment of adolescent headache. *Headache, 28*, 612-617.

Zaichkowsky, L., & Zaichkowsky, L. (1984). The effects of a school-based relaxation training program on fourth grade children. *Journal of Clinical Child Psychology, 13*, 81-84.

CHAPTER 15

The Assessment of Coping in Chronically Ill Children: Implications for Clinical Practice

ANTHONY SPIRITO, LORI J. STARK,
and LENORA G. KNAPP
Rhode Island Hospital/Brown University Program
in Medicine

The field of pediatric medicine has evolved from primarily acute care of infectious diseases to the prevention and long-term management of chronic illness. Many pediatric disorders, such as certain types of cancer, no longer result in early death and may be treated successfully by aggressive treatment over several years. Other diseases, such as diabetes, do not pose an imminent threat but require lifelong daily management. Despite these differences in sequelae, all illnesses present children with the difficult task of coping with a multitude of stressors.

Stressors associated with chronic illness include receiving the diagnosis, building relationships with health care providers, dealing with the symptoms of the illness and various treatment procedures, being separated from family for hospitalizations, confronting potential disfigurement or impairment, and dealing with the possibility of shortened life expectancy. A child's ability to cope and adapt to these stressors may affect both the course of the illness and the child's psychological adjustment (Holroyd & Lazarus, 1982). Although early studies (e.g., Pless, Roghmann, & Haggerty, 1972) described chronically ill children as being at risk for emotional maladjustment, the prevailing consensus from more recent studies is that most such children are psychologically normal (see Varni, 1983, for a review). Although these data would imply that most children are able to adapt to the stressors associated with a chronic illness, the naturalistic coping mechanisms utilized to achieve this positive outcome have yet to be investigated fully.

Assessment of children's perceptions of medical stressors and their spontaneous coping responses to these events is an important task for pediatric psychology. Investigations with chronically ill children may provide normative information on aspects of chronic illness that distress children, as well as on the coping strategies they employ and find effective in dealing with such stressors (Spirito, Stark, & Tyc, 1989). This, in turn, may improve the design of psychological interventions intended to enhance children's coping with stressful medical procedures (Peterson, 1989) and may broaden the application of coping interventions beyond medical procedures to other aspects of adjustment to chronic illness, as discussed above (Spirito, Stark, & Tyc, 1989).

The purpose of the present chapter is to review research on chronically ill children's coping with illness-related stressors, to discuss assessment tools utilized in these studies, and to provide a framework for the integration of these findings into the clinical practice of the pediatric psychologist. Investigations of acutely ill children undergoing medical procedures are reviewed elsewhere in this volume (e.g., Miller, Sherman, Combs, & Kruus, Chapter 8). Only studies that examined children actually experiencing a medical stressor are reviewed here, because they are considered more relevant to clinical practice than studies in which children were asked to recall or imagine a medical-related stressor (e.g., Brown, O'Keeffe, Sanders, & Baker, 1986). Also not covered here are the interviews and scales that have examined coping responses in healthy children (e.g., Band & Weisz, 1988; Compas, Malcarne, & Fondacaro, 1988), but have not been used with a chronically ill population (see Knapp, Stark, Kurkjian, & Spirito, in press, for a review).

In the present chapter, the Lazarus and Folkman (1984) definition of coping as "constantly changing cognitive and behavioral efforts to manage specific external and/or internal demands that are appraised as taxing or exceeding the resources of the person" (p. 144) has been employed. According to this widely accepted conceptualization (see Compas, Worsham, & Ey, Chapter 1, this volume), coping is a dynamic process as opposed to a static trait. This definition allows for variation in the frequency and type of coping strategies used across time and across different medically related situations. Such a conceptualization is consistent with the observation that the same child may cope in one way with a discrete medical procedure (e.g., wanting a parent to hold his or her hand, and talking to the parent as a distraction technique), but may employ a very different strategy for dealing with the news that his or her medical condition is deteriorating (e.g., withdrawing and refusing to talk to anyone, including a parent). Thus, the Lazarus and Folkman (1984) conceptualization of coping appears to hold the most promise for translating research findings into the everyday clinical practice of pediatric psychologists who work with chronically ill children.

SPONTANEOUS COPING IN RESPONSE TO SURGERY OR INVASIVE MEDICAL PROCEDURES

Observational Scales

Direct observation appears most useful as a description of overt coping behavior occurring in response to a stressful situation. Two groups of investigators have developed direct observation scales specifically for use in examining how chronically ill children cope with medical procedures (Hubert, Jay, Saltoun, & Hayes, 1988; Ritchie, Caty, & Ellerton, 1988).

Ritchie et al. (1988) used the Children's Coping Strategies Checklist (CCSC), an observational system consisting of 40 items divided into six subscales, to assess how hospitalized preschool children with both acute and chronic illness cope with medical procedures. Four of the subscales (27 items) represent cognitive and behavioral coping strategies: information seeking (e.g., asking a question), direct action (e.g., choosing finger to be pricked), inhibition of action (e.g., clenching fists or teeth), and seeking or accepting help or comfort from others (e.g., saying, "Hold my hand"). Adequate interrater reliability was reported, but coefficient alphas calculated for the subscales were only in the moderate range. No validity data were reported. Ritchie et al. (1988) reported that the most common coping strategies used by chronically ill children to deal with medical procedures were information seeking (watching the procedure), inhibition of action (tense compliance), and direct action (tension reduction, active participation, and active self-protection).

The CCSC is notable because its developers conducted preliminary studies (e.g., Ritchie, Caty, & Ellerton, 1984) and are continuing to work on instrument development. High interrater reliability and categorization of coping strategies on a conceptual basis are also positive features. However, the rather low internal consistency of the original subscales suggests the need to refine items to be more consistent with the subscale conceptualizations. In addition, several of the behaviors classified as "coping" on the subscale assessing direct action, such as aggressive acts against others, have been conceptualized as "distress" behaviors by other investigators (e.g., Hubert et al., 1988). The inclusion of such responses as coping may hinder comparisons of findings across studies.

The Behavioral Approach–Avoidance and Distress Scale (BAADS) was employed to measure the behavior of pediatric cancer patients undergoing painful medical procedures (Hubert et al., 1988). For the Approach–Avoidance subscale, which is used to measure coping behaviors, observers rate the child's coping behavior on a 5-point scale: 1 = "turns away/tries to escape or change situation" (high avoidance), 3 = "watches but does not participate verbally or nonverbally," and 5 = "looks/touches/questions/ initiates involvement" (high approach). Interrater reliability data were not reported, but internal consistency was high for the scale. Concurrent validity was demonstrated by a significant relationship between the Approach–Avoidance subscale and distress behaviors. Specifically, children whose coping was characterized by more approach than avoidant behaviors displayed less distress than those who used avoidant strategies. This was true during both preparation and the actual procedure, and is consistent with studies of acutely ill patients (Peterson, 1989). No age differences were revealed with respect to coping behavior. The virtue of this scale is its straightforward approach to measuring a construct (approach–avoidance) that has been shown in many studies to characterize the behavior of children undergoing medical procedures (Peterson, 1989). Presumably, interrater reliability should be relatively easy to establish for the scale.

Implications for clinicians. The utility of observational scales may be limited by the circumscribed range of coping strategies that can be measured and by the types of stressors for which direct observation is appropriate. Also, it is difficult to infer reliably what cognitive strategies may be indicated by children's overt behaviors. However, because young children (7 years of age or under) are less able to respond appropriately to interview and self-report measures, clinicians must rely on observational scales to assess the coping behaviors of young children.

Interviews

Interviews designed to assess coping with medical procedures such as surgery (LaMontagne, 1984, 1987) or dental treatment (Curry & Russ, 1985) are rare. Only one study (Siegel, 1981) has used chronically ill children in its sample. The Coping Strategies Interview (CSI; Siegel, 1981) consists of seven questions about what children thought (cognitions) and did (behaviors) immediately prior to, during, and after an invasive medical procedure (e.g., bone marrow aspiration), as well as what kinds of things they thought or did that made them feel better or worse. Children are also asked whether they switched strategies if the original coping strategy was unsuccessful. Finally, any suggestions that they would give to another child to help lessen pain and fear about undergoing a similar procedure are elicited. To aid recall of the procedure, children are instructed to close their eyes and remember their thoughts and behaviors as if they are "running a movie" through their heads.

Children's responses on the CSI are coded according to the following coping categories: distraction–external, distraction–internal, distraction–imagery, reinterpretation of sensations, fantasy, mental rehearsal, relevant information seeking, irrelevant information seeking, positive self-statements, negative self-statements, catastrophizing thoughts, affective expression, affective inhibition, relaxation, solicitation of help/emotional support, physical activity, seeking active termination of procedure, passive acceptance, or no strategy reported. Siegel (1981) found that "successful copers" (e.g., children who were rated by medical staff as cooperative, exhibiting a low level of anxiety, and good tolerance of physical discomfort) tended to rely on relevant information seeking as a coping response, whereas "unsuccessful copers" were more likely to engage in negative self-statements. "Successful copers" also used a greater variety of coping strategies than "unsuccessful copers."

Although Siegel (1981) presents many details on the interview itself, psychometric properties of the scale have not been reported. Given the number of categories that can be coded, interrater reliability needs to be assessed. Nonetheless, the fact that the scale can be administered immediately after experiencing a medical procedure represents a strength of the measure, as it may enhance the accuracy of the information obtained. In addition, the different types of questions asked in the interview, including the affective outcome of the coping strategy, add to its comprehensiveness.

Implications for clinicians. The interview approach to assessment has intuitive appeal to clinicians because it can be easily integrated into their daily clinical work. Moreover, interview formats enable a clinician to obtain more in-depth information (i.e., cognitive strategies) than that available through observational systems. Such data may be needed to tailor interventions to the specific needs of a patient and to monitor the efficacy of interventions designed to reduce distress during painful medical procedures.

COPING WITH ASPECTS OF CHRONIC ILLNESS

Most studies of coping by pediatric patients have focused on responses to medical procedures and have involved young children. Coping with other chronic illness stressors has been neglected, as has research with older children and adolescents. Chronic illness involves many stresses, such as hospital admissions, acute and chronic pain secondary to disease states, and limitations on daily activities. Understanding how cognitive and behavioral coping strategies affect adjustment to these aspects of chronic illness is an important but very underinvestigated area. Mattsson (1972) has suggested that realistic cognitive understanding of the illness, release and control of emotions, compensatory physical activities, selective use of denial, and family support are adaptive coping mechanisms in the chronically ill child. However, empirical data on such coping strategies are limited. Studies examining these strategies are discussed in this section.

Interviews

Ross and Ross (1984b) interviewed (1) healthy children, and (2) children with chronic headaches, stomachaches, or earaches; juvenile rheumatoid arthritis; leukemia; and sickle cell disease, about their pain experiences. Patients were asked open-ended questions, such as "Did you do anything all by yourself to help the pain?" and "When you had the pain, was there anything you tried to do yourself so that it wouldn't hurt so much?" Although psychometric data on the interview questions were not presented, Ross and Ross (1984a) demonstrated that open-ended questions (e.g., "Was there anything you tried to do yourself so that it wouldn't hurt so much?") elicited a much lower frequency of reported usage of coping strategies than did specific questions (e.g., "Did you try not to think about the pain?"). Although findings specific to chronically ill patients were not separately analyzed, distraction, thought stopping, and relaxation were the most common self-initiated pain strategies reported by the sample as a whole. Because Ross and Ross (1984b) did not emphasize the assessment of coping in their study, the questions they used to assess coping in their interview are rather limited. Nonetheless, their companion article (Ross & Ross, 1984a) on interviewing children provides important information for both clinicians and researchers on the structure and manner in which interviews with children about pain should be conducted (Spirito & Stark, 1987).

Worchel, Copeland, and Barker (1987) employed an interview format to assess strategies for gaining control used by childhood cancer patients. Questions on behavioral control pertained to medical treatments (e.g., "Do you hold a parent's hand?", "Do you use deep breathing?", "Do you try to get the medical staff to stop and/or wait?"). Cognitive control questions related to illness (e.g., "How often do you talk about your illness to other people?"). Informational control consisted of questions such as "How often do you like to ask questions about your illness?" Moderate internal consistency was reported for the three types of control (behavioral, cognitive, and informational). Worchel et al. (1987) reported that more frequent use of behavioral control strategies was associated with poor adjustment as measured by self-report of depression and somatic complaints, as well as by ratings of the nursing staff on behavior and compliance. Cognitive control strategies (i.e., thinking about the disease) were related to nurses' ratings of passive noncompliance. No relationship was demonstrated between informational control strategies and adjustment. The Worchel et al. (1987) interview consists only of questions about different types of control; thus, the types of coping strategies assessed are limited. As in other scales that use just a few questions to assess one construct (e.g., Ritchie et al., 1988), internal consistency is difficult to achieve. One advantage of the structure of questions used is their applicability to a wide range of activities and issues associated with a chronic illness.

Band (1990) asked children with diabetes what they thought or did to help themselves with, for example, dietary restrictions, insulin injections, and blood glucose testing. Data were coded into three control categories: primary control (i.e., efforts to modify the events, a categorization similar to problem-focused coping), secondary control (i.e., efforts to influence the child's psychological state, comparable to emotion-focused coping), and relinquished control (i.e., a failure to cope). Each child also rated the "goal" of the coping strategy ("How does _____ help or make things better?"). Each strategy was then classified as either instrumental (a specific behavior), cognitive, or social–emotional (an interpersonal behavior), resulting in a 2 (primary vs. secondary) × 3 (instrumental vs. cognitive vs. social–emotional) matrix with six possible categories. For example, injecting insulin to prevent a reaction would be coded as "instrumental strategy, primary control," whereas sticking to a diet in order to feel good about oneself would be coded as "instrumental strategy, secondary control."

Interrater reliability for the classification scheme was high. Internal consistency of primary–secondary control was moderately high. Validity data were not reported. Children were more likely to use primary control than were older children. Children who tended to rely on primary-control styles of coping were rated as displaying better medical adjustment by their physician or nurse practitioner than those who used secondary-control strategies more frequently. Band's (1990) coding system for coping is noteworthy for its two-dimensional categorization, which is more sophisticated than that used by other investigators. Despite the level of complexity, interrater reliability for the coding system was high. The format can also be applied to other chronic illness tasks, making the interview of considerable interest to both clinicians and researchers.

Implications for clinicians. The Band (1990) and Worchel et al. (1987) studies examined children with different chronic illnesses (which involve different disease-related tasks) using different assessment systems. The lack of uniformity in the definition of coping strategies across studies is problematic when one is attempting to draw specific conclusions regarding the coping of pediatric patients. Nonetheless, the findings from these two studies are consistent in that older and more cognitively sophisticated patients rely more heavily on cognitive strategies. The Ross and Ross (1984b) study found that children were much less likely to report using a coping strategy for pain when open-ended questions were asked than when specific questions were posed. These data suggest that a combination of open-ended and specific questions (in either an interview or a self-report measure) may be the best procedure for clinicians to use.

Self-Report

Gil, Williams, Thompson, and Kinney (in press) used a self-report measure to assess how children and adolescents coped with sickle cell disease pain. The Coping Strategies Questionnaire (CSQ; Rosenstiel & Keefe, 1983), a scale developed to assess adults' strategies for coping with pain, was the primary measure used in the study. The CSQ has 13 subscales with six items on each subscale. Respondents rate how often they use each strategy, on a Likert scale from 0 (never) to 7 (always). Factor analysis of children's responses revealed three factors, labeled Coping Attempts (diverting attention, reinterpreting pain, ignoring pain sensations, calming self-statements, and increased behavior activity), Negative Thinking (catastrophizing, fear self-statements, anger self-statements, and isolation), and Passive Adherence (resting, taking fluids, praying and hoping, heat/cold/massage). Children with high scores on the Negative Thinking and Passive Adherence subscales were less active, required more health care services, and were more psychologically distressed when confronted with a painful episode. Children who used a higher number of coping strategies were more active and required less frequent health care services. The CSQ is unique among the scales/interviews discussed thus far in its attention to scale development and psychometrics. Further studies will be needed to confirm its appropriateness for use with children and adolescents.

Implications for clinicians. The Gil et al. (in press) study is noteworthy because it assesses how children cope with disease-related pain, an important aspect of the chronic illness experience that has not been investigated in other studies. When a clinician is assessing disease-related pain, it will be necessary to survey a broader array of coping strategies than when studying procedure-related pain, where approach–avoidance strategies may suffice. Paper-and-pencil instruments are appealing, because the ease of administration of such scales minimizes the amount of professional time that must be devoted to the task of assessment. Brevity of assessment is especially important in clinical practice, where the pediatric psychologist working with chronically ill children and their families often needs to address a variety of symptoms, behaviors, and issues. Although Gil et al. (in press) used a scale designed to assess pain coping strategies, it exemplifies the utility of self-report scales in examining coping. The ease of administration and the amount of information obtained through self-report measures suggest that this approach may be valuable in assessing coping with other aspects of a chronic illness beyond pain and medical procedures.

CURRENT RESEARCH PROGRAM

The literature review above is remarkable for the small number of studies conducted with chronically ill children and the infrequent use of self-report measures with this population. The paucity of research in this area is surprising, given the interest in chronic illness among pediatric psychologists and the need for easy-to-administer assessments in the pediatric setting. In response to this gap in the literature, we embarked on a research program designed to study coping in chronically ill children. Our major interest was in assessing the coping strategies of a large sample of chronically ill children, in order to gain better understanding of normative coping in this population. Consequently, we designed a measure that assessed a broad range of cognitive and behavioral strategies, but was sufficiently brief to facilitate assessment of coping in clinical practice. The devised measure, the Kidcope, assesses 10 common cognitive and behavioral coping strategies utilized by children and adolescents (see Table 15.1). The frequency (not at all, sometimes, a lot of the time, almost all the time) and the perceived efficacy (not at all, a little, somewhat, pretty much, very much) of each strategy is determined by the child's or adolescent's self-report. Age-appropriate versions of the Kidcope have been developed for younger (ages 7-12 years) and older (ages 13-18 years) children. Properties of the scale have been described elsewhere (Spirito, Stark, & Williams, 1988; Spirito, Stark, Grace, & Stamoulis, in press). Healthy children were employed as subjects in the initial development of the measure, and the normative data are of interest in examining how chronically ill children cope with everyday stressors compared to healthy children.

Kidcope Findings: Chronically Ill Children's Coping Strategies

After completing initial studies of the Kidcope with healthy children (Spirito et al., in press) and adolescents (Stark, Spirito, Williams, & Guevremont, 1989), as well as psychiatrically disturbed populations (Spirito, Overholser, & Stark, 1989), we began a cross-sectional study of the use and perceived efficacy of coping strategies among chronically ill children. Children with a variety of illnesses, such as cancer, congenital heart disease, diabetes, and hemophilia, were interviewed with the Kid-

Table 15.1. Kidcope Items

Category	Examples of Responses
Distraction	"I just tried to forget it," "I did something like watch TV or play a game to forget it."
Social withdrawal	"I stayed by myself," "I kept quiet about the problem."
Cognitive restructuring	"I tried to see the good side of things."
Self-criticism	"I blamed myself for causing the problem."
Blaming others	"I blamed someone else for causing the problem."
Problem solving	"I tried to fix the problem by thinking of answers," "I tried to fix the problem by doing something or talking to someone."
Emotional regulation	"I yelled, screamed, or got mad," "I tried to calm myself down."
Wishful thinking	"I wished the problem had never happened," "I wished I could make things different."
Social support	"I tried to feel better by spending time with others like family, grownups, or friends."
Resignation	"I didn't do anything because the problem couldn't be fixed."

cope while hospitalized or during an outpatient clinic visit. Children were asked to select and describe a health-related problem that had occurred in the previous month and to rate the degree to which the situation produced feelings of anxiety, sadness, and anger. They then completed the Kidcope by indicating how often they used the different coping strategies to deal with the identified problem and how effective the coping strategies were in alleviating distress. The hospitalized children were also asked to respond to a self-generated, hospital-related stressor. In addition, all children were asked to select a common, everyday problem that had occurred in the past month and to complete the Kidcope for that problem. The latter task was designed to examine the specificity of coping strategies for medically related versus everyday problems.

Preliminary findings indicated sex differences in chronically ill children's coping with medically related stressors (Spirito, Stark, & Tyc, 1989). Across all of the different stressors chosen (e.g., painful procedures, limitations on activities imposed by the disease, being admitted to the hospital), females used more coping strategies than males. Examination of the use of specific coping strategies revealed that females employed emotional regulation more often than did males. These findings suggest the importance of considering sex differences when examining the coping strategies used by chronically ill children.

In another study of coping by pediatric patients (Spirito, Stark, Williams, Stamoulis, & Axelson, 1988), the coping of children referred for psychological evaluation (because of emotional problems associated with their disease) was compared to that of nonreferred chronically ill children. A problem related to the disease was chosen by each child as the focus of his or her coping responses on the Kidcope. Patients referred for psychological evaluation used distraction, social withdrawal, and wishful thinking more frequently than the nonreferred children.

Kidcope Findings: Effects of Hospitalization

Another question of interest is how chronically ill children cope with the stress of hospitalization. In order to examine this question, chronically and acutely ill children and adolescents were interviewed during a hospital admission (Stark, Spirito, & Tyc, 1991). Diagnoses for the chronically ill group included cancer, diabetes, asthma, sickle cell anemia, and cystic fibrosis. Patients in the acutely ill group were admitted for orthopedic surgery, appendicitis, abdominal pain, and other acute problems. These patients selected a problem related to their hospitalization and were then asked to complete the Kidcope in response to this problem. The stressors were categorized into (1) a specific aspect of hospitalization (e.g., trouble sleeping at night, bad food, lack of privacy), (2) a disease-related problem (i.e., some concern about their illness triggered by the hospitalization), or (3) pain-related concerns (e.g., discomfort secondary to disease state or a medical procedure while hospitalized).

Among the chronically ill children, 50% selected some aspect of the hospitalization as a problem, 33% described pain as the problem, and 17% selected some aspect of their diagnosis. Of the pain problems reported, 39% were associated with disease state and 61% were secondary to medical procedures. Thus, when asked to select their own medically related stressor, only 20% of hospitalized children and adolescents selected pain associated with a medical procedure. These results indicate the need to broaden research efforts beyond pain associated with invasive medical procedures to include other illness-related stressors. In regard to coping strategies, several main effects were noted. For example, both problem solving and wishful thinking were used more frequently by older children, anxious children, and sad children. Acutely ill children were more likely to use distraction, self-blame, and wishful thinking as coping strategies than chronically ill children. There was also an age by chronic/acute illness interaction effect for social withdrawal, self-blame, and wishful thinking. Young, acutely ill children used social withdrawal more than chronically ill adolescents, young chronically ill, and acutely ill adolescents. Chronically ill adolescents used self-blame and wishful thinking less often than acutely ill adolescents, young acutely ill, and young chronically ill.

Strengths and Weaknesses of the Kidcope

The Kidcope is unique in respect to a number of qualities of scale development, including multiple studies with different populations (i.e., physically and psychologically healthy, chronically ill, and psychiatrically disturbed) and different age groups. Concurrent validity data reported with adolescents are promising; as for other coping measures reviewed, however, more extensive work is indicated.

One strength of the Kidcope—its brevity—is also a weakness. Because each item is meant to represent an independent coping strategy (e.g., distraction vs. problem solving), test-retest reliability has been calculated item by item rather than for the total score. Thus, reliability coefficients are lower than those for scales including multiple items. Also, the fact that the Kidcope is based on a process model of coping implies that high test-retest correlations may not be achievable, as coping strategies for the same problem may vary over time (Mash & Terdal, 1988). Other types of reliability measures (e.g., internal consistency) may be more suitable to process measures. Unfortunately, because each item of the Kidcope is independent, alpha coefficients are not appropriate for this measure. Although this is a relative weakness of the measure, the findings on test-retest reliability are similar to those found in other studies of process measures (see Spirito, Stark, & Williams, 1988).

Implications for clinicians. Checklist assessments may be especially useful to clinicians, because they are brief and easy to administer. The Kidcope can be used to assess coping across a number of stressful situations, and offers information regarding the frequency and perceived efficacy of a wide variety of cognitive and behavioral coping strategies. Because normative data have been collected on the Kidcope, information on spontaneous coping strategies used by a variety of chronically ill children is available. Such data would be useful in evaluating coping, because the data presented in this chapter suggest that chronically ill and acutely ill children differ in their perceptions of stressors and in the coping strategies they employ. It should be noted that the Kidcope was designed to be a screening measure and is not intended to provide a comprehensive assessment of coping. Although its brevity is appealing, the instrument should be supplemented by interviews and/or direct observations to obtain an in-depth assessment of coping by children and adolescents.

SUGGESTIONS FOR CLINICAL PRACTICE

We close this chapter with thoughts on how clinicians may assess coping in chronically ill children. We do so for several reasons. First, because the majority of chronically ill children are psychologically healthy (see Varni,

1983), traditional assessment measures of psychopathology may not be appropriate for this population. Thus, assessment of coping strategies may offer a more appropriate focus. Second, the experience garnered by clinicians in assessing coping strategies may provide important stimuli for developing hypotheses about chronically ill children's coping that can be tested in clinical research programs. Third, encouraging clinicians to assess coping in day-to-day practice may result in improvements in the care of chronically ill children. For example, reactive effects from a coping assessment may lead to a patient's identifying a potential intervention (e.g., distraction) for himself or herself. Reactive effects have an added advantage: Patients can take credit for their ability to master the difficult situation almost entirely themselves, which in turn may enhance feelings of self-efficacy.

This section focuses on relevant clinical information that can be obtained by systematically assessing the coping of chronically ill pediatric patients through either observation, interview, or questionnaire techniques. The following recommendations are drawn from three sources: the limited research literature, our own research program, and clinical experience. Given the limited knowledge base currently existing in this area, future research is needed to validate the utility of these approaches in assessing coping as part of an overall treatment program for chronically ill pediatric patients.

Assessing an Individual's Coping Strategies

For presenting problems such as invasive medical procedures, a child can be observed directly. In most cases, the coding system described by Hubert et al. (1988) should be sufficient. If these observations provide sufficient information to permit the clinician to devise an effective intervention, no further assessment is indicated. However, for other facets of a chronic illness, interviews will usually be necessary for assessing cognitive coping strategies. At least two areas related to coping should be addressed in a structured interview with the patient. First, the clinician should ask what the child does or thinks at the time he or she is trying to cope with the medically related stressor in question. These questions can be adapted from the CSI (Siegel, 1981). Because pain associated with disease state is a commonly described illness-related stressor for chronically ill children, it is also important to have interview questions specific to this type of pain. The questions used by Ross and Ross (1984b) are recommended for this part of the interview. Second, the clinician should inquire about some other illness-related stressor that is not problematic for the child, in order to determine whether he or she possesses an adequate repertoire of coping strategies.

The administration of a specific coping measure is recommended after the interview. This will be most helpful in cases where the responses to the open-ended interview questions reveal very little information—a common occurrence when interviewing children about self-initiated coping strategies (Ross & Ross, 1984a). In such cases, a screening measure that is applicable to most disease-related stressors and that prompts children to consider a number of cognitive and behavioral strategies (e.g., the Kidcope) will be advantageous. At other times, a measure devised to tap a specific subject area (e.g., pain) may be required, or an existing measure may need to be adapted to address the problem. For example, when the Kidcope is being used for a pain-related problem, the addition of three items adapted from Rosenstiel and Keefe (1983) is recommended: (1) "I try to think of it [the pain] as a different feeling, like being numb, or as if the pain is not part of my own body," (2) "I think of the future when I won't have pain; I think someday I will find someone (e.g., a doctor) who can help my pain," and (3) "I take medicine, lie down, use a heating pad, ice pack".

The coping strategies employed by parents when they themselves are placed in stressful medical situations may influence the advice they are providing for their children. A parent's coping style is also likely to affect the behaviors reinforced, ignored, or punished in a child's coping repertoire. Consequently, there may be times when formally assessing the coping strategies of parents is useful. The Coping Strategies Inventory (Tobin, Holroyd, Reynolds, & Wigal, 1989) is a useful instrument for assessing coping strategies used by adults in a variety of situations. Adults' coping with pain can be assessed via the CSQ (Rosenstiel & Keefe, 1983).

Future Directions: Screening Coping Strategies

The screening of coping strategies used by chronically ill children serves two purposes: triage and prevention. In a large and busy clinical service, resources available for psychological intervention may be limited. Consequently, the most intensive intervention efforts must be reserved for patients with substantial behavioral and emotional upset secondary to their illness. Brief screening devices, such as the Kidcope, allow routine assessments to be conducted in pediatric clinics. These may result in the early identification of children who are having difficulty coping and the implementation of preventive interventions. Rather than assuming that children can or cannot find ways to cope with illness-related stressful experiences, clinicians can directly assess the types of strategies available through a brief screening measure. Chronically ill children who have a limited number of coping strategies can be targeted for early intervention, perhaps in a group format. Research with healthy and chronically ill children suggests that having a wide variety of coping strategies available is associated with adaptive functioning (Knapp et al., in press). This is consistent with the notion that chronically ill children need to adjust to the different types of external and internal demands they will encounter in the course of their disease and treatment (Holroyd & Lazarus, 1982).

Those children who are not able to generate any coping strategies should be targeted first in prevention efforts. Providing information on the ways other children cope with the different medically related situations encountered in the treatment of their disease is an example of an educational intervention. These children can then be followed to determine which coping strategies they have found successful for different types of situations commonly encountered in the disease course (e.g., school readjustment or responding to teasing by peers in childhood cancer patients). Unfortunately, what may be clearly evident to the clinician may not be so evident to a patient or his or her parents. Thus, when a child has successfully dealt with a stressor, it will often be necessary for the clinician to elaborate on reasons for success, such as the use of certain coping strategies (e.g., distraction). Reinforcing the connection may encourage the use of similar coping strategies at the next occurrence of a similar stressor. To facilitate this process, the patient can be asked to generate some alternative behaviors or cognitions that he or she might try when placed in potentially stressful situations that are anticipated in the future.

When is the best time to screen coping strategies? A logical time for an initial screening is shortly after the diagnosis of an illness. By this time, the child has usually been exposed to a number of disease-related and treatment-related stressors. If the child demonstrates increased difficulty in managing these stressors over time, then the child should be assessed again to determine whether his or her coping strategies have changed in response to different demands or aversiveness of the disease or treatment. Screening at milestones in the disease course (e.g., the shift from active treatment to remission in cancer patients) and/or developmental transition stages (e.g., the onset of adolescence in children with diabetes) is also recommended.

Changes in a pediatric patient's disease status or developmental stage may require changes in the types of coping strategies used to deal with the disease. Interviewing the child a number of times over the course of the illness helps the clinician to determine whether coping strategies are changing. Clinical experience suggests that chronically ill children continue to employ the same types of coping strategies when confronted with repetitive stressful medical procedures, but that for a substantial portion of these children these strategies lose their effectiveness over time. The need for more intensive training in the use of certain pre-existing coping strategies or in specific cognitive–behavioral self-control strategies can be gauged with this assessment approach. Finally, regardless of the point in the course of the disease at which coping is assessed, it is best to observe or interview children in at least two different situations. First, it is useful to do an assessment of the child when no major stressor is immediately anticipated, to determine whether coping strategies are available under optimal circumstances. Second, an assessment immediately before the child is about to be exposed to a stressor (e.g., an invasive medical procedure, hospitalization) will help determine whether the coping strategies are available to the child under stressful conditions.

CONCLUSION

Although most researchers and clinicians agree that coping is an important construct in understanding adaptation in chronic illness, the scanty empirical literature on the topic highlights the gap between theory and research. Assessment of coping in clinical practice is also limited. We hope that this chapter will stimulate pediatric psychologists to conduct more formal assessments of coping in clinical practice. Findings from the literature are difficult to summarize because of the different classification schemes and assessment approaches used. Whether a coping strategy is maladaptive or adaptive cannot be inferred from the empirical literature (except for the literature on medical procedures, which indicates that active coping is adaptive; Peterson, 1989), but must be decided on an individual basis. A major goal of future research will be to determine whether certain coping strategies are inherently adaptive for different types of disease-related stressors encountered by the chronically ill child. Many of the ideas described in this chapter can be considered not only for their clinical utility, but also for their potential to generate research hypotheses that may be tested in single-subject methodologies or more formal research programs.

REFERENCES

Band, E. B. (1990). Children's coping with diabetes: Understanding the role of cognitive development. *Journal of Pediatric Psychology, 15,* 27–42.

Band, E. B., & Weisz, J. R. (1988). How to feel better when it feels bad: Children's perspectives on coping with everyday stress. *Developmental Psychology, 24,* 247–253.

Brown, J. M., O'Keeffe, J., Sanders, S. H., & Baker, B. (1986). Developmental changes in children's cognition to stressful and painful situations. *Journal of Pediatric Psychology, 11,* 343–357.

Compas, B. E., Malcarne, V. L., & Fondacaro, K. M. (1988). Coping with stressful events in older children and young adolescents. *Journal of Consulting and Clinical Psychology, 56,* 405–411.

Curry, S. L., & Russ, S. W. (1985). Identifying coping strategies in children. *Journal of Clinical Child Psychology, 14,* 61–69.

Gil, K., Williams, D., Thompson, R., & Kinney, T. (in press). Sickle cell disease in children and adolescents: The relation of child and parent pain coping strategies to adjustment. *Journal of Pediatric Psychology.*

Holroyd, K. A., & Lazarus, R. S. (1982). Stress, coping and somatic adaptation. In C. Goldberger & S. Breznitz (Eds.), *Handbook of stress: Theoretical and clinical aspects* (pp. 21–35). New York: Free Press.

Hubert, N., Jay, S., Saltoun, M., & Hayes, M. (1988). Approach–avoidance and distress in children undergoing preparation for painful medical procedures. *Journal of Clinical Child Psychology, 17,* 194–202.

Knapp, L., Stark, L. J., Kurkjian, J., & Spirito, A. (in press). Assessing coping in children and adolescents: Research and practice. *Educational Psychology Review.*

LaMontagne, L. L. (1984). Children's locus of control beliefs as predictors of preoperative coping behavior. *Nursing Research, 33,* 76–85.

LaMontagne, L. L. (1987). Children's preoperative coping: Replication and extension. *Nursing Research, 36,* 163–167.

Lazarus, R. S., & Folkman, S. (1984). *Stress, appraisal, and coping.* New York: Springer.

Mash, E. J., & Terdal, L. G. (1988). Behavioral assessment of childhood disturbance. In E. J. Mash & L. G. Terdal (Eds.), *Behavioral assessment of childhood disorders* (2nd ed., pp. 3–78). New York: Guilford Press.

Mattsson, A. (1972). Long-term physical illness in childhood: A challenge to psychosocial adaptation. *Pediatrics, 50,* 801–811.

Peterson, L. (1989). Coping by children undergoing stressful medical procedures: Some conceptual, methodological, and therapeutic issues. *Journal of Consulting and Clinical Psychology, 57,* 380–387.

Pless, I., Roghmann, K., & Haggerty, R. (1972). Chronic illness, family functioning, and psychological adjustment. *International Journal of Epidemiology, 1,* 271–277.

Ritchie, J., Caty, S., & Ellerton, M. (1984). Concerns of acutely ill, chronically ill, and healthy preschool children. *Research in Nursing and Health, 7,* 265–274,

Ritchie, J., Caty, S., & Ellerton, M. (1988). Coping behaviors of preschool children. *Maternal Child Nursing Journal, 17,* 153–171.

Rosenstiel, A., & Keefe, F. (1983). The use of coping strategies in low back pain patients: Relationship to patient characteristics and current adjustment. *Pain, 17,* 33–40.

Ross, D., & Ross, S. (1984a). The importance of type of question, psychological climate, and subject set in interviewing children about pain. *Pain, 19,* 71–79.

Ross, D., & Ross, S. (1984b). Childhood pain: The school-aged child's viewpoint. *Pain, 20,* 179–191.

Siegel, L. J. (1981, April). *Naturalistic study of coping strategies in children facing medical procedures.* Paper presented at the annual meeting of the Southeastern Psychological Association, Atlanta.

Spirito, A., Overholser, J., & Stark, L. J. (1989). Common problems and coping strategies: II. Findings with adolescent suicide attempters. *Journal of Abnormal Child Psychology, 17,* 213-221.

Spirito, A., & Stark, L. J. (1987). Childhood pain: The assessment and importance of self-report. *Behavioral Medicine Abstracts, 8,* 1-4.

Spirito, A., Stark, L. J., Grace, N., & Stamoulis, D. (in press). Common problems and coping strategies in childhood and early adolescence. *Journal of Youth and Adolescence.*

Spirito, A., Stark, L. J., & Tyc, V. (1989). Common coping strategies employed by children with chronic illness. *Newsletter of the Society of Pediatric Psychology, 13*(1), 3-8.

Spirito, A., Stark, L. J., & Williams, C. (1988). Development of a brief checklist to assess coping in pediatric patients. *Journal of Pediatric Psychology, 13,* 555-574.

Spirito, A., Stark, L. J., Williams, C., Stamoulis, D., & Axelson, D. (1988, April). *Coping strategies utilized by referred and nonreferred pediatric patients and a healthy control group.* Poster presented at the annual meeting of the Society of Behavioral Medicine, Boston.

Stark, L. J., Spirito, A., & Tyc, V. (1991). *Coping strategies used by chronically ill and acutely ill hospitalized children.* Manuscript submitted for publication, Rhode Island Hospital.

Stark, L. J., Spirito, A., Williams, C. A., & Guevremont, D. C. (1989). Common problems and coping strategies: I. Findings with normal adolescents. *Journal of Abnormal Child Psychology, 17,* 203-212.

Tobin, D., Holroyd, K., Reynolds, R., & Wigal, J. (1989). The hierarchical factor structure of the Coping Strategies Inventory. *Cognitive Therapy and Research, 13,* 343-361.

Varni, J. W. (1983). *Clinical behavioral pediatrics.* Elmsford, NY: Pergamon Press.

Worchel, F., Copeland, D., & Barker, D. (1987). Control-related coping strategies in pediatric oncology patients. *Journal of Pediatric Psychology, 12,* 25-38.

Coping with Aversive Medical Treatments

LYNNDA M. DAHLQUIST
Baylor College of Medicine
Texas Children's Hospital

Since the early work of Vernon, Foley, Sipowicz, and Schulman (1965), who proposed that inadequate information about the hospital setting is a major cause of psychological distress during pediatric hospitalization, the importance of helping children during hospitalization and stressful medical procedures has been widely acknowledged in the health care literature (Elkins & Roberts, 1983; Melamed, 1977; Melamed & Siegel, 1975). Most children's hospitals now routinely provide patients with some sort of preparation before surgery, and many clinics also use psychological methods, such as distraction or relaxation, during the execution of uncomfortable procedures. However, the research foundations for the preparation programs currently in widespread use are surprisingly limited. Recent advances in the field suggest that the process of helping children cope with aversive medical procedures may not be as straightforward as it once appeared. Some preparation strategies may be ineffective for certain children or may even have harmful effects.

This chapter presents an overview of current intervention research designed to decrease children's distress during aversive medical procedures. This review is designed to be selective rather than comprehensive, and to illustrate clinical applications, highlight new empirical findings, identify areas of controversy, and suggest directions for future research.

TYPES OF INTERVENTION STRATEGIES

The psychological strategies currently available to help children cope with stressful medical procedures can be grouped into three primary categories, based on the object or goal of the intervention: informational, environmental, and coping skills training. The objectives of informational programs are (1) to correct misconceptions a child might have about a medical procedure; (2) to facilitate the development of a trusting relationship between the child and the medical staff (Elkins & Roberts, 1983; and (3) make uncomfortable aspects of the medical procedure more predictable, which should thereby decrease anxiety and enhance the child's tolerance of and habituation to aversive medical stimuli (Dahlquist & Czyzewski, 1989; Siaw, Stephens, & Holmes, 1986; Staub, Tursky, & Schwartz, 1971). Environmental interventions are designed to change the nature of the medical procedure in a way that facilitates the child's coping. For example, the child may be allowed to participate in part of the procedure, or distracting activities may be included in the medical setting. In contrast, coping skills training interventions typically involve teaching the child specific coping strategies (e.g., imagery, relaxation, or deep breathing) to use during stressful medical procedures.

In the following sections, examples of each of these intervention approaches are presented. Informational and environmental interventions are presented relatively briefly, with an emphasis on current issues. Cognitive–behavioral coping skills interventions are discussed in greater detail and are illustrated with examples from my colleagues' and my investigations.

INFORMATIONAL INTERVENTIONS

Verbal Explanation

The most straightforward way to communicate information about a medical procedure is to tell a child what will happen. With children (and with adults), such verbal information appears to be most effective when "sensory" as well as "procedural" information is included (Johnson, Kirchoff, & Endress, 1975; Johnson & Rice, 1974). For example, Johnson et al. (1975) compared three different methods of preparing 84 children from 6 to 11 years of age for orthopedic cast removal. One group heard a tape recording consisting of "sensory" information about cast removal, such as the noise of the saw, the vibrations when a cast is cut, and the appearance of the skin under the cast. The second group heard a tape of equal length describing the cast removal procedure (i.e., the room in which cast removal would take place; the use of the saw, spreaders, and scissors; and X-ray procedures). A control group received no tape-recorded information. Blind observer ratings of the children's distress and pulse rates obtained during the actual cast removal indicated that the distress of children in the sensory information group was significantly lower than the distress of children in either the procedural information group or the control group.

It should be noted, however, that sensory information inevitably includes some procedural information (i.e., "When the doctor cuts the cast with the saw [procedural information], you will hear a noise that sounds like this . . ." [sensory information]). Therefore, it is probably most accurate to conclude that sensory plus procedural information is more effective than procedural information alone in decreasing distress associated with a medical procedure.

Demonstration

Relying solely on verbal explanation can be problematic for young children, who may not understand complicated verbal explanations or may have difficulty visualizing unfamiliar procedures. Exposure to the actual medical stimuli through demonstration or role play is often necessary.

The "tell–show–do" method is a simple way to provide concrete information that is routinely recommended in the pediatric dentistry literature (Ingersoll, 1982). This approach involves three steps: (1) *Tell* the child what will happen in simple, developmentally appropriate language; (2) *show* how the procedure works on a doll or yourself; (3) when you are certain that the child understands, *do* the procedure.

Although these procedures have intuitive appeal and are widely employed in hospital settings, there has been relatively little empirical study of their effectiveness (Elkins & Roberts, 1983). One of the few empirical studies of a verbal information, demonstration, and role-play approach was conducted by Twardosz, Weddle, Borden, and Stevens (1986). They randomly assigned 60 children (ages 3 to 12) who were scheduled for minor surgery to one of three conditions. One group of children participated in a 20- to 30-minute preoperative class involving 2 to 10 children each, which was conducted by a nurse. The class included "information about hospital procedures and resulting sensations; instructions about how to behave during these procedures; the opportunity to ask and answer questions; interaction with a supportive nurse and other children; role-play with puppets, medical instruments, and hospital clothing; and a tour of the operating and recovery rooms" (Twardosz et al., 1986, p. 15). The second group individually viewed a 20-minute videotape of a preoperative class conducted by the same nurse in the same setting as the preoperative class. A nurse verified that the children actually watched the tape, and was available to answer questions. The third group of children were visited by a floor nurse who explained what would happen before and after surgery.

The children who participated in the preoperative class showed significantly fewer negative behaviors (e.g., crying, yelling, and noncompliance) during a preoperative injection and during the trip to surgery than did the children who viewed the taped class. The children who received the nurse's visit demonstrated fewer negative behaviors than the videotape group but more negative behavior than the group receiving the preoperative class.

Although the results of this study demonstrated the potential benefits of preoperative classes, the mechanisms accounting for the effects remain unclear. It is possible that the *in vivo* exposure of the preoperative class provided more or different information than could be conveyed on a videotape. On the other hand, the exposure to the unfamiliar environment and staff members may have served a desensitizing function, reducing anxiety without necessarily increasing information. The measurement of both information acquisition and self-reported anxiety or physiological arousal in future studies would help clarify these mechanisms.

The "tell–show–do" approach appears to be particularly appropriate for children with special educational needs. For example, my colleagues and I (Dahlquist, Gil, Kalfus, Blount, & Boyd, 1984) used a "tell–show–do" approach combined with a reward program to prepare a 14-year-old autistic girl for gynecological examinations. The intervention consisted of several components. First, because the girl's verbal skills were significantly delayed, verbal explanations were presented at a level appropriate for the average 6- or 7-year-old. Second, to accommodate her short attention span, the exam was broken down into eight short, simple steps. Because her responsiveness to social interaction was very limited, a female therapist demonstrated each step with concrete objects and pictures. The patient then practiced each step and was rewarded by her therapist and a female pediatrician for compliance with each step. Sips of soda and puzzle play were used as rewards. For example, the first step simply involved undressing and lying on the examination table, whereas the final step involved remaining still and using deep breathing while the pediatrician inserted and removed the speculum. When all of the steps of the exam had been demonstrated and practiced, a female and then a male physician successfully conducted complete exams. The patient also successfully underwent pelvic exams with different physicians 11 and 24 weeks after intervention.

This case clearly illustrates the potential reductions in psychological distress and increases in cooperation that can result if a child is provided with adequate, developmentally appropriate information regarding medical procedures. Although this intervention did take several hours of therapist time, the overall cost remained much lower than the cost of the alternative considered by the health care team—namely, general anesthesia.

Modeling

Modeling approaches are most often employed when a medical procedure is complex, when multiple procedures are involved, and/or when specific information about the behavior expected of the child is of concern. The effectiveness of peer modeling in conveying information about a medical procedure and in reducing children's fears and disruptive behavior associated with medical procedures has been well documented by the extensive work of Melamed and her associates (see Elkins & Roberts, 1983; Melamed, 1977). More recent research in this area, therefore, has been focused on the refinement of modeling strategies to maximize their effectiveness. Primary emphasis has involved the timing of modeling interventions and individual differences in response to intervention.

The timing of surgery preparation appears to be an important determinant of effectiveness. For example, Faust and Melamed (1984) compared a hospital-relevant peer modeling film with a control film for two different presurgery time periods: (1) hospital admission and preparation the night before surgery, and (2) hospital admission and preparation the same day as surgery. They found that the children who viewed the peer modeling film the night before surgery showed heart rate increases during the film, but decreased palmar sweating and self-reported anxiety. However, the children who saw the peer modeling film the same day as surgery showed increased palmar sweating and almost no decrease in anxiety after the film. Faust and Melamed speculated that the children admitted the same day as surgery did not benefit from preparation because they had little time to use the information from the film to help cope with their fears. However, the control film appeared to have a beneficial, distracting effect for these children: they demonstrated decreased sweating and reduced self-report of hospital fears after viewing the distracting film. Therefore, when only limited time is available for preparation, modeling may not be helpful. Distraction may be the treatment of choice in this case.

Striking differences in children's responses to modeling preparation have also been found, depending on the children's age and previous experience. For example, Klorman, Hilpert, Michael, LaGana, and Sveen (1980) reported two studies in which peer modeling was not effective in reducing the dental fears and disruptive behavior of children who had previously undergone dental restorations. In the first study, 60 children, with a mean age of 8, viewed either a coping modeling film of an initially anxious child who nonetheless copes well with the procedure, a mastery modeling film of a child who is fearless throughout the procedure, or a control film. However, following film viewing, groups did not differ on dentists' ratings of nervousness or on observed frequency of anxious and uncooperative behaviors.

Speculating that the lack of effects indicated that the modeling films were not powerful enough, Klorman et al. (1980) modified the films by adding a simulated postdental treatment interview in which the peer model either emphasized his lack of fear or discomfort during the dental treatment (mastery model) or explained how he had coped with his anxiety during the treatment (coping model). However, even with these efforts to increase the credibility and salience of the modeling films, no significant effects were found. The experienced pedodontic patients who viewed the revised modeling films did not differ from control subjects on either dentist ratings or observed behavior. In contrast, when the same three films were shown to a separate sample of similar-age children who had never before experienced a dental restoration or extraction, significant effects were found (Klorman et al., 1980). Subjects who viewed the modeling films demonstrated significantly lower levels of disruptive behavior than did subjects who viewed a control film. Thus, the Klorman et al. (1980) studies suggest that medical preparation involving peer modeling may only be effective with naive patients and may have no effect on the fears or cooperative behavior of children who have had prior dental experience.

More recent research suggests that peer modeling may even have a detrimental effect on experienced children. Melamed, Dearborn, and Hermecz (1983) provided 58 children from 4 to 17 years of age with either a slides and tape surgery preparation involving peer models or an unrelated control film. They found that the surgery preparation film led to the acquisition of greater information in prepared subjects, but the acquisition of more information was not necessarily beneficial. Children under age 8 who had previous surgery experience appeared to be sensitized by the hospital relevant film. Their self-report of medical fears increased following viewing of the hospital film. In contrast, experienced young children showed decreased anticipatory medical concerns when shown an unrelated film. Similar results were obtained by Faust and Melamed (1984) in a study of 66 surgery patients between the ages of 4 and 17. Children with previous surgery experience demonstrated increased palmar sweating following a hospital-relevant preparatory film, whereas children without previous surgery experience had decreased sweating after the hospital relevant film.

The differential responses to modeling films of naive and experienced children makes sense in terms of the likely bases for their apprehensions about medical procedures. The medical fears of naive, inexperienced children are likely to be based on erroneous information or the "unknown" aspects of the medical procedure. Peer modeling appears to enhance the knowledge of naive children effectively, and thereby to reduce anxiety and disruptive behavior. However, as Melamed et al. (1983) argued, presenting children "with information about what will occur through the eyes of peer models does not necessarily provide new information for those children who have already had a previous hospitalization for surgery" (p. 523). Experienced children already have information from past experience regarding the impending medical procedure, and this information may well be the basis for their fears. Providing them with *more* information may simply remind them of what they have to fear. Therefore, alternative intervention strategies are needed to address the concerns of experienced children.

ENVIRONMENTAL INTERVENTIONS

Distraction

Although the work of Melamed and colleagues suggests that distracting films may be beneficial for experienced children, only a few studies have specifically examined the utility of distraction to facilitate children's coping with stressful medical procedures. Kelley, Jarvie, Middlebrook, McNeer, and Drabman (1984) provided a 4-year-old girl and a 6-year-old girl with cartoons as distractors during hydrotherapy for burns. They found significant correlations between intervals of no observed pain behaviors and the amount of cartoon viewing for both subjects. However, a star chart reward system for reducing pain behaviors was also employed in their study. Thus, it is impossible to isolate the specific effects of distraction from their data.

Distraction techniques also have been used in conjunction with chemotherapy treatment. Kolko and Rickard-Figueroa (1985) provided three children (ages 11 to 17) with access to video games during chemotherapy treatments in a combined multiple-baseline and ABAB withdrawal design. During the distraction condition, all subjects demonstrated significant reductions in self-reported distress in the 24 hours prior to chemotherapy, in observed behavioral distress during the 5 minutes prior to chemotherapy, and in self-reported distress during the chemotherapy treatment. Although the subjects' actual behaviors during venipunctures and chemotherapy administration were not observed, the obtained improvements in anticipatory distress and chemotherapy-related symptoms are encouraging. Video game distraction also has been shown to reduce children's self-reported nausea during chemotherapy (Redd et al., 1987). In both a repeated-measures analysis of variance design and an ABAB withdrawal design, 9- to 20-year-old subjects reported lower levels of nausea during video game playing.

Video games appear to be an ideal distractor for children. They require considerable attention (and thereby interfere with attention to the stressful medical procedure), and most children enjoy playing video games. Further research is needed to evaluate the effectiveness of video game distraction for children under the age of 9 during chemotherapy procedures, and for children of all ages undergoing other stressful medical procedures.

Interesting descriptive results have been reported with audiotape distraction for children undergoing cardiac catheterization (Caire & Erickson, 1986). For example, tapes of nursery rhymes appeared to calm infants during the procedure; babies stopped crying when the tapes began and resumed crying at the end of the tapes. For older children, benefits appeared mixed. Some children agreed to listen to rock music or relaxation tapes and were rated by staff members as benefiting from the tapes. Others refused to try the tapes or became increasingly agitated during the catheterization.

Fowler-Kerry and Lander (1987) further evaluated the merits of auditory distraction in an experimental study. Using an impressive sample of 200 children from 4 to 6 years of age, they found that distraction in the form of music played through headphones during an injection resulted in lower self-reported pain than a headphone-only or a no-treatment control condition. However, cooperation and distress behaviors during the injection were not assessed. Further research is needed to determine whether music distraction can effectively reduce uncooperative behavior during medical procedures.

The results of these few studies suggest that distraction may have beneficial effects during stressful medical procedures. However, considerably more work is needed to determine the effectiveness of distraction with children of different ages undergoing different medical procedures. and to evaluate the relative effectiveness of different types of distractors (e.g., auditory vs. visual). In addition, the long-term benefits of distraction interventions need to be evaluated. Stark et al. (1989) obtained initial reductions in disruptive behavior during dental treatment in four 4- to 7-year-old children who were exposed to visual distraction (posters) and auditory distraction (audiotaped stories). However, their well-controlled multiple-baseline design revealed that anxious and disruptive behavior increased in subsequent dental visits, despite the continued use of distraction.

Perceived Control

Previous research has shown that distress associated with noxious stimuli can be reduced when the individual perceives that he or she has control over the administration of the aversive stimulus (Bowers, 1968; Glass, Singer, & Friedman, 1969; Staub et al., 1971). Tarnowski, McGrath, Calhoun, and Drabman (1987) speculated that providing a child control over a painful medical procedure could possibly serve as an effective distress management intervention that would not involve extensive therapist time. They observed distress behaviors in a 12-year-old boy with second-degree burns over 25% of his body under two conditions: (1) self-mediated debridement, when the child was allowed to remove skin tissue on his arm and hand; and (2) therapist-mediated debridement, when all tissue removal was performed by the physical therapist.

Tarnowski et al. (1987) found that this youngster showed significantly fewer distress behaviors when he conducted the debridement himself than when the physical therapist conducted debridement of the same body parts. They speculated that his lower distress levels may have been due to the fact that he was distracted from his pain by the act of debriding, or that by being "in control" he was able to modulate his pain and physiological arousal, and therefore showed fewer behavioral indications of distress. However, there also appeared to be a serious drawback to this intervention: The termination of control over debridement seemed to result in increased distress. When therapist-mediated debridement was resumed, the patient demonstrated higher than baseline levels of distress. These findings are consistent with the results of Staub et al. (1971), who found that increased control over the timing and intensity of aversive stimulation results in increased pain tolerance, but that when this control is removed, diminished pain tolerance results.

The principle of allowing a child some control over the timing of painful medical procedures appears to have promise, especially for procedures such as burn debridement, where it is feasible for the child actually to conduct part of the painful activity. However, there are potential dangers associated with allowing the child some control, especially if control will be withdrawn in the future. Furthermore, it is also possible that the child will refuse to perform the painful activity or will delay performing the painful activity when given control. Refusal or delay may result in avoidance of pain, which can easily negatively reinforce uncooperative behavior.

TRAINING IN COGNITIVE-BEHAVIORAL COPING STRATEGIES

Cognitive-behavioral coping skills training first emerged in the preparation literature in response to the argument that informational and modeling techniques did not necessarily adequately prepare children to initiate coping efforts themselves (Peterson & Shigetomi, 1981). Specific training in cognitive coping strategies was hypothesized to provide children with superior abilities to handle the discomfort and fears of medical procedures. Therefore, early studies of cognitive-behavioral coping skills training focused on demonstrating the effectiveness of the technique and on comparing the relative efficacy of informational and coping skills training approaches.

Although specific procedures varied across studies, most investigators taught children a cognitive-behavioral coping skills "package" involving deep breathing exercises, muscle relaxation, positive self-statements, and relaxing or coping imagery. Without exception, training in cognitive-behavioral coping strategies resulted in beneficial effects (e.g., lower physiological arousal and greater cooperation) during dental treatment (Klingman, Melamed, Cuthbert, & Hermecz, 1984; Nocella & Kaplan, 1982; Siegel & Peterson, 1980, 1981) and prior to surgery (Peterson & Shigetomi, 1981). Early studies also showed that cognitive-behavioral coping skills training was at least as effective as modeling and sensory information in reducing physiological arousal and disruptive behavior of inexperienced children during dental procedures (Siegel & Peterson, 1980, 1981) and elective surgery (Peterson & Shigetomi, 1981). These studies further suggested that coping skills training may be superior to sensory information in reducing anticipatory arousal (Siegel & Peterson, 1980), and more effective than peer modeling in reducing distress during surgery (Peterson & Shigetomi, 1981).

In the only study to examine the potential mechanisms by which coping skills training is effective, Klingman et al., (1984) found that active rehearsal of coping skills may be necessary for maximum effectiveness. They showed a videotape in which peer models actively prompted subjects to practice controlled breathing and imagery distraction (participant modeling) or a videotape in which these skills were simply demonstrated by the peer models (symbolic modeling) to 38 children from 8 to 13 years of age with high self-reported fear of dental restorations. Both films also included information about the dental procedures.

The children in the participant modeling condition retained more information, reported more frequent use of imagery during the film, and reported greater reductions in dental fears than the symbolic modeling subjects. The children who had been encouraged to practice coping skills actively also demonstrated lower levels of disruptive behavior during actual dental treatment. When experienced and first-time patients were compared, the experienced children appeared to benefit more. Their self-reported dental fears were reduced after viewing either film; by contrast, naive subjects showed reductions in overall fears after film viewing, but their specific dental fears did not decrease until after the dental treatment experience.

More recent studies have focused on the generalizability of cognitive-behavioral coping skills training to the significant distress experienced by children who are required to undergo repeated stressful medical procedures, such as those procedures involved in cancer or burn treatment. These children are "experienced" with the medical procedure, and therefore can be expected to have realistic fears about the pain or discomfort they will experience. Procedural or sensory information is unlikely to be of help, and, as suggested by the modeling literature, may even sensitize these children.

Cognitive-behavioral coping skills training programs typically teach the child a variety of coping strategies and allow the child to choose the specific coping skills he or she prefers to use. The specific skills taught in such programs include the following:

1. Deep breathing exercises (deep inhalation and slow exhalation) (Dahlquist, Gil, Armstrong, Ginsberg, & Jones, 1985; Elliott & Olson, 1983; Jay, Elliott, Katz, & Siegel, 1987; Jay, Elliott, Ozolins, Olson, & Pruitt, 1985).
2. Attention distraction (e.g., focusing on stimuli other than the medical procedure, such as counting ceiling tiles or doing mental arithmetic) (Elliott & Olson, 1983).
3. Emotive imagery involving reconceptualizing the medical setting or the pain stimulus; for example, a child might imagine himself or herself as a superhero undergoing a painful test of his or her superpowers, or the child might imaginally transform the burning sensation of an injection to an icy, numbing, cold sensation (Elliott & Olson, 1983; Jay et al., 1985, 1987).
4. Relaxing imagery (Dahlquist et al., 1985; Elliott & Olson, 1983; Jay et al., 1985, 1987).
5. Behavioral rehearsal (Jay et al., 1985, 1987) or imaginal rehearsal (Dahlquist et al., 1985).
6. Progressive muscle relaxation (Dahlquist et al., 1985).
7. Rewards for using coping strategies (Dahlquist et al., 1985; Elliott & Olson, 1983; Jay et al., 1985, 1987).

The skills are taught by the therapist during sessions typically lasting approximately 45 minutes. The therapist also is present during the actual medical procedure, serving as a "coach" to prompt the child to use the coping strategies and praising the child's efforts to cope.

The effects of cognitive-behavioral coping skills training sessions have been extremely impressive. For example, using a multiple baseline design. Elliott and Olson (1983) obtained up to 52% reductions in observed distress behaviors in four children (ages 5 to 9) undergoing hydrotherapy for burns. Approximately 50% reductions in observed distress were documented by Jay et al. (1985) with five pediatric cancer patients (ages 3 to 7) undergoing bone marrow aspiration (BMA) or lumbar puncture (LP). We (Dahlquist et al., 1985) obtained similar levels of behavioral distress reductions (46–68% decreases) in 11- to 14-year-old children undergoing chemotherapy.

Because of the limited sample sizes of many of the studies of cognitive-behavioral treatment for children undergoing repeated invasive medical procedures, the generalizability of treatment effects across subjects has emerged as an important question. Jay et al. (1987) attempted to evaluate the generalizability issue by applying a modification of the cognitive–behavioral package used by Jay et al. (1985) to a larger sample of pediatric cancer patients (ages 3 to 13). They compared the effectiveness of the cognitive–behavioral package with that of two other interventions: (1) 0.3 mg/kg of oral Valium administered 30 minutes before a BMA, and (2) an "attention control" condition involving 30 minutes of cartoon viewing. Fifty-six subjects were evaluated over the course of three consecutive BMAs. All subjects received all three experimental treatments, but in different order.

When the children were in the behavior therapy condition, they consistently exhibited less behavioral distress, reported lower levels of pain, and had lower pulse rates than when in the attention control (cartoon) condition. When the subjects received Valium, they only differed from the attention control condition on the blood pressure measure. Thus, cognitive–behavioral coping skills training appears to be effective in reducing the behavioral distress of a wide range of children. In addition, it appears to be more effective than Valium in reducing behavioral distress.

Methodological Issues

The behavior therapy condition in the Jay et al. (1987) study resulted in distress scores only 18–25% lower than those in the control condition. This finding suggests that the behavior therapy package used by Jay et al. (1987) may have been less effective than the approaches used in previous work (i.e., Elliott & Olson, 1983; Jay et al., 1985), or that treatment effectiveness may vary depending on subject characteristics. It is also likely that the control condition was distracting and therefore may have actually had some therapeutic benefit. The inclusion of baseline monitoring in the absence of any intervention would have allowed these issues to be evaluated by Jay et al. (1987) and is strongly recommended for future studies.

Another important methodological consideration that is lacking in nearly all of the studies of coping skills training for medical procedures is a check on whether or not subjects actually used the coping skills they were taught. We (Dahlquist et al., 1986) specifically asked subjects whether they had done anything special to help themselves feel better during a medical examination, but only 11 of the 30 subjects in the study who had been taught coping skills reported attempting to relax or use coping statements during the exam. The children who said they used the coping skills did show approximately 50% lower levels of behavioral distress than subjects who did not report using coping strategies, but the large number of subjects who did not use the skills weakened the overall impact of the intervention. Future research should include similar manipulation checks to determine which skills, if any, children use during medical procedures. In addition, it may be crucial to reward children for using the coping strategies.

Treatment Matching

Another factor that may influence the effectiveness of coping skills training interventions is the "fit" between the intervention strategy and the child's preferred coping style (Peterson, 1989). It has been argued that children who tend to cope by avoiding information may do best if assisted in "perfecting" this style by learning more effective avoidant techniques such as distraction. On the other hand, their avoidant behavior may need to be challenged and redirected to a more active coping strategy through shaping, modeling, and/or desensitization. Or it may simply be best to provide no preparatory intervention for these children, if they are already experienced with the procedure. As Peterson (1989) so clearly summarizes, these questions remain "among the most pressing research concerns in the field today" (p. 385).

Facilitating Long-Term Clinical Improvement

Although the immediate effects of cognitive–behavioral treatment programs have been very impressive, the results of the few studies that have examined maintenance of effects have been disappointing. Both Elliott and Olson (1983) and Jay et al. (1987) found that distress reductions did not continue in subsequent medical treatment sessions when the therapist (coach) was not present. When the therapist was absent, subjects returned to baseline levels of distress. Thus, we appear to have the technology to provide immediate reductions in children's distress, but we have yet to develop the methodology needed to help children continue to cope with aversive medical procedures once psychological treatment is terminated.

Two explanations are proposed to account for the failure to obtain long-term maintenance of treatment gains. First, children may need more extensive training and practice before they can use cognitive–behavioral coping strategies to calm themselves during stressful medical procedures. If so, several sessions of cognitive–behavioral therapy should prove much more effective than the single 45-minute therapy session typically employed in the literature. On the other hand, children may not be able to use cognitive–behavioral coping strategies without the assistance of an adult coach. If this premise is accurate, one would not expect maintenance of distress reductions in the absence of the therapist coach.

A longitudinal study of three cancer patients receiving chemotherapy venipunctures (Dahlquist et al., 1985) provides some support for the potential benefits of repeated instruction and practice in cognitive-behavioral coping strategies. Following baseline observation, my colleagues and I conducted four treatment sessions involving training in deep breathing exercises and tension-release relaxation involving six muscle groups. Over the course of training, muscle groups were gradually collapsed until each child was able to initiate whole-body relaxation cued by a word (such as "relax") and by breathing deeply. Subjects also were taught to use positive coping statements (e.g., "I can handle this") and to imagine a pleasant scene while relaxing. Sessions were audiotaped so that subjects could practice relaxation techniques between sessions.

All subjects showed significant decreases in distress during chemotherapy venipunctures, which were maintained over several chemotherapy administrations while the children received ongoing coaching in coping strategies. Observed distress scores decreased by 46% for subject 1, by 60% for subject 2, and by 68% for subject 3. Corresponding decreases in self-reported distress ranged from 9% to 22%. Although we did not plan to study maintenance of effects in the absence of the therapist/coach, the last two chemotherapy observations for subject 1 occurred while he listened to a relaxation tape without receiving *in vivo* coaching, and the last observation for subject 3 occurred in the absence of coaching or any other intervention. Both of these subjects maintained low distress levels without coaching.

Although these data represent only short-term posttreatment maintenance of treatment gains (since only one or two medical procedures were evaluated), they are encouraging nonetheless, in light of the failure of other investigators to obtain maintenance for even a single procedure (Elliott & Olson, 1983; Jay et al., 1987). These findings suggest that maintenance may be achieved after multiple training and coaching sessions (in this case, three or six sessions) and/or that maintenance may be facilitated by providing relaxation tapes to use during stressful procedures.

These issues were explored in a subsequent case study (Dahlquist, 1989) The subject of this investigation was an 8-year-old boy who experienced significant anxiety during chemotherapy, which was evidenced by vomiting a minute *before* chemotherapy venipunctures. Because of the extensive amount of time required to train a child and to be present for *in vivo* coaching, an attempt was made in this study to decrease treatment costs by eliminating the need for live coaching. Three 1-hour therapy sessions involving intensive training in condensed tension–release progressive muscle relaxation, relaxing breathing, and distracting imagery and home practice were conducted. However, as Figure 16.1 indicates, after an initial improvement, the boy's performance deteriorated: He vomited 2 minutes before the needle was inserted for chemotherapy.

Because the child appeared skilled in relaxation strategies in the therapy sessions (i.e., he was able to spontaneously execute the relaxation sequence and to achieve visible relaxation in his face and limbs), his continued difficulties during chemotherapy appeared to reflect a generalization problem rather than lack of ability. To facilitate generalization, therefore, he was instructed to listen to relaxation tapes before and during chemotherapy venipunctures. However, this intervention also was not effective (see Figure 16.1.)

In the third phase of treatment, *in vivo* therapist coaching in distracting imagery and relaxation strategies was introduced along with rewards for improved vomiting latencies. As illustrated in Figure 16.1, significant

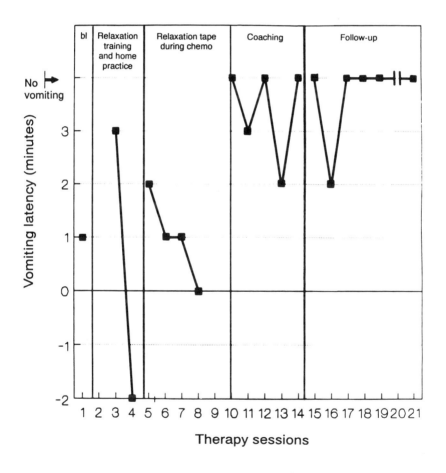

Figure 16.1. Vomiting latencies over the course of psychological treatment. Note: Negative values indicate that vomiting occurred *before* needle insertion. Positive values indicate vomiting that occurred *after* needle insertion.

improvements were obtained with coaching. For the first time in 5 months, the boy did not vomit at the start of chemotherapy. His self-reported nausea also decreased significantly. Only three more episodes of vomiting that could not clearly be attributed to the emetic effects of chemotherapy occurred. When live coaching was discontinued (session 15), his improvements maintained over the subsequent six chemotherapy administrations and at one-year follow-up. Although *in vivo* therapist coaching was confounded with the institution of a reward system, thus making it impossible to determine the relative efficacy of these two individual components, the findings were nonetheless promising. Significant reductions in anticipatory symptoms were achieved only when the multiple-session cognitive–behavioral package was combined with *in vivo* therapist coaching and rewards. More importantly, treatment gains were maintained when active therapist intervention was discontinued.

In a subsequent case study (Dahlquist, 1989), the effectiveness of multiple-session cognitive–behavioral treatment and live coaching was replicated with a 5½-year-old boy who demonstrated high levels of behavioral distress during chemotherapy venipunctures. Ten therapy sessions were conducted in which relaxing breathing, distracting imagery, and rewards for attempting to use coping strategies were employed. *In vivo* therapist coaching was provided during chemotherapy initiation following each behavior therapy session. Treatment was terminated when the subject was able to undergo a BMA without crying or interfering with the procedure. Follow-up observations of several different chemotherapy treatments were obtained at 9, 10, and 13 weeks following the termination of psychological treatment by a naive observer who had been trained to 85% agreement with the Observation Scale of Behavioral Distress (OSBD); Elliott, Jay, & Woody, 1987; Jay, Ozolins, Elliot, & Caldwell, 1983) distress scores. The resulting mean OSBD scores demonstrated 70–87% reductions in distress.

The successful outcomes of the cases described above suggest that in order to achieve long-term maintenance of distress reduction, children may simply need several sessions of cognitive–behavioral therapy accompanied by live coaching. If the number of sessions provided is adequate, a child will have the skills necessary to calm himself or herself during subsequent medical procedures. In our current research program at Texas Children's Hospital, we have been exploring this premise. In our treatment program, children with cancer are taught the following cognitive–behavioral coping skills: (1) relaxing deep breathing, (2) progressive muscle relaxation involving eight muscle groups, (3) relaxing imagery, and (4) positive self-statements. After each therapy session, the therapist coaches the child through the actual medical procedure (i.e., BMA, LP, or chemotherapy administration).

We are currently studying the number of cognitive–behavioral therapy sessions needed to achieve significant behavioral distress reductions during the repeated invasive medical procedures involved in chemotherapy, as well as the number of sessions needed to achieve maintenance in the absence of therapist coaching. Our initial findings suggest that more than four sessions of treatment may be needed. For example, Figure 16.2 presents the observed distress behaviors of a 6-year-old boy undergoing chemotherapy injections. As the figure demonstrates, his distress decreased during coaching, but maintenance was not achieved after two sessions of cognitive–behavioral therapy and therapist coaching. A trend toward maintenance was achieved in session 9, after three more intervention sessions; however, more intensive intervention still appeared needed. The 9-year-old child in Figure 16.3 received four sessions of

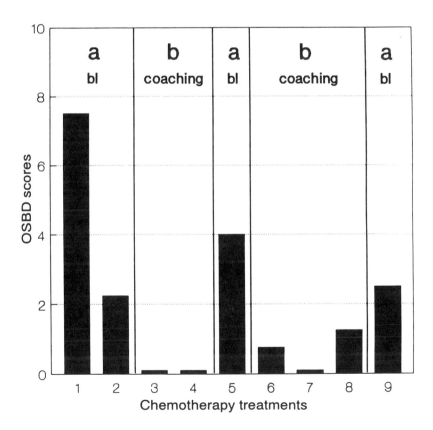

Figure 16.2. Mean Observation Scale of Behavioral Distress (OSBD) scores during chemotherapy injections across baseline and coaching conditions.

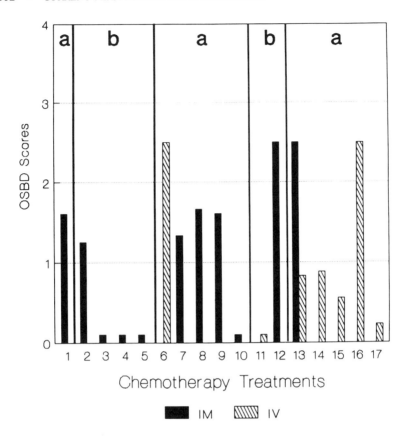

Figure 16.3. Mean OSBD scores during chemotherapy injections across baseline and coaching conditions.

cognitive–behavioral therapy with therapist coaching, which resulted in significant decreases in distress, but he too returned to baseline levels of distress when the coach was withdrawn. Maintenance was not achieved with two additional therapy and coaching sessions.

The 10-, 7-, and 5-year-old subjects presented in Figures 16.4, 16.5, and 16.6 each received six sessions of cognitive–behavioral therapy with therapist coaching. All subjects demonstrated decreased distress during therapist coaching, but long-term maintenance of distress reduction varied across subjects. These data suggest that six-session cognitive–behavioral intervention with therapist coaching may be effective in decreasing behavioral distress during chemotherapy injections, and that some (e.g., the children in Figures 16.4 and 16.5), but not all, children may maintain

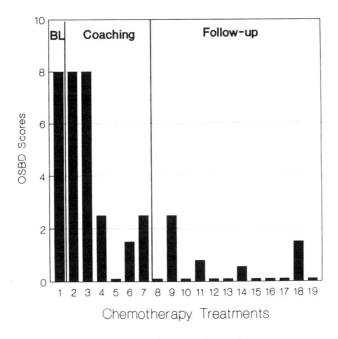

Figure 16.4. Mean OSBD scores during chemotherapy injections across baseline, coaching, and follow-up conditions.

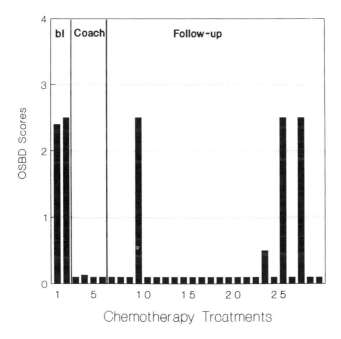

Figure 16.5. Mean OSBD scores during intramuscular and intrathecal chemotherapy administrations across baseline, coaching, and follow-up conditions.

decreased distress levels following intervention. Ongoing coaching may be necessary for subjects similar to the child in Figure 16.6.

These pilot data suggest that there are individual differences in children's ability to benefit from cognitive–behavioral intervention. In other words, it may be too difficult for some children to exert the self-control necessary to remain calm independently. They may need the structure provided by an adult who is present during the procedure to help them remain calm. If adult participation in a coaching role is indeed necessary, issues of cost-effectiveness must be taken into consideration. In most clinical settings, personnel limitations may make it difficult to provide ongoing coaching for all children during every invasive procedure. Financial support for such services (if they must be provided by psychologists) may also be prohibitive. Therefore, it is important to consider possible cost reduction strategies, such as the use of parents as coaches.

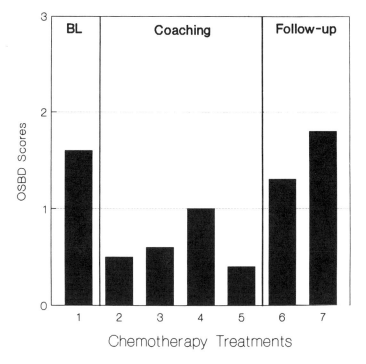

Figure 16.6. Mean OSBD scores during intrathecal chemotherapy treatments across baseline, coaching, and follow-up conditions.

THE ROLE OF PARENTS DURING STRESSFUL PROCEDURES

Parental Presence

There is considerable controversy in the literature regarding the effects of parental presence during stressful medical procedures. Shaw and Routh (1982) found that both 18-month-old and 5-year-old children whose mothers were present during routine immunizations cried longer and continued to fuss more after an injection than did same-aged children whose mothers were not present during the injection. Similar findings were reported by Gross, Stern, Levin, Dale, and Wojnilower (1983) with 4- to 10-year-old children: Regardless of age, children whose mothers were present exhibited significantly more crying before a blood test than did children whose mothers were absent. Gonzales et al., (1989) also observed more crying in children over the age of 4 years whose parents were present during a routine injection, but not in younger children.

The results of these studies are understandable in light of the typical child's history, in which crying usually results in attention and comfort from the mother and the elimination of the aversive stimulus. When the mother does not eliminate the aversive stimulus (in these cases, the blood test or injection), an extinction contingency appears to be established, resulting in increased responding (crying). If the aversive medical procedures could be repeated several times under the same stimulus conditions, one would expect the child's crying to eventually extinguish. However, medical personnel rarely have the time or patience to allow such extinction to occur.

Rather, the data typically are used to argue that increased cooperation from children could be obtained if procedures were conducted without the parent present. Indeed, this is often routine practice (and may be justified) in dental settings, where procedures cannot easily be repeated and where crying would interfere with the execution of the procedure. Ethical considerations, however, call into question the advisability of routinely separating children from their parents during a procedure if the children's crying is merely uncomfortable for staff members, but poses no serious harm. Many children prefer to have their parents present during difficult medical procedures (Gonzales et al., 1989). It is possible that subjective distress increases when parents are not present, even if crying is inhibited.

There is also some evidence that separation from parents may actually increase the children's overt behavioral distress during a medical procedure. For example, we (Dahlquist et al., 1986) compared three preparatory strategies, an attention control condition (story reading or brief discussion with an adult), and a no-treatment control for children undergoing throat cultures and throat examinations. We found that children with a history of negative medical experiences showed higher levels of behavioral distress during the medical exam after brief attention control contact alone with the experimenters than did either no-treatment control subjects or subjects who were separated briefly from their parents and provided with information and/or coping skills training. We speculated that separation from parents prior to a medical procedure was anxiety-provoking for all the children. Children in the preparatory conditions were provided with content that may have helped reduce their anxiety, but the children in the attention control condition did not receive any intervention that would be expected to decrease anxiety and therefore demonstrated higher distress during the exam. Thus, one cannot assume that simply removing the parent from the setting will necessarily reduce a child's distress during a medical procedure. In fact, separation prior to procedures may increase the child's anxiety and result in greater degrees of behavioral distress during the actual procedure.

The studies reviewed above suggest that parents may play an important role in mediating children's distress during stressful medical procedures. However, the process by which parents affect children's distress has only been investigated in a few studies.

Parental Affect

One way in which parents may influence children's distress during medical procedures is by modeling fearful or distressed behavior. For example, higher levels of child distress during exams and cancer procedures have been reported when parents engage in behaviors that appear to communicate anxiety, such as agitation (Bush, Melamed, Sheras, & Greenbaum, 1986) and apology (Blount et al., 1989; Blount, Sturges, & Powers, 1990).

Parental Discipline Practices

There is also some evidence that general parental discipline practices may influence child distress during aversive medical treatment. For example, Dolgin and associates (Dolgin & Katz, 1988; Dolgin, Katz, McGinty, & Siegel, 1985) found that children with anticipatory nausea and vomiting associated with chemotherapy were more anxious, and had parents who reported relying more on threat of punishment and less on modeling and reassurance, than children with no anticipatory symptoms. Similar findings have been documented with general pediatric patients and with hospitalized and surgical pediatric patients. Bush and Cockrell (1987) documented higher levels of distress during routine medical exams in children whose mothers reported using punishment. In a study of hospitalized and surgical pediatric patients, Zabin and Melamed (1980) found that lower levels of child state anxiety were associated with reported parental use of positive reinforcement, modeling, and reassurance, whereas higher child state anxiety was correlated with reported parental use of punishment, force, and reinforcement of dependency. Thus, it appears that punitive discipline styles are associated with increased child distress during exams and hospitalization, and that reinforcement of dependency is related to fearful behavior.

In addition, parents may differentially attend to, and thereby reinforce, distress behaviors during the actual medical procedure. For example, Blount et al. (1989, 1990) found that adult behaviors that involved paying attention to child distress, such as reassurance, giving control to the child, and criticism, were associated with child distress behaviors during BMA and LP. Similarly, lower levels of parental ignoring were associated with higher levels of child distress during medical exams (Bush et al., 1986). On the other hand, when parents attended to positive behaviors and specifically directed children to use a coping strategy (e.g., deep breathing) or attempted to distract the children, lower levels of child distress were reported during exams (Bush et al., 1986) and during BMA and LP procedures (Blount et al., 1989, 1990).

Integrating Parental Influences

In a recent study of parent–child interactions while children with cancer underwent BMA and LP procedures (Cox, Dahlquist, & Fernbach, 1987), we attempted to integrate some of the parental variables reported in the literature to influence child distress. Sixty-six children with cancer and their parents were evaluated during a routine BMA or LP. The following variables were assessed:

1. Parental state–trait anxiety.
2. Parenting style as measured by the Parenting Dimensions Inventory (PDI; Slater & Power, 1987), an 84-item questionnaire that assesses three global dimensions of parenting: "support" (e.g., nurturance, sensitivity to the child's input, and nonrestrictive attitudes), "control" (e.g., amount of rule setting, type of discipline used, and demands for maturity), and "structure" (e.g, consistency and organization of the household).
3. Observed parent–child interactions during the medical procedure, which were coded via the Dyadic Prestressor Interaction Scale (DPIS; Bush et al., 1986).

4. Parental Likert-type ratings of child distress before and during the procedure.
5. Observed child distress as measured by the OSBD.

Several interesting patterns of relationship emerged between parental variables and child variables, which appear to have implications for children's coping with aversive medical procedures. First, parental anxiety appeared to be an important variable. Parental anxiety was related to parenting style and to parental behavior during the BMA or LP, but for young (2- to 7-year-old) children only. Anxious parents of young children were more agitated and less reassuring during the medical procedure, and reported using discipline practices that were less consistent, less organized, less nurturant, less reliant on rule setting, and more punitive. Parents with high state anxiety scores also tended to perceive their children as more anxious prior to the BMA or LP.

When child distress was examined, both the age of the child and the phase of the medical procedure emerged as important factors. Few significant relationships were found for older children, suggesting that parental influences during aversive procedures may be less important in children over the age of 7. However, parent discipline practices were significantly related to the distress of young children. Parents of young children who reported using less rule setting and less consistent, less organized, and more permissive discipline practices perceived their children as more anxious prior to the medical procedure. In addition, young children of parents who reported less responsive and less nurturant discipline styles demonstrated higher levels of behavioral distress during the anticipatory phase of the medical procedure. Parenting variables were not significantly related to child distress during the painful phase of the medical procedure (perhaps because the pain of the procedure may be the most important determinant of child distress at this point in time). Finally, children with higher levels of anticipatory distress exhibited more attachment and exploratory behavior; their parents demonstrated more reassurance and more agitation, but also tended to demonstrate more frequent ignoring of their children.

Although the correlational nature of these data does not allow for inferences regarding cause and effect, the pattern of results suggests several hypotheses worthy of further study. First, there appears to be a pattern of parenting attitudes that is associated with greater anxiety on the part of a parent as well as greater distress in a child. Whether ineffective parenting precedes or results from anxiety in the child or parent is unclear. However, at the very least, it appears that non-nurturing, punitive, inconsistent, insensitive, disorganized, or overly permissive discipline styles are likely to be associated with greater distress in young children undergoing stressful medical procedures. Children of parents who report ineffective parenting practices may be particularly at risk for developing problems coping with aversive medical procedures. Training in more effective parenting strategies may prove to be a helpful and perhaps crucial intervention for these parents.

In addition, there appears to be a maladaptive pattern of interaction between distressed young children and their parents during medical procedures. These youngsters appear to attempt to engage their parents in some sort of interaction before the medical procedure, but their parents appear either to ignore or to respond ineffectually to them. The more the parents ignore the children, the more the children may try to elicit some sort of comfort or protection from the parents, thus perpetuating a vicious cycle. In our clinical work with childhood cancer patients and their families, my colleagues and I have found that many parents feel overwhelmed during their children's medical procedures. They report feeling uncertain about how to help their children and therefore leave it to the physician or nurse to take charge of the situation, or they report feeling so stressed themselves that most of their energy is directed at keeping their own emotions under control. Thus, the parents' lack of response or inconsistent response to the children is quite understandable. The key to helping these children cope with stressful medical procedures may therefore lie in helping their *parents* cope more effectively with the procedure.

Preparing Parents

One approach that may help reduce parental distress and facilitate their coping with children's medical procedures is to include parents in the preparation program. Peterson and Shigetomi's (1981) preparation program, described earlier, indirectly involved parents; they were present during intervention procedures and were encouraged to discuss the hospital experience with their children and to help their children cope with hospitalization. Although it was unclear what the parents actually did to help the children, parents in the coping skills condition rated themselves as more competent and less anxious after surgery, whereas parents in the modeling condition rated themselves as more anxious and less competent.

Zastowny, Kirschenbaum, and Meng (1986) extended the work of Peterson and Shigetomi (1981) by specifying and expanding the role parents should play in helping their children cope with hospitalization. Thirty-three 6- to 10-year-old children who were scheduled for elective surgery and their parents were randomly assigned to one of three preparation programs conducted 1 week prior to admission. All of the children and their parents viewed a 22-minute videotape of a puppet positively describing his positive hospitalization experience, and participated in a hospital tour. Participants were then assigned to one of the following conditions:

1. *Information only:* Parents were instructed to spend an additional hour the following week in one-on-one activity with their children to facilitate a positive response to stress.

2. *Anxiety reduction:* Parents viewed a film describing Melzack's (1973) conceptualization of stress and attended a lecture describing ways to reduce their own distress reactions by recognizing signs of stress, using relaxation, and reconceptualizing stressful events in less negative ways. Parents were instructed to work at reducing their own distress in the upcoming week, and to spend an hour in special time with their children in which they should communicate their own confident, relaxed attitude about the impending hospitalization and surgery.

3. *Coping skills:* Parents viewed a videotape that presented Melzack's stress model and Meichenbaum's (1975) stress inoculation (coping skills) procedures. They then viewed a videotape that portrayed a parent and child coping with various stressors associated with hospitalization. Parents were given a practice booklet outlining steps in coping with various hospital experiences, to work through at least three times with their children over the next week. The parents' role as coping coaches for their children was emphasized.

Zastowny et al. (1986) found that both the coping skills and anxiety reduction conditions resulted in lower child self-report of medical fears and lower parental distress ratings before and after hospitalization. However, only the coping skills condition resulted in fewer overt problem behaviors, as documented by parental diaries.

Another approach to parent-oriented intervention is the stress inoculation program developed by Jay and Elliott (1990). Their program consists of (1) a modeling film providing information about childhood cancer treatment and an adult coping model who models positive coping strategies during a BMA and LP; (2) approximately 15 minutes of training in positive coping self-statements; and (3) a 15-minute audiotaped relaxation session.

Jay and Elliott (1990) found that parents of leukemia patients who participated in the stress inoculation program reported lower anxiety immediately before and more positive self-statements immediately after their children underwent a BMA or LP than did parents who merely watched their children receive training in cognitive–behavioral coping skills. However, parental physiological arousal, distress behavior during the medical procedure, and interactions with the children did not differ between groups. Jay and Elliott (1990) speculated that both conditions provided modeling of parent coping behavior, and both therefore may have had beneficial effects on parental behavior and arousal. No-treatment control conditions may be necessary to address this issue in future studies. In addition, it will be important to evaluate whether changes in parental anxiety and coping efforts affect the children's subjective or overt expressions of distress during the medical procedure.

Parents as Coaches

Another way to alter maladaptive parent-child interactions during medical procedures, as we have noted (Cox et al., 1987), is to teach parents specific ways to interact with their children during the medical procedure. Although ways to coach children were implied in the parent interventions employed by Jay and Elliott (1990), the only study to date in which parents were specifically taught to coach their children during a medical procedure was conducted by Manne et al. (1990). They taught 23 parents of 3- to 9-year-old cancer patients to help their children distract attention away from venipunctures by blowing on a party blower while the parents counted slowly to pace the children's breathing. Parents also were taught to administer stickers as rewards for holding still and using the party blower during the venipuncture. A psychologist helped the parents coach the children during the first venipuncture, provided less assistance during the subsequent venipuncture, and observed but did not intervene during the third and final venipuncture.

The results of this relatively simple intervention were very encouraging: Parents who participated in the coaching training reported less anxiety during the venipunctures, and their children demonstrated greater reductions in behavioral distress during venipunctures, than did parents and children assigned to an attention control condition. Furthermore, the beneficial effects appeared to be maintained over three consecutive venipunctures.

The potential use of parents as coaches during stressful medical procedures is an important issue that warrants further study. If parents can serve as effective coaches for their children, a number of benefits may be expected. Parental anxiety is likely to decrease as the role of a parent in the medical setting becomes less ambiguous and as a child's level of distress improves. Parent coaching should also interrupt negative patterns of parent-child interaction, which appear to be related to increased child distress. The possibility also exists that new coaching behaviors may generalize outside the medical setting, thus improving the overall quality of parenting skills. Finally, the use of parents as coaches may substantially decrease the cost of psychological care for children with chronic illnesses requiring repeated stressful medical treatments.

SUMMARY

Verbal information, demonstration, and modeling interventions appear to be effective methods for imparting information regarding medical procedures, and appear to be extremely useful in decreasing anxiety and facilitating cooperation in children who are unfamiliar with the medical procedure. However, children who already have experience with medical procedures, particularly children whose previous experience was negative, may not benefit from or may be sensitized by informational programs. Recent research suggests that distraction or training in cognitive–behavioral coping strategies is effective in reducing the distress of experienced children undergoing repeated stressful medical procedures. However, current treatment strategies are time-consuming and costly. Further research is needed to decrease the cost of treatment and to increase the generalizability and maintenance of intervention effects.

Recent studies of individual differences in children's responses to stressful medical procedures suggest that child coping style, parent anxiety, parent discipline style, and parent-child interactions during stressful medical procedures may all affect a child's coping with a procedure. Thus, future efforts to help children cope with aversive medical procedures may need to consider matching psychological interventions to a particular child's coping style, and also may need specifically to involve parents.

REFERENCES

Blount, R. L., Corbin, S. M., Sturges, J. W., Wolfe, V. V., Prater, J. M., & James, L. D. (1989). The relationship between adult's behavior and child coping and distress during BMA/LP procedures: A sequential analysis. *Behavior Therapy, 20*, 585-601.

Blount, R. L., Sturges, J. W., & Powers, S. W. (1990). Analysis of child and adult behavioral variations by phase of medical procedure. *Behavior Therapy, 21*, 33-48.

Bowers, K. S. (1968). Pain, anxiety, and perceived control. *Journal of Consulting and Clinical Psychology, 32*, 596-602.

Bush, J. P., & Cockrell, C. S. (1987). Maternal factors predicting parenting behaviors in the pediatric clinic. *Journal of Pediatric Psychology, 12*, 505-518.

Bush, J. P., Melamed, B. G., Sheras, P. L., & Greenbaum, P. E. (1986).

Mother-child patterns of coping with anticipatory medical stress. *Health Psychology, 5,* 137-157.

Caire, J. B., & Erickson, S. (1986). Reducing distress in pediatric patients undergoing cardiac catheterization. *Children's Health Care, 14,* 146-152.

Cox, C., Dahlquist, L. M., & Fernbach, D. (1987, March). *Parenting and children's distress during invasive medical procedures.* Paper presented at the annual meeting of the Society of Behavioral Medicine, Washington, D.C.

Dahlquist, L. M. (1989). Cognitive-behavioral treatment of pediatric cancer patients' distress during painful and aversive medical procedures. In M. C. Roberts & C. E. Walker (Eds.), *Casebook in child and pediatric psychology* (pp. 360-379). New York: Guilford.

Dahlquist, L. M., & Czyzewski, D. (1989). Pediatric behavioral medicine. In M. Hersen (Ed.), *Innovations in child behavior therapy* (pp. 156-190). New York: Springer.

Dahlquist, L. M., Gil, K. M., Armstrong, F. D., DeLawyer, D., Greene, P., & Wuori, D. (1986). Preparing children for medical examinations: The importance of previous medical experience. *Health Psychology, 5,* 249-259.

Dahlquist, L. M., Gil, K. M., Armstrong, F. D., Ginsberg, A., & Jones, B. (1985). Behavioral management of children's distress during chemotherapy. *Journal of Behavior Therapy and Experimental Psychiatry, 16,* 325-329.

Dahlquist, L. M., Gil, K. M., Kalfus, G. R., Blount, R. L., & Boyd, M. S. (1984). Enhancing an autistic girl's compliance with gynecological examinations. *Clinical Pediatrics, 23,* 203.

Dolgin, M. J., & Katz, E. R. (1988). Conditioned aversions in pediatric cancer patients receiving chemotherapy. *Journal of Developmental and Behavioral Pediatrics, 9,* 82-85.

Dolgin, M. J., Katz, E. R., McGinty, K., & Siegel, S. E. (1985). Anticipatory nausea and vomiting in pediatric cancer patients. *Pediatrics, 75,* 547-552.

Elkins, P. D., & Roberts, M. C. (1983). Psychological preparation for pediatric hospitalization. *Clinical Psychology Review, 3,* 275-295.

Elliott, C. H., Jay, S. M., & Woody, P. (1987). An observation scale for measuring children's distress during medical procedures. *Journal of Pediatric Psychology, 12,* 543-551.

Elliott, C. H., & Olson, R. A. (1983). The management of children's distress in response to painful medical treatment for burn injuries. *Behaviour Research and Therapy, 21,* 675-683.

Faust, J., & Melamed, B. G. (1984). Influence of arousal, previous experience, and age on surgery preparation of same day of surgery and in hospital pediatric patients. *Journal of Consulting and Clinical Psychology, 52,* 359-365.

Fowler-Kerry, S., & Lander, J. R. (1987). Management of injection pain in children. *Pain, 30,* 169-175.

Glass, D. C., Singer, J. E., & Friedman, L. N. (1969). Psychic cost of adaptation to an environmental stressor. *Journal of Personality and Social Psychology, 12,* 200–210.

Gonzalez, J. C., Routh, D. K., Saab, P. G., Armstrong, F. D., Shifman, L., Guerra, E., & Fawcett, N. (1989). Effects of parent presence on children's reactions to injections: Behavioral, physiological, and subjective aspects. *Journal of Pediatric Psychology, 14,* 449–462.

Gross, A. M., Stern, R. M., Levin, R. B., Dale, J., & Wojnilower, D. A. (1983). The effect of mother–child separation on the behavior of children experiencing a diagnostic medical procedure. *Journal of Consulting and Clinical Psychology, 51,* 783–785.

Ingersoll, B. D. (1982). *Behavioral aspects in dentistry.* New York: Appleton-Century-Crofts.

Jay, S. M., & Elliott, C. H. (1990). A stress inoculation program for parents whose children are undergoing painful medical procedures. *Journal of Consulting and Clinical Psychology, 58,* 799–804.

Jay, S. M., Elliott, C. H., Katz, E., & Siegel, S. (1987). Cognitive–behavioral and pharmacologic interventions for children's distress during painful medical procedures. *Journal of Consulting and Clinical Psychology, 55,* 860–865.

Jay, S. M., Elliott, C. H., Ozolins, M., Olson, R. A., & Pruitt, S. D. (1985). Behaviourial management of children's distress during painful medical procedures. *Behaviour Research and Therapy, 23,* 513–520.

Jay, S. M., Ozolins, M., Elliott, C. H., & Caldwell, S. (1983). Assessment of children's distress during painful medical procedures. *Health Psychology, 2,* 133–147.

Johnson, J. E., Kirchoff, K. T., & Endress, M. P. (1975). Altering children's distress behavior during orthopedic cast removal. *Nursing Research, 24,* 404–410.

Johnson, J. E., & Rice, V. H. (1974). Sensory and distress components of pain: Implications for the study of clinical pain. *Nursing Research, 23,* 203–209.

Kelley, M. L., Jarvie, G. J., Middlebrook, J. L., McNeer, M. F., & Drabman, R. (1984). Decreasing burned children's pain behavior: Impacting the trauma of hydrotherapy. *Journal of Applied Behavior Analysis, 17,* 147–158.

Klingman, A., Melamed, B. G., Cuthbert, M., & Hermecz, D. A. (1984). Effect of participant modeling on information acquisition and skill utilization. *Journal of Consulting and Clinical Psychology, 52,* 414–422.

Klorman, R., Hilpert, P. L., Michael, R., LaGana, C., & Sveen, O. B. (1980). Effects of coping and mastery modeling on experienced and inexperienced pedodontic patients' disruptiveness. *Behavior Therapy, 11,* 156–168.

Kolko, D. J., & Rickard-Figueroa, J. L. (1985). Effects of video games on the adverse corollaries of chemotherapy in pediatric oncology patients: A single-case analysis. *Journal of Consulting and Clinical Psychology, 53,* 223–228.

Manne, S. L., Redd, W. H., Jacobsen, P. B., Gorfinkle, K., Schorr, O., & Rapkin, B. (1990). Behavioral intervention to reduce child and parent distress during venipunctures. *Journal of Consulting and Clinical Psychology, 58*, 565–572.

Meichenbaum, D. (1975). Self-instructional methods. In F. H. Kanfer & A. P. Goldstein (Eds.), *Helping people change* (pp. 357–392). Elmsford, NY: Pergamon Press.

Melamed, B. G. (1977). Psychological preparation for hospitalization. In S. Rachman (Ed.), *Contributions to medical psychology* (Vol. 1, pp. 43–74) Oxford: Pergamon Press.

Melamed, B. G., Dearborn, M., & Hermecz, D. A. (1983). Necessary considerations for surgery preparation: Age and previous experience. *Psychosomatic Medicine, 45*, 517–525.

Melamed, B. G., & Siegel, L. (1975). Reduction of anxiety in children facing hospitalization and surgery by use of filmed modeling. *Journal of Consulting and Clinical Psychology, 43*, 511–521.

Melzack, R. (1973). *The puzzle of pain.* New York: Basic Books.

Nocella, J., & Kaplan, R. M. (1982). Training children to cope with dental treatment. *Journal of Pediatric Psychology, 7*, 175–178.

Peterson, L. (1989). Coping by children undergoing stressful medical procedures: Some conceptual, methodological, and therapeutic issues. *Journal of Consulting and Clinical Psychology, 57*, 380–387.

Peterson, L., & Shigetomi, C. (1981). The use of coping techniques to minimize anxiety in hospitalized children. *Behavior Therapy, 12*, 1–14.

Redd, W. H., Jacobsen, P. B., Die-Trill, M., Dermatis, H., McEvoy, M., & Holland, J. (1987). Cognitive/attentional distraction in the control of conditioned nausea in pediatric cancer patients receiving chemotherapy. *Journal of Consulting and Clinical Psychology, 55*, 391–395.

Shaw, E. G., & Routh, D. K. (1982). Effect of mother presence on children's reaction to aversive procedures. *Journal of Pediatric Psychology, 7*, 33–42.

Siaw, S. N., Stephens, L. R., & Holmes, S. S. (1986). Knowledge about medical instruments and reported anxiety in pediatric surgery patients. *Children's Health Care, 14*, 134–141.

Siegel, L. J., & Peterson, L. (1981). Maintenance effects of coping skills and sensory information on young children's response to repeated dental procedures. *Behavior Therapy, 12*, 530–535.

Siegel, L. J., & Peterson, L. (1980). Stress reduction in young dental patients through coping skills and sensory information. *Journal of Consulting and Clinical Psychology, 48*, 785–787.

Slater, M. A., & Power, T. G. (1987). Multidimensional assessment of parenting in single-parent families. In J. P. Vincent (Ed.), *Advances in family intervention, assessment, and theory* (Vol. 4, pp. 197–228). Greenwich, CT: JAI Press.

Stark, L. J., Allen, K. D., Hurst, M., Nash, D. A., Rigney, B., & Stokes, T. F. (1989). Distraction: Its utilization and efficacy with children undergoing dental treatment. *Journal of Applied Behavior Analysis, 22*, 297–307.

Staub, E., Tursky, B., & Schwartz, G. E. (1971). Self-control and predictability: Their effects on reactions to aversive stimulation. *Journal of Personality and Social Psychology, 18,* 157–162.

Tarnowski, K. J., McGrath, M. L., Calhoun, M. B., & Drabman, R. S. (1987). Pediatric burn injury: Self- versus therapist-mediated debridement. *Journal of Pediatric Psychology, 12,* 567–579.

Twardosz, S., Weddle, K., Borden, K., & Stevens, E. (1986). A comparison of three methods of preparing children for surgery. *Behavior Therapy, 17,* 14–25.

Vernon, D. T. A., Foley, J. M., Sipowicz, R. S., & Schulman, J. L. (1965). *The psychological responses of children to hospitalization and illness: A review of the literature.* Springfield, IL: Charles C Thomas.

Zabin, M., & Melamed, B. G. (1980). The relationship between parental discipline and children's ability to cope with stress. *Journal of Behavioral Assessment, 2,* 17–38.

Zastowny, T. R., Kirschenbaum, D. S., & Meng, A. L. (1986). Coping skills training for children: Effects on distress before, during and after hospitalization for surgery. *Health Psychology, 5,* 231–247.

CHAPTER 17

Multiple-Level Interventions in Pediatric Psychology Settings: A Behavioral–Systems Perspective

LARRY L. MULLINS
University of Oklahoma Health Sciences Center
JEFFREY GILLMAN and CYNTHIA HARBECK
Ohio State University
Children's Hospital, Columbus, Ohio

By its very nature, the clinical practice of pediatric psychology involves the consideration of multiple interrelated causal factors and influences. The process of coping with stressful chronic conditions is a multifaceted and complex task for both child and family. Whether the presenting individual is a mentally retarded encopretic child in the clinic or a severely burned adolescent in the hospital, evaluation and treatment will take place in a complex system and can involve numerous change agents and change strategies. The social, cultural, medical, family, and ethical milieu will certainly shape the manner in which such a child's stressful problems are addressed. And, at some point in time, the pediatric psychologist will become a part of that system. He or she may be shaped as much by that system as he or she shapes it in an attempt to reconcile the presenting problem. The purpose of the current chapter is to review an emerging behavioral–systems perspective in pediatric psychology—one that views stress and coping as a complex, interactional process.

Consider the following example. A 13-year-old Native American was admitted to a burn unit with second- and third-degree burns over 40% of his total body surface area. Apparently he had been spending the night in an abandoned house with friends when a kerosene lantern was knocked over. Allegations were made that drug use was involved in this incident. In addition, child welfare workers indicated that this adolescent had been previously placed in a group home after abuse charges had been filed against the parents. The attending physician requested pediatric psychology services for "pain management."

Would pain management be the only service provided for this identified patient? Most likely not. Indeed, the brief scenario depicted above would provide a vast array of assessment and intervention opportunities. Treatment of this patient would warrant a careful and thorough assessment of multiple cultural, social, institutional, familial, and intrapersonal factors before pain management could be addressed. Many different individuals might play a role in the disposition of this case, including physicians, nurses, social workers, psychologists, physical and occupational therapists, parents, siblings, grandparents, drug counselors, and tribal elders. And each of these individuals and the systems they represent would have the potential to influence one another and thus the care of the identified patient.

The traditional leaning of many pediatric psychologists has been toward behavioral and cognitive–behavioral models, which tend to focus largely on individual behavior and intrapersonal functioning (e.g. Kaufman, Holden, & Walker, 1989; O'Leary, 1984). Such models have been employed successfully for many types of child behavior problems. At the same time, shortcomings in both our conceptual models and our treatment interventions have been acknowledged. The new conceptual *Zeitgeist* for pediatric psychology in the 1990s would appear to be systems theory and an ecological–systems perspective on child and family functioning (e.g., Bronfenbrenner, 1986; Kanfer & Schefft, 1988). In particular, child health psychology has witnessed an expansion of a systems perspective (Dolgin & Jay, 1989; Mash, 1989).

Evidence for this conceptual shift is also apparent in the writings of a number of prominent pediatric and child psychologists. Peterson and Harbeck (1988) include a section on systems aspects of pediatric psychology practice in their recent book, whereas Henggeler and Borduin (1990) premise their entire book on complex systems formulations as applied to therapeutic change in children and adolescents. Roberts and Magrab (1991) have presented in the *American Psychologist* a family-centered, community-based model of care for children with special needs. Their model is predicated on systems tenets, with an emphasis on interdisciplinary care, ecological framework, community resources, and preservation of family culture.

What factors account for this growing trend toward utilization of systems models? Increasingly, both normal development and responses to health-related problems are seen as processes of stress, coping, and adaptation. Such models are typically multivariate or multifactorial in nature (e.g., Folkman & Lazarus, 1985; Hanson, Henggeler, & Burghen, 1987; LaGreca, 1987; Wallander et al., 1989). These models typically involve multiple levels of influences, including disease and illness parameters, socioeconomic/utilitarian resources, family variables such as cohesion and adaptation, intrapersonal coping resources, cognitive appraisal mechanisms, and external life stressors. Such models thus include variables from different domains and contextual realms, each of which influences and is influenced by the others. Concomitantly, research tools that allow for assessment of strength and directionality of such multiple influences have been developed and utilized, such as path analyses and structural equation modeling.

Systems approaches to behavior change are certainly not new, and have guided the work of family therapists for two to three decades. It is probably safe to say, however, that the theory and practice that have been parts of that movement have rarely been data-driven. Systems theorists have often used nonscientific language, and many of their concepts can not be operationalized. Use of parables, metaphors, and talk of "magic" has often obscured proposed conceptual models and interventions. Case study formats have typically been utilized in lieu of rigorous research design, with rare exceptions. In fact, an empirical approach to family therapy and systems theory has often been met with derision from and rejection by adherents of these approaches (e.g., Colapinto, 1979).

More recent systems formulations, however, have been characterized by the inclusion of an empirical approach to pediatric psychology problems, with an integration of existing data and previously supported behavior change strategies (e.g., Brunk, Henggeler, & Whelan, 1987). Mash (1989) refers to this approach as the "behavioral–systems perspective," a term that perhaps comes closest to capturing the essence of pediatric psychology's scientific approach to the study of human behavior, coupled with the more contemporary heuristic of systems theory. Mash (1989) proposes an amalgamation of systems or ecological frameworks that view child disorders as a constellation of interrelated response systems. He further proposes the view that the same behaviors may have different sets of initiating circumstances, and that intervention may have multiple influences on the entire set of relationships within the family system.

Initial reports would suggest that systems approaches can lend themselves to empirical scrutiny and are clinically potent. For example, in a meta-analysis of 20 studies comparing family therapy to no-treatment groups or alternative therapy, measures of family interaction or behavior of the identified patient indicated that family therapy was relatively more effective than no treatment or alternative treatments (Hazelrigg, Cooper, & Borduin, 1987). Increasingly, empirical studies report that family systems interventions are more effective than individual-oriented treatment for particular problems (e.g., Dadds, Schwartz, & Sanders, 1987).

The broad goal of this chapter is to present an emerging model of pediatric psychology practice that is particularly relevant to stress and coping with chronic conditions. Such an approach incorporates contemporary systems theory, empirically proven behavior change strategies, multiple-level interventions, and interdisciplinary and transdisciplinary efforts. Given the recency of such approaches, theory, research, and practice have not yet been fully assimiliated (Mash, 1989). Thus, the caveat is offered that much of what follows is heuristic in nature. In the remainder of this chapter, we first focus briefly on the nature of systems and multiple-level approaches, followed by an overview of proposed consultation and intervention models. Next, a pragmatic clinical perspective is offered, reviewing issues related to the process of interdisciplinary approaches in the pediatric context. Finally, future directions for multiple-level interventions from a behavioral–systems perspective are set forth.

SYSTEMS THEORY AND SYSTEMS REFORMULATIONS

A complete overview of contemporary systems models is certainly beyond the scope of this chapter. However, certain key elements should be reviewed that will allow for a basic understanding of systems tenets, as well as the ways in which a systems perspective differs from other models of thought.

Systems approaches have existed for many years and have been applied to various disciplines (e.g., von Bertalanffy, 1968). In the past 20 years, numerous therapists have debated the applications of systems theory to mental health problems. Such debate has often been controversial, even within the subdiscipline of family therapy. Although many formulations of systems theory have been proposed, a number of central tenets have been summarized (Henggeler & Borduin, 1990; Minuchin, 1985). These principles include the following:

1. Systems exist as organizing structures at different levels of human interaction and human context, including families as well as institutions.
2. Each system has multiple interrelated parts, with a history of interaction and expectation of future interaction.
3. Systems tend toward a homeostatic balance; changes in one part of the system inevitably result in changes in other parts of the system.
4. Rules, both implicit and explicit, govern a system; some rules allow for change, and other rules serve to maintain order.

5. Patterns of interaction within the system are not linear, but circular.

Thus, the systems approach emphasizes multiple causes for given behaviors, reciprocal influences, and interaction within the ecological context. Such an approach reflects a major paradigmatic shift away from the linear, reductionistic approach that has typified efforts to understand the nature and causes of human behavior.

Although the systems approach may appear to be a dramatic departure from more traditional perspectives, Mash (1989) points out that certain elements of systems theory are inherent in behavioral approaches. Skinner (1948) wrote of the importance of families and communities in terms of behavioral theory. Social learning approaches have long emphasized reciprocal determinism and person–environment influences (e.g., Bandura, 1969). Many of the parent training programs that rely heavily on behavioral principles also include other contextual variables, such as the quality of the parent–child relationship (e.g., Eyberg & Robinson, 1982). In contrast to a focus on the parent–child dyad, couples therapy focuses on the spouse dyad and frequently combines behavioral techniques such as reinforcements with systems concepts such as communication issues. Therefore, the current focus on systems perspectives by pediatric psychologists can be conceptualized in many regards as a logical extension of previous models to a more explicit, empirically driven systems orientation and approach to understanding human behavior.

Although the expansion of systems concepts appears to be increasingly recognized, there are a few additional works that have particular relevance to the practice of pediatric psychology. Of particular relevance is the previously mentioned work of Henggeler and Borduin (1990). In what may be considered a rapprochement of traditional family therapy and contemporary cognitive–behavioral and developmentally based perspectives, Henggeler and Borduin offer what they refer to as the "multisystemic model." The multisystemic model is distinguished by its focus upon the following:

1. Multiple interrelated systems, including peers, school, social support, and genetically based individual differences.
2. Consideration of developmental variables, including cognitive abilities, developmental stage of the family, and language development.
3. Inclusion and integration of "nonsystemic" therapeutic interventions, including cognitive–behavioral strategies and behavior management techniques.

The multisystemic model provides a synthesis of theoretical perspectives—one that may be quite effective in dealing with the problems encountered in the pediatric context. Henggeler, Borduin, and colleagues provide considerable evidence that the multisystemic treatment model is a potent intervention for individuals and families with quite serious psychological difficulties, including inner-city delinquents (Borduin et al., 1990; Henggeler et al., 1986) and families of abused and neglected children (Brunk et al., 1987). Empirical evidence for a multisystemic model of insulin-dependent diabetes mellitus has also been gathered (e.g., Hanson & Henggeler, 1984, Hanson, Henggeler, & Burghen, 1987; see also Hanson, Chapter 10, this volume).

Wynne, McDaniel, and Weber (1986) provide another perspective relevant to pediatric psychology practice. They offer extensive recommendations on the application of systems theory to various contexts, including the mental health system, medical context, community systems, and military and business systems. Wynne et al. propose a move away from the therapist as a provider simply of family therapy services, and toward a perspective of "systems consultation." As a systems consultant, the therapist is able to take what is referred to as a "meta-" position, from which he or she can selectively evaluate the multiple subsystems related to a given problem, can shift professional roles between and among such subsystems, and can establish multiple-level treatment interventions. Such a perspective is certainly in keeping with our perception of the role of the pediatric psychologists—that is, as a multiple-systems consultant intervening at select levels of the system.

In summary, systems approaches offer an emerging framework for intervention in the context of pediatric psychology. Few would argue that the complexity of the pediatric environment offers considerable challenge, and that consultation and intervention efforts will call for careful evaluation of the contexts of which the problem is a part. In the next section, we present an overview of specific consultation and intervention models, particularly as they relate to the systems perspective and multiple-level interventions.

PEDIATRIC PSYCHOLOGY CONSULTATION AND INTERVENTION MODELS

To date, relatively little has been written about consultation models that incorporate a behavioral–systems approach. The traditional types of consultation models employed by pediatric psychologists in their work have been described elsewhere (Drotar, 1978; Roberts, 1986; Stabler, 1988). These models vary from two or more professionals working separately with the same patient, to close collaboration (with face-to-face contact) among the patient, family, physician, psychologist, and other professionals (Stabler, 1988). Such models vary considerably in the extent to which they address systems issues and multiple-level interventions.

One of the most frequently utilized consultation models in the medical setting is the "independent-functions model" described by Roberts (1986), which has also been called the "noncollaborative approach" (Drotar, 1978) and the "coordination of multiservices" (Stabler, 1979). In this model, the psychologist assesses or treats the patient and has little interaction with other professionals. For example, the psychologist may be asked to assess the level of anxiety and depression in a patient experiencing recurrent abdominal pain. The psychologist may do a thorough assessment and communicate the results to the patient and referral agent, while the physician completes the medical assessment. The referral agent and psychologist may have no communication other than a brief phone call, progress notes in the medical chart, and a final report. Although this model may be less time-consuming, by definition it involves very limited coordination and integration among care providers.

In the "indirect-psychological-consultation model" (Roberts, 1986), the psychologist indirectly provides services to a patient and family. The physician retains primary responsibility for the patient and communicates information about the patient to the psychologist, who then offers recommendations. Also included under this model are the seminars, conferences, and in-service training that a psychologist may provide to educate and train medical personnel in understanding psychological issues. This model has also been referred to as "process-educative" (Stabler, 1979). Such a model is also limited in the extent to which multiple systems affecting the patient are addressed.

A third commonly utilized model is the "collaborative-team model" (Roberts, 1986), which is similar to the "process consultation model" described by Stabler (1979). In this model, the physician and psychologist function as equals, each contributing his or her unique perspective and sharing jointly in decision making. This type of relationship frequently occurs when the psychologist becomes part of a "team" of professionals working on a particular service (e.g., oncology, pulmonary). For example, a physician may manage the medical treatment for an oncology patient; the social worker may help the family find needed resources, such as housing near the hospital; and the psychologist may work with the patient and family to improve pain management, decrease anxiety, and increase communication in the family. This situation differs from that described in the independent-functions model, in that the team members frequently communicate with one another and have face-to-face meetings to discuss the family's situation and treatment plan.

In this model, the patient and family members may also be viewed as part of the team and share in decision making. Although a disadvantage of this model is the apparent cost involved in professional time for team meetings and care conferences, the benefits of an integrated plan, increased communication, and increased team cohesion make the use of this model very important in complicated cases. The collaborative-team model is perhaps the most systems-oriented model thus elucidated. Most descriptions of this model, however, do not detail the interrelationships between and among team members and the larger systems of which patient, family, and caregivers are a part, or the types of conflicts and problems that arise in attempts to orchestrate treatment efforts.

Although much less frequently noted in the pediatric psychology literature, Wynne et al.'s (1986) "metasystem consultation model" bears further mention. In this model, the psychologist may view the entire system of patient, family, and staff from a "meta-" position and decide which levels need intervention. For example, a psychologist may notice that a previously well-integrated and effective team (e.g., the cystic fibrosis team) has gradually become less efficient in the delivery of care. The psychologist may further notice that the staff has experienced many patient deaths in recent months. He or she thus recommends that the staff members meet with a psychologist or consultant to discuss their reactions to this experience, as a way of coping with professional stress and reducing staff burnout. As in the indirect-consultation model, the psychologist may not intervene with a particular patient. Yet in addition to providing education, the psychologist utilizing a metasystems orientation may focus an intervention on increasing the staff's general effectiveness and ability to act as an integrated team. Perhaps the most important difference between this model and those previously mentioned is the emphasis upon interventions targeting systems of individuals at different levels (e.g., the interdisciplinary team), and not just the individual and the family unit.

An alternative model for consultation in hospital settings has been proposed by Kolb, Rubin, and McIntyre (1979). They organize their approach by first analyzing the various subsystems of the larger hospital system, including (1) people, (2) authority, (3) information, (4) task, (5) policy/culture, and (6) environment. For each of these subsystems, the consultant must elucidate (1) the problem definition, (2) the proposed solution, and, perhaps most importantly, (3) the effects on other subsystems. Such organization allows for individual assessment of the various hospital subsystems, and also for the impact that change in one system will have upon others as intervention proceeds. Such a model is furthermore distinguished by its specification of administrative policy issues, lines of authority and power, and institutional policy. Although the pediatric psychologist may not be targeting this aspect of the system for intervention, failure to take such issues into consideration may attenuate the potency of attempted interventions. An example of this would be the case of a physician and a physical therapist devising a rehabilitation program for a pediatric burn patient without taking into account the parent's and child's willingness to follow such a program, or the need for coordination with other staffs, (e.g., nursing). Lack of communication among subsystems may then compromise patient goals. Mullins (1989) has further detailed how administrative policy, institutional culture, and subsystem conflict can readily compromise the interdisciplinary team's efforts.

UTILIZING CONSULTATION
AND INTERVENTION MODELS

Although no single model is most effective or appropriate in all settings (Roberts, 1986: Roberts & Wright, 1982), it would appear that in situations where it can be implemented, the collaborative-team model may result in the most highly coordinated care for the patient. Indeed, none of these models has been tested empirically. Yet it seems logical to suggest that models of consultation that incorporate broad systems perspectives are most likely to result in comprehensive assessment and understanding of the many factors that play a role in most pediatric problems. In other words, the behavioral–systems perspective advocates the simultaneous consideration and integration of multiple care providers at multiple levels of involvement across time and settings.

It is also reasonable to assume that the consultation model may change over time. The collaborative-team model may work best when a patient is on a hospital unit, whereas after the patient is discharged an independent-functions model may be most pragmatic. An initial focus may be upon educating staff members about multiple levels of influence and intervention in the pediatric setting. As efforts among caregivers become better coordinated and integrated, there may follow a shift to a team that shares values (i.e., interdisciplinary), and eventually to a team that transcends traditional role boundaries.

Other factors must be considered in the selection of a clinical consultation and intervention model. It is important to point out that collaboration may not always be requested or valued by the referral agent, who may only desire limited contact from the psychologist and limited treatment efforts. When the issue of seeking consultation from other professionals arises, the physician seeking such consultation has traditionally viewed the consultee as a resource who provides expert advice but rarely interacts with the other health-care professionals on the caregiving team (Stabler, 1988). Such a lack of interaction and communication may lead to a less than desirable outcome—that is, a diminished likelihood of comprehensive care and multiple-level interventions.

Previous research has found that physicians' satisfaction with consultation services is correlated with the agreement between the referral agents' perceptions of patients' psychological problems and the consultants' feedback (Olson et al., 1988). It is expected that congruence between the consultation model a physician expects and the consultation model a psychologist utilizes will also have a large impact on the physician's satisfaction with consultation/liaison services. Therefore, the systems-oriented psychologist may need to obtain a balance between meeting the referral agent's expectations, and educating him or her about other roles a psychologist can effectively play.

It is equally important for systems-oriented psychologists to be aware of limits of involvement. The above-described consultation models include the levels of the patient, the family, the extended family, the hospital staff, community resources, and even national policies and resources. It is important to consider each of these levels when assessing and intervening with a particular patient. However, it is also clear that psychologists need not and often cannot intervene at each of these levels with each patient. Time constraints, limited resources, training, and interest frequently dictate that a pediatric psychologist intervene with the patient, family, and hospital staff, rather than with entire communities or cultures. For example, in the case example given at the beginning of the chapter, the psychologist would have to appreciate the culture of the Native American family and the limited resources of the child welfare system, but the psychologist would probably decide to intervene at the interpersonal and familial level, rather than to treat entire cultures or state systems. In the section to follow, practical considerations in implementing a multiple-level systems approach are discussed.

THE PRAGMATIC ASPECTS OF MULTIPLE-LEVEL INTERVENTIONS

Although the various models of consultation provide a working structure for the psychologist, the actual process of conducting clinical work follows a more dynamic course. This is particularly true with regard to the introduction and implementation of a multiple-level format for patient care. Although we cannot begin to address the huge range of assessment and intervention possibilities across contexts and with different clinical problems, practicing pediatric psychologists must face a number of common issues.

Pediatric psychology often differs from other subdisciplines of clinical psychology in the extent to which physicians' referral and control over patient care guides the course of treatment, particularly in inpatient settings. At the outset, it is important to understand that the setting in which this is typically initiated, the pediatric medical center, functions within the context of a power hierarchy. At the top of this hierarchy are specialty physicians, with nonspecialty physicians and nonphysicians occupying lower rungs on this ladder, and therefore lower levels of both responsibility for and control over patient care.

This tradition of medical hierarchies, and medicine's historical method of conducting consultation services, are what provide the pediatric psychologist with his or her initial challenge in the development of multiple-level interventions. It is also our contention that the pediatric psychologist is in a unique position, by virtue of his or her broad-based training in both individual and systemic functioning, to alter and reshape this tradition of medical colleagues. The ensuing discussion focuses on the practical issues involved in the development of multiple-level interventions.

The development of a multiple-level intervention may be clinically conceptualized as the examination and integration of a series of concentric circles. At the center of these circles is the pediatric patient, who is surrounded by a succession of caregiving levels. At the next level is the nuclear family circle, which is closely followed by the extended family circle. The next circle is occupied by the first of many professional caretakers—namely, the physician. This is followed by a series of additional caretakers which may include other health professionals, teachers, members of the clergy, and so on. Beyond these levels exist additional levels of systems, including institutional systems (e.g., hospital, group home), societal systems, and cultural systems.

For the pediatric psychologist, the entrance to this system is often provided by the physician who is managing the health care of the child, who is at the center of the system. This introduction can occur when the physician seeks the consultation of the psychologist for a host of issues relative to adjustment and coping, including acceptance of a new diagnosis, problems with adherence to medical regimens, pain assessment and management, or communication problems between the professional staff and the child and/or parents.

Tasks of the Pediatric Psychologist

In response to the request for consultation, the psychologist is faced with a series of five preparatory tasks, each of which serves as a means of understanding the successive levels of the system outlined above. By successfully addressing each of these tasks, the consulting psychologist is afforded the opportunity to integrate this understanding by means of a final task, that being the shared development and implementation of a comprehensive treatment plan. Through this final task, the psychologist is able to help educate and integrate a variety of independently functioning caregivers into a collaborative treatment team.

The first of these tasks involves an assessment of the stated reasons—and, perhaps just as important, the unstated reasons—for initiation of the referral. The process of this assessment is, in and of itself, a collaborative effort between the referring physician and the consulting psychologist. Such assessment also serves as an important modeling tool by which to educate the physician about this process of interdisciplinary care. This process begins with the consultant's and physician's discussing in some detail the specific questions being asked and services being requested (for a detailed review of this process, see Gillman & Mullins, in press). A primary goal at this stage is the development of a common conceptual model for understanding the identified problem(s). To address this first step, the consultant and physician may jointly consider the following basic questions:

1. What is the nature of the child's problem? In what specific ways is this manifested (e.g., behaviorally, affectively, cognitively, and/or physiologically)? Has an underlying physiological/medical etiology been identified? What has the family been told? What does the child seem to understand about the problems?

2. When did the problem begin? How has it changed over time?

3. For whom is it a problem? Is the child or family distressed, or is the staff distressed by the child?

4. Who is currently involved in the care of the child (e.g., staff, family, teachers, etc.), and what steps have they taken to address the problem?

5. What would the referral source like to see accomplished? What level of responsibility is the psychologist being asked to assume?

6. Has the possibility of a pediatric psychology consult been discussed with the parents? Have the parents and child offered consent?

Apart from its obvious clinical importance, developing a common conceptual framework has several other significant implications. First, many ethical issues are involved in accepting certain types of referrals, and these must be clarified for each professional. Second, an accurate and shared conceptualization of the referral question has a direct bearing on the relationship between the referring physician and the psychologist. This is a crucial point; as we have noted earlier, recent research in pediatric settings indicates that referral source satisfaction is often a function of the congruence between the pediatrician's perception of the problem and feedback from the psychologist about the nature and treatment of the problem (Olson et al., 1988). In turn, this will logically play an important role in the pediatrician's willingness to accept and implement the findings and recommendations offered by the psychology consultant.

The second task is akin to more traditional assessment. This task consists of assessing the parents and developing a trusting, supportive relationship with them. We recommend beginning with the parents rather than the child, since successful intervention almost invariably relies on the implicit and explicit support, understanding, and active involvement of the parents (Gillman & Mullins, in press). Furthermore, Munson (1986) notes that it is crucial to assess and closely monitor the dynamics of the child's family, since these patterns of interaction often play a very salient role in the development and maintenance of illness, and may also play a similar role in the facilitation of "wellness."

Since the parents are the ones who play the most critical role in communicating to the child various expectations and beliefs about (as well as the willingness to participate in) intervention strategies, it is mandatory that a strong alliance be developed with the parents. It is the responsibility of the psychologist to initiate a dialogue with the parents that contains strong elements of collaboration, education, and hopefulness. This is no small task, since the perception of many family members is that they are passive recipients of care. A major goal of the psychologist is to teach them methods of becoming "active partners" in the process of helping their child. For example, this may include teaching parents assertion skills with medical staff, or training them to coach their child's use of coping strategies.

The third task consists of assessing the child and developing a therapeutic relationship with him or her. Just as parents often respond to medical interventions with a passive stance, so too does the child. Moreover, just as the parents are often bewildered, angered, or distressed by the psychologist's involvement, the child is likely to share such feelings. In order to elicit the child's cooperation and active participation in this process, the psychologist must convey warmth and support; a willingness to listen; and a respect for the child's levels of developmental functioning, coping resources, and conceptions about what is happening to him or her. Furthermore, the psychologist must engage the child in a process of interacting with caregivers at all levels, with the goal of teaching proactive rather than reactive functioning to the medical context.

The fourth preparatory task involves the assessment of the larger or more distant levels of caregivers and systems, in terms of their potential attributes and liabilities in ultimately contributing to the intervention program. These caregivers may include nurses, medical students and residents, occupational and physical therapists, child life specialists, nutritionists, members of the clergy, and teachers. Each of these professionals possesses a set of specific skills that can be utilized in the development of a comprehensive, integrated intervention program. As part of this portion of the assessment process, the psychologist will certainly need to examine the relationships between and among these various subsystems of care, paying particular attention to their overlap of roles, ability to function in a collaborative manner, and the quality and effectiveness of communications among them. To the extent that these team members disagree in terms of role function, goals, and perception of the problem, the likelihood of success is diminished.

The fifth major task is that of educating the referral source about specific, practical, empirically sound intervention strategies (Stabler, 1988). The specifics of these recommendations will obviously depend upon the assessment of the child, parents, and other subsystems. However, a word of caution is warranted. As stated earlier, a critical element in determining physician satisfaction is the "degree of fit" between the referring agent's conceptual framework and the feedback that is presented in the form of recommendations. Stabler (1988) cogently points out that this can best be accomplished by educating the referring physician regarding the rationale for utilizing a comprehensive, multisystemic intervention and a scientific, data-oriented approach. Our experience has generally been that when the physician has been appropriately educated by the psychologist regarding the orchestration of multiple systems into an integrated model of intervention, he or she is very frequently willing to be an active collaborator in this process.

Care Conferences

It has previously been suggested that one of the most significant factors in the development of an effective, well-integrated treatment plan is that of shared consent among care providers (Gillman & Mullins, in press). In other words, it is critical that all participants be in full agreement with the program, and that they understand its direction, its specific parameters, and the process by which it will be conducted, and their specific roles. In order to maximize the opportunity for the development of shared consent, we suggest that the input of all participants be used in developing the plan. This is often best accomplished through team meetings or a care conference that includes all participants. It is frequently helpful to meet with the treatment team alone for the first half of the conference for planning purposes, and then to meet with the parents and child.

During such a conference, the psychologist's role may include the following: (1) helping the staff to share in a productive manner their perceptions of the problem; (2) educating the team regarding psychosocial factors and their effect on both the child's and family's functioning; (3) clarifying for others the child's and family's perceptions of the current situation; and (4) helping the care providers to communicate with the family, as well as with one another, in a smooth, reciprocal manner. In addition, the psychologist may take the lead in developing an effective, empirically based treatment plan. This plan may include behavioral management contingencies, suggested psychotherapy for the patient and family, involvement with social services, pain management, and so forth. Sometimes developing a contract among the patient, parents, and staff is helpful in clarifying future expectations and consequences. It is always helpful to document the plan in writing, and later to distribute it to all staff members involved. The psychologist may also need to mention the implementation of the treatment plan and to educate staff members who were unable to attend the care conference about the treatment plan.

After the initial care conference, effective communication remains important. The psychologist may wish to arrange a series of brief meetings to assess progress. In this way, coordination of efforts can be maintained and problems resolved in a productive manner.

Such a team of individuals from different disciplines has been described most often as the "interdisciplinary team." Interestingly, this term has given way to the "transdisciplinary team" (Fisher, Burd, & Kerbeshian, 1985). The major task of the transdisciplinary team is to establish a set of goals and working relationships that transcend traditional, discipline-specific goals and strategies. Each discipline may offer unique skills, yet superordinate goals must be defined. By contrast, the interdisciplinary approach encourages cooperation and reinforcement of each discipline's goals, yet roles often remain strictly defined. The transdisciplinary approach encourages "role release"—that is, the letting go of traditional strict role definitions when intervention takes place.

These recommendations can provide a basic framework for a multisystemic or behavioral–systems approach to problems of coping and stress in children. The following case example further explicates this process by detailing the management of multiple interrelated systems.

CASE EXAMPLE

Let us consider the case outlined at the beginning of this chapter in greater detail. As noted earlier, a 13-year-old Native American, John, was admitted to the burn unit of Children's Hospital with second- and third-degree burns covering 40% of his total body surface area. On the seventh day after admission, his attending physician consulted the psychology staff, requesting assistance with pain management during dressing changes and debridement procedures. After receiving the consultation request, the psychologist first contacted the referring physician to clarify the reasons for the request. According to the physician, the nursing staff had initiated the request because John tried to delay dressing changes by whining, manipulating the staff, and not following directions. The physician also mentioned his own concern that John was not talking about the events surrounding the injury, and that he might be feeling guilty about his role in this accident. A review of John's medical chart revealed that John had received no visitors aside from his mother, who had come the first night after he was admitted. At the conclusion of their conversation, it became clear that the physician was quite concerned that John's psychological status and his oppositional behaviors were significantly compromising his recovery. It was the physician's desire for the psychologist to investigate this possibility and to take responsibility for addressing these issues.

Because John's mother was unavailable for a meeting at the hospital, the psychologist contacted her by telephone at home. During this conversation, the psychologist described his role in the treatment process as that of helping children and their families cope with the many stressors involved in the hospitalization process. In addition, he explained to John's mother that an important part of his job was to help facilitate a close working relationship among the child, parents, physicians, and other health care providers. During the conversation, the mother anxiously inquired about her son's progress and stated that she had not been to the hospital after the first evening because she did not have transportation. She stated that she would be available the following day, as a friend had agreed to transport her. The next day John's mother did not arrive for the meeting; she was recontacted and stated that her ride had become unavailable. The psychologist arranged for the social worker to contact John's mother and arrange transportation. The mother did come to the next meeting, appearing uncomfortable in the hospital setting. She reported a great deal of guilt over John's burn injury, stating that she and John had grown more distant since the parents had separated 2 years earlier. She also expressed a great deal of defensiveness about her parenting skills, stating that she had been "doing the best she could."

It appeared during this interview that John's mother possessed very limited information about his injury and progress, and that she was extremely concerned that she would lose custody of him because of his injury. (As noted at the beginning of the chapter, John had been placed in a group home at an earlier time after his parents had been charged with and found guilty of abuse.) The psychologist indicated that he did not know any details about this possibility, but that he would keep her informed of any such information. It was the psychologist's recommendation to John's mother that she could and should be an active participant in his care. Several methods for this were described to her in detail, including maintaining frequent and regular contact either by phone or in person with the medical staff, as well as with John himself. Furthermore, she was informed that any and all of her questions were welcome and would be answered to the best of the staff's ability. In addition, it was suggested that she be a participant in a care conference that would be organized in order to discuss John's progress, current concerns, and future goals.

After the mother had an opportunity to meet with John, the psychologist came to John's room and met with both him and his mother. The mother introduced the psychologist as the individual who would be working with them and assisting with issues of pain management, anxiety, and the general distress of hospitalization. The mother encouraged John to speak openly with the psychologist and explained that she would be respectful of the issues of confidentiality. John was initially responsive and superficially cooperative with the psychologist in responding to questions, but volunteered very little information spontaneously. John reported that the debridement procedure was the most difficult part of the hospitalization, and stated that being immersed in the tank was the most painful part of the debridement process. John appeared to have very minimal understanding of his injury and the recovery process. He expressed a belief that the staff was cruel and angry with him because he cried during painful procedures. He acknowledged that he would very much like to have more control, but did not know how he could do this. The psychologist began by explaining in general terms about pain management, as well as the use of assertive communication with the staff. John was also told that the psychologist would be seeing him on a daily basis in order to provide ongoing support, and that he would be a member of a team of professionals whose goal was to help support John through this recovery process.

The third stage of this intervention involved meeting with the various staff members involved with John's care. They were invited to share their perceptions of John's needs, his strengths and coping skills, and the particular problems they were experiencing with him. Furthermore, information was elicited concerning their positions on John's care schedule and their perceptions about decisions or choices John could make regarding scheduling, therapy procedures, and other areas of control. It was pointed out during these conversations that John was experiencing a profound sense of loss of control, as was his mother. A major focus of these discussions was on helping determine methods by which both the mother and John could be involved with and in control of various aspects of the recovery process. During these discussions, it became clear that John's primary nurse was threatened by the involvement of the psychology staff, and that she was also very angry with John's mother. This nurse expressed her belief that providing unconditional nurturance and responding quickly to each of John's requests would be the most kind and supportive way of assisting John. These beliefs placed this particular nurse in conflict with other staff members, who were supportive of a program that entailed clear limit setting and use of contingent rewards for age-appropriate expression of needs.

The psychologist then requested a brief meeting with the attending physician in order to share these observations about John, his family situation, and various staff subsystems. The psychologist offered a number of general recommendations, with a specific focus on the need for consistent expression of messages to John by all caregivers. It was pointed out that such consistency might be compromised by different levels of understanding on the part of various staff members. It was then suggested that a two-part care conference be held in order for the physician to explain John's immediate and long-term medical needs; for the staff members to share their perceptions of John's current status; for all parties to develop a commonly agreed-upon intervention program; and for the team to involve both John and John's mother in this process. Furthermore, the psychologist explained to the physician recommendations for pain management, including increasing John's pain medication, scheduling and tracking his progress, and including John in the decision-making processes.The physician was also informed that John would receive individual therapy for guilt, depression, and adjustment to disability. The physician agreed to these recommendations, but felt that he himself did not have sufficient time to meet with the staff and with John. He did agree to have the resident physician present for the care conference.

The care conference was scheduled during the first hour of the second shift, in order to enable staff members from each shift to attend. John's primary nurse and new staff members were especially encouraged to attend. The psychologist, resident physician, social worker, physical therapist, nutritionist, and three members of the nursing staff attended the conference. During the first half of the meeting, the staff discussed John's medical progress, goals, current problems, and future plans. Additional concerns were discussed, including John's decreasing weight and his refusal to eat meals unless one of his favorite nurses sat with him. The psychologist offered recommendations for a pain management program, which included progressive muscle relaxation, guided imagery, and the use of increased medication prior to the debridement process. It appeared to the staff members that each of them reacted to John's delaying tactics in very different ways, and that at times this might unintentionally have reinforced his efforts at delaying the debridement. The staff agreed to handle these tactics in a uniform manner, in part by offering John choices, involving him in the dressing changes, and reinforcing his use of the various coping strategies that the psychologist would be working on with him. Furthermore, the psychologist agreed to attend John's morning dressing changes during the ensuing 2 weeks to observe and offer suggestions to the staff. A behaviorally focused feeding program was also recommended, which emphasized John's earning time with the staff by means of completing meals and snacks. Plans were also made to develop a daily schedule with the support of the nursing staff; such scheduling would further increase John's sense of control. Finally it was voted that the psychologist would provide individual therapy for depression and adjustment throughout the course of hospitalization. The staff unanimously agreed to implement this program, contingent upon both John's and his mother's agreement.

During the second half of the care conference, John and his mother were invited to join the staff. They were encouraged to ask questions and share their comments regarding the hospitalization. John was surprisingly open in expressing his anxiety about taking oral pain medications, since he had a pill phobia. It was suggested that these pain medications could be given through his intravenous hookup, which would eliminate this source of stress. John's mother was very tearful and distressed throughout the course of the conference. It was suggested that the social worker be available to speak with her by phone on a daily basis when she was unable to come to the hospital. This would afford her a continuing source of information and support. At the conclusion of this meeting, both John and his mother agreed to the recommendations that were offered. It was further agreed that a written plan of these interventions would be developed and posted at John's bedside and in his hospital chart. A follow-up care conference was scheduled for 2 weeks later.

Soon after the interventions were implemented, it became apparent that John's primary nurse was sabotaging the feeding program on her shift. She was sitting with John during his meals and coaxing him to eat. Meals began to take longer, although John's intake did not increase. The physician spoke with the nurse individually to educate her about the importance of John's nutrition, and the psychologist again contacted her to explain the rationale for the feeding program. The primary nurse explained that she would not follow the feeding program because she thought it was "cruel"; however, she agreed to meet with the head nurse about the situation, as she realized that John would have a nasal–gastric tube placed soon if he did not begin to maintain weight. After much discussion, it was agreed that the primary nurse would be unable to assist with the agreed-upon plan for John, and she was reassigned to other patients. Shortly after this, John's oral intake gradually began to increase.

At the end of the 2 weeks, the follow-up care conference was held to assess John's progress. John was beginning to maintain his weight and was cooperative during dressing changes. It was decided to continue both the pain management and the feeding program for 2 additional weeks, and then to fade them gradually. A final care conference was held 3 days prior to John's discharge. Plans were made for medical follow-up appointments. The social worker for the burn unit agreed to assist John's mother with transportation, and to meet with her and John at each visit to monitor progress. She also agreed to inform other involved staff members if future problems arose.

The *types* of services provided by the pediatric psychologist in this example may not have been dramatically different from those offered by any well-trained pediatric psychologist. However, John's case illustrates an approach that views coping as a dynamic set of interchanges between individuals and systems, and multiple influences among factors. In an intervention of this sort, systems on a number of levels are orchestrated in order to achieve a given goal. We believe that when such an ecological framework guides service provision, it will facilitate optimal coping and adaptation.

FUTURE DIRECTIONS

As medical technology has expanded and psychosocial aspects of medical conditions have become more complex, the demand for systems-oriented interdisciplinary approaches to medical problems and for multiple-level interventions appears to be increasing. It can perhaps be argued that pediatric psychologists have always employed a variety of assessment and treatment tools in their clinical work, and have typically involved multiple subsystems as a part of their change strategies. However, the conceptual model that guides and provides a framework for intervention appears to be shifting. Behavioral and cognitive models are now being increasingly integrated with ecological and family systems perspectives to understand the process of stress and coping. Clinics for chronic diseases (e.g., cystic fibrosis, diabetes, juvenile rheumatoid arthritis), as well as interdisciplinary pain clinics, are predicated upon such models. Family therapy approaches, merged with behavioral treatment approaches, also seem to be increasingly utilized.

Another trend for pediatric psychologists is occurring within the realm of empirical inquiry. Pediatric psychologists are learning to appreciate and utilize systems theory, while retaining their use of cognitive-behavioral interventions and the demand for a sound empirical approach to treatment. It is this desire for empirically based treatment that may promote further interdisciplinary and multiple-level interventions in the context of stress and coping. With new statistical tools, we can now subject interventions based on a systems model to empirical examination. Numerous questions can be addressed: When are multiple-level interventions necessary? Which consultation models are most effective in which settings? In what part of the system is it most effective to intervene? Sound research is required to demonstrate to our colleagues the value of multiple-level interventions. We anticipate that this research will further our understanding of psychosocial aspects of medical conditions, and will also help shape psychologists' future role in medical settings.

REFERENCES

Bandura, A. (1969). *Principles of behavior modification*. New York: Holt, Rinehart & Winston.

Borduin, C. M., Blaske, D. M., Mann, B. J., Treloar, L., Henggeler, S. W., & Fucci, B. R. (1990). *Multisystemic treatment of juvenile offenders: A replication and extension*. Manuscript submitted for publication.

Bronfenbrenner, U. (1986). Ecology of the family as a context for human development: Research perspectives. *Developmental Psychology, 22,* 723-742.

Brunk, M. A., Henggeler, S. W., & Whelan, J. (1987). A comparison of multisystemic therapy and parent training in the brief treatment of child abuse and neglect. *Journal of Consulting and Clinical Psychology, 55,* 171-178.

Colapinto, J. (1979). The relative value of empirical evidence. *Family Process, 18,* 427-441.

Dadds, M. R., Schwartz, E., & Sanders, M. R. (1987). Marital discord and treatment outcome in behavioral treatment of child conduct disorders. *Journal of Consulting and Clinical Psychology, 55,* 396-403.

Dolgin, M. J., & Jay, S. M. (1989). Pain management in children. In E. J. Mash & R. A. Barkley (Eds.), *Treatment of childhood disorders* (pp. 383-404). New York: Guilford Press.

Drotar, D. (1978). Training psychologists to consult with pediatricians: Problems and prospects. *Journal of Clinical Child Psychology, 7,* 57-60.

Eyberg, B. M., & Robinson, E. A. (1982). Parent-child interaction training: Effects on family functioning. *Journal of Clinical Child Psychology, 11,* 130-137.

Fisher, W., Burd, L., & Kerbeshian, J. (1985). Integrating developmental, pharmacological and psychological diagnoses and management through the transdisciplinary team process. *Rehabilitation Literature, 46,* 268-271.

Folkman, S., & Lazarus, R. S. (1985). If it changes it must be a process: Study of emotion and coping during these stages of a college examination. *Journal of Personality and Social Psychology, 48,* 150-170.

Gillman, J., & Mullins, L. L. (in press). Professional and pragmatic issues in pediatric pain. In. J. P. Bush & S. Harkins (Eds): *Children in pain: Clinical and research issues from a developmental perspective*. New York: Springer-Verlag.

Hanson, C. L., & Henggeler, S. W. (1984). Metabolic control in adolescents with diabetes: An examination of systems variables. *Family Systems Medicine, 2,* 5-16.

Hanson, C. L., Henggeler, S. W., & Burghen, G. A. (1987). Social competence and parental support as mediators of the link between stress and metabolic control in adolescents with insulin-dependent diabetes mellitus. *Journal of Consulting and Clinical Psychology, 55*, 529–533.

Hazelrigg, M. C., Cooper, H. M., & Borduin, C. M. (1987). Evaluating the effectiveness of family therapies: An integrative review and analysis. *Psychological Bulletin, 101*, 428–462.

Henggeler, S. W., & Borduin, C. M. (Eds.). (1990). *Family therapy and beyond: A multisystemic approach to treating the behavior problems of children and adolescents.* Pacific Grove, CA: Brooks/Cole.

Henggeler, S. W., Rodick, J. D., Borduin, C. M., Hanson, C. L., Watson, S. M., & Urey, J. R. (1986). Multisystemic treatment of juvenile offenders: Effects on adolescent behavior and family interaction. *Developmental Psychology, 22*, 132–141.

Kanfer, F. H., & Schefft, B. K. (1988). *Guiding the Process of therapeutic change.* Champaign, IL: Research Press.

Kaufman, K., Holden, E. W., & Walker, C. E. (1989). Future directions in pediatric and clinical child psychology. *Professional Psychology: Research and Practice, 20*, 148–152.

Kolb, D. A., Rubin, I. M., & McIntyre, J. M. (1979). *Organizational psychology: An experiential approach.* Englewood Cliffs, NJ: Prentice-Hall.

LaGreca, A. (1987). Children with diabetes and their family: Coping and disease management. In T. Field, P. McCabe, & N. Schneiderman (Eds.), *Stress and coping across development* (Vol. II). Hillsdale, NJ.: Lawrence Erlbaum.

Mash, E. J. (1989). Treatment of child and family disturbance: A behavioral-systems approach. In E. J. Mash & R. A. Barkley (Eds.), *Treatment of childhood disorders.* (pp. 3–38) New York: Guilford Press.

Minuchin, P. P. (1985). Families and individual development: Provocations from the field of family therapy. *Child Development, 56*, 289–302.

Mullins, L. L. (1989). Hate revisited: Power, envy and greed in the rehabilitation setting. *Archives of Physical Medicine and Rehabilitation, 70*, 740–744.

Munson, S. (1986). Family-oriented consultation in pediatrics. In L. C. Wynne, S. H. McDaniel, & T. T. Weber (Eds.), *Systems consultation: A new perspective for family therapy* (pp. 219–239). New York: Guilford Press.

O'Leary, K. D. (1984). The image of behavior therapy: It's time to take a stand. *Behavior Therapy, 15*, 219–233.

Olson, R. A., Holden, E. W., Friedman, A., Faust, J., Kenning, M., & Mason, P. J. (1988). Psychological consultation in a children's hospital: An evaluation of services. *Journal of Pediatric Psychology, 18*, 479–492.

Peterson, L., & Harbeck, C. (1988). *The pediatric psychologist: Issues in professional development and practice.* Champaign, IL: Research Press.

Roberts, M. C. (1986). *Pediatric psychology: Psychological interventions and strategies for pediatric problems.* New York: Pergamon.

Roberts, M. C., & Wright, L. (1982). Role of the pediatric psychologist as consultant to pediatricians. In J. Tuma (Ed.), *Handbook for the practice of pediatric psychology* (pp. 251–289). New York: Wiley.

Roberts, R. N., & Magrab, P. R. (1991). Psychologist's role in a family centered approach to practice, training and research with young children. *American Psychologist, 46,* 144–148.

Skinner, B. F. (1948). *Walden two.* New York: Macmillan.

Stabler, B. (1979). Emerging models of psychologist–pediatrician liaison. *Journal of Pediatric Psychology, 4,* 307–313.

Stabler, B. (1988). Pediatric consultation–liaison. In D. K. Routh (Ed.), *Handbook of pediatric psychology* (pp. 538–536). New York: Guilford Press.

von Bertalanffy, L. (1968). *General systems theory.* New York: Braziller.

Wallander, J. L., Varni, J. W., Babani, L., Banis, H. T., DeHaan, C. B., & Wilcox, K. T. (1989). Disability parameters, chronic strain, and adaptation of physically handicapped children and their mothers. *Journal of Pediatric Psychology, 14,* 25–42.

Wynne, L. C., McDaniel, S. H., & Weber, T. T. (Eds.). (1986). *Systems consultation: A new perspective for family therapy.* New York: Guilford Press.

Index